CRC Series in Membrane-Linked Diseases

MALIGNANT HYPERTHERMIA
A Genetic Membrane Disease

CRC Series in Membrane-Linked Diseases

S. Tsuyoshi Ohnishi and Tomoko Ohnishi, Series Editors
Philadelphia Biomedical Research Institute
and
University of Pennsylvania School of Medicine

Membrane Abnormalities in Sickle Cell Disease and in Other Red Blood Cell Disorders (1994)

Malignant Hyperthermia: A Genetic Membrane Disease (1994)

Cellular Membrane: A Key to Disease Processes (1992)

Forthcoming Titles

Central Nervous System Trauma

Prostaglandin Derivatives as Membrane Protecting Agents

Mitochondrial Genetic Diseases

CRC Series in Membrane-Linked Diseases

MALIGNANT HYPERTHERMIA
A Genetic Membrane Disease

Edited by
S. Tsuyoshi Ohnishi, Ph.D.
Director
Philadelphia Biomedical Research Institute
King of Prussia, Pennsylvania

Tomoko Ohnishi, Ph.D.
Research Professor
Department of Biochemistry and Biophysics
and the Johnson Research Foundation
University of Pennsylvania School of Medicine
Philadelphia, Pennsylvania

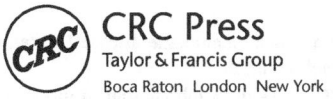
CRC Press
Taylor & Francis Group
Boca Raton London New York

CRC Press is an imprint of the
Taylor & Francis Group, an **informa** business

CRC Press
Taylor & Francis Group
6000 Broken Sound Parkway NW, Suite 300
Boca Raton, FL 33487-2742

© 1994 by Taylor & Francis Group, LLC
CRC Press is an imprint of Taylor & Francis Group, an Informa business

First issued in paperback 2019

No claim to original U.S. Government works

ISBN-13: 978-0-367-44962-9 (pbk)
ISBN-13: 978-0-8493-8093-8 (hbk)

Visit the Taylor & Francis Web site at
http://www.taylorandfrancis.com

and the CRC Press Web site at
http://www.crcpress.com

Library of Congress Card Number 93-5727

Library of Congress Cataloging-in-Publication Data

Malignant hyperthermia : a genetic membrane disease / edited by S.
  Tsuyoshi Ohnishi, Tomoko Ohnishi.
      p.   cm. -- (CRC series in membrane-linked diseases.)
   Includes bibliographical references and index.
   ISBN 0-8493-8093-6
1. Malignant hyperthermia.   I. Ohnishi, S. Tsuyoshi.
II. Ohnishi, Tomoko.   III. Series.
   [DNLM: 1. Malignant Hyperthermia.   WO 184 M25o 1993]
RD82.7.M3M333   1993
617.9'6--dc20
DNLM/DLC
for Library of Congress   93-5727
                                                                            CIP

DEDICATION

To those who died of Malignant Hyperthermia and to their families.

TABLE OF CONTENTS

Preface x
The Editors... xii
Contributors xiv
Introduction xvii

PART I: PROLOGUE

Chapter 1
"If Only Dantrolene Had Been Available Then . . . ".................... 3
Betty L. Martin

Chapter 2
"I Am Punching the Walls. My Hands Are Bleeding.
I Want Daniel!"... 7
George Massik

Part 2: The History and Accomplishments of the
Malignant Hyperthermia Association of the
United States (MHAUS)... 10
Suellen Gallamore, George Massik

Chapter 3
"Why Him? Why Us?"... 15
Alison Winks

Part 2: History of the British Malignant
Hyperthermia Association 18

PART II: HISTORY OF MALIGNANT HYPERTHERMIA RESEARCH

Chapter 4
The Early History of Malignant Hyperthermia — a Personal
Perspective 23
Werner Kalow

Chapter 5
The Discovery of Malignant Hyperthermia in Pigs — Some
Personal Recollections... 29
Gaisford G. Harrison

Chapter 6
How Was the Abnormal Calcium Release from the
Sarcoplasmic Reticulum Identified? 45
S. Tsuyoshi Ohnishi

**PART III: CURRENT UNDERSTANDING ON THE MECHANISM OF
MALIGNANT HYPERTHERMIA**

Chapter 7
Clinical Features of Malignant Hyperthermia in Man..................... 69
Scott R. Schulman, Gerald A. Gronert

Chapter 8
The Porcine Hyperthermia and Stress Syndromes 81
Gaisford G. Harrison

Chapter 9
Canine Malignant Hyperthermia/Canine Stress Syndrome 105
Peter J. O'Brien

Chapter 10
Drug-Induced Hypermetabolic Syndromes............................. 117
*Stanley N. Caroff, Stephan C. Mann, Kenneth Sullivan,
Wayne Macfadden*

Chapter 11
Free Calcium Concentration in Skeletal Muscle of Malignant
Hyperthermia Susceptible Subjects: Effects of Ryanodine............... 133
Jose Rafael Lopez-Padrino

Chapter 12
Malignant Hyperthermia and Free Radicals............................. 151
Gary G. Duthie, John R. Arthur

PART IV: DIAGNOSIS OF MALIGNANT HYPERTHERMIA

Chapter 13
The North American Protocol for the Caffeine Halothane
Contracture Test in the Diagnosis of Malignant Hyperthermia 171
Beverley A. Britt

Chapter 14
Measurement of Calcium-Induced Calcium Release Activity in
the Sarcoplasmic Reticulum Membrane with Special Reference
to Diagnosis of Malignant Hyperthermia 199
Makoto Endo

Chapter 15
Measurement of Calcium Accumulation by Sarcoplasmic
Reticulum in Whole Homogenate — a Potential Diagnostic
Test for Malignant Hyperthermia Susceptibility 211
Khay S. Cheah, A. M. Cheah, J. E. Fletcher, H. Rosenberg

Chapter 16
Noninvasive Screening for Malignant Hyperthermia by Means
of the Lymphocyte Test 225
Beverley A. Britt, Amira Klip, Peter J. O'Brien, Barbara I. Kalow

Chapter 17
A Noninvasive Diagnosis of Malignant Hyperthermia: Direct
Thermometry of Intramuscular Temperature............................251
S. Tsuyoshi Ohnishi, Kenneth K. Sadanaga

**PART V: NEW DEVELOPMENTS IN MALIGNANT
HYPERTHERMIA RESEARCH AND MOLECULAR GENETIC
DIAGNOSIS OF MALIGNANT HYPERTHERMIA**

Chapter 18
The Genetic Basis of Malignant Hyperthermia 259
David H. MacLennan, Michael S. Phillips, Yilin Zhang

Chapter 19
Demonstration of the Mutation Associated with Porcine
Stress Syndrome...273
Xia Zhang, Hua Shen, C. Robert Cory, Peter J. O'Brien

Chapter 20
Molecular Genetic Diagnosis of Human
Malignant Hyperthermia...293
Kirk Hogan

Index 321

PREFACE

Your Death Was Not Wasted!

Malignant hyperthermia (MH) is a unique disease.
This is not an ordinary disease, because in many cases
The "patients" may not experience any symptoms
Throughout their lifetimes.
They are quite healthy, and do not even know
That they are genetically susceptible to the disease.
The disease occurs only when the "patients"
Are exposed to inhalational anesthesia in the operating room.
Yes!
The disease occurs because the patients do not know
That they are "patients".
If they had known, the disease could have been avoided.

MH is a sad disease.
A patient went into the operating room for minor surgery,
Hoping to get back to work or school within a few days.
He had a plan to go to a medical school.
She was expecting to wear a beautiful dress on her next birthday.
The family members kissed and sent them off to the operating room,
Expecting to see the happy smile of their loved one soon.
Yet, this did not happen.
Out of the clear blue sky,
The patient suddenly developed a high fever,
Rigid muscles, difficulty in breathing, and
Death!
Leaving the family in turmoil and total agony.

MH is an example of a disease
In which family members of the victims
Developed a campaign to educate physicians.
Because of their determination to stop
The misery which they had experienced,
The campaign has been a tremendous success.
Look!
Today, hospitals store dantrolene,
The specific life saver for MH.
Physicians are aware of what to do
If MH suddenly occurs on their patients.

MH is a disease for which a concerted effort was made.
Physicians, anesthesiologists, veterinary scientists,
Physiologists, biochemists, biophysicists, and molecular biologists
Have identified the cause of this disease,
Have developed methods of diagnosing the disease
Before sending a patient to a potential death bed.
We are reaching the stage
Where the susceptibility to this disease could be diagnosed,
Not by painful muscle biopsy, but by
A simple lab test!

MH has created much tragedy,
But our future will be bright.
We pray for the repose of those who died of MH.
Your death was not wasted.
Because of the determination of your family,
Because of scientists who pledged to stop the misery,
We have won!
The day is coming
When no more death will happen
On the bed of the operating room.

S. Tsuyoshi Ohnishi

THE EDITORS

S. Tsuyoshi Ohnishi, Ph.D., is Director of the Philadelphia Biomedical Research Institute, King of Prussia, Pennsylvania, and is Visiting Professor of Hahnemann University School of Medicine, Philadelphia, Pennsylvania.

Dr. S. T. Ohnishi graduated from Kyoto University, Kyoto, Japan, in 1954 with a B.S. degree in Physics. He obtained his Master's Degree in Chemistry in 1956 and his Ph.D. from Nagoya University in 1959. He was a Post Doctoral fellow at Nagoya University (Biophysics) from 1960 to 1962, and Visiting Scientist fellow between 1963 and 1965 at the University of Tokyo School of Medicine (Pharmacology). He served as Associate Professor at Waseda University, Tokyo, from 1956 to 1967, Visiting Associate Professor at the Johnson Foundation, University of Pennsylvania, from 1967 to 1968, Assistant Professor at the Medical College of Pennsylvania from 1969 to 1972, Associate Professor at Hahnemann University School of Medicine from 1973 to 1984, and Research Professor at the same university in 1985. He was Director of the Membrane Research Institute from 1985 to 1989, and Director at the Philadelphia Biomedical Research Institute from 1989 to present.

Dr. S. T. Ohnishi was Visiting Professor at Hokkaido University, Japan, in 1979 and Visiting Professor at Mayo Medical School in 1982. He was an Invited Research Scientist at MIT, Boston, in 1983.

He is a member of the American Society of Biological Chemistry, the Biophysical Society, the Society of Neuroscience, and the American Hematological Society.

In the early 1960's, he pioneered the discovery that a muscle protein actin exists in biological membranes. Working with Dr. Setsuro Ebashi at the University of Tokyo, Dr. Ohnishi developed the murexide method to measure the concentration of calcium ions in physiological media and demonstrated that the sarcoplasmic reticulum takes up calcium ions at a rate rapid enough to account for the speed to muscle relaxation. He developed a spectrophotometer using a rotating sector-semiconductor switching circuit, and the technology has been widely used since. He contributed to the development of the concept of "membrane-acting" antisickling agents. In the early 1980's, he demonstrated that irreversibly sickled cells can be formed *in vitro* when the red blood cells from sickle cell anemia patients were exposed to repeated cycles of sickling and unsickling. He also determined that the cause of Malignant Hyperthermia is the abnormally high calcium release from the sarcoplasmsic reticulum of genetically susceptible subjects.

Dr. S. T. Ohnishi has made over 50 presentations and invited lectures in national and international meetings. He has published 120 papers and is a co-author of three books. He has been the recipient of 20 research grants from the National Institutes of Health, National Science Foundation, and other private foundations. His current research interest is investigating the role of antioxidants in ischemia-reperfusion injury, malaria, cancer, and AIDS.

Tomoko Ohnishi, Ph.D., is Research Professor at the University of Pennsylvania School of Medicine and the Johnson Research Foundation.

Dr. Ohnishi graduated from Kyoto University in 1956 with a B.S. degree in Biochemistry and obtained her Ph.D. in 1962 from Nagoya University. She was a Visiting Scientist fellow between 1961 and 1963 and worked in the Osaka University School of Medicine (Biochemistry). She was Research Associate at Wenner-Gren Institute, University of Stockholm, Sweden, from 1965 to 1966; Visiting Professor at Phillips University, Marburg/Lahn, Germany, in 1966; and Research Associate at Cornell University from 1966 to 1967. Dr. Tomoko Ohnishi was Visiting Assistant Professor at the Johnson Research Foundation, University of Pennsylvania, from 1967 to 1971, and Assistant Professor at the same Foundation from 1971 to 1977. She served as Research Associate Professor at the University of Pennsylvania Department of Biochemistry and Biophysics from 1977 to 1984. She is currently Research Professor at the same department and also of the Johnson Research Foundation.

Dr. Ohnishi received the International Cell Research Award to attend the international conference and workshop in Stockholm in 1965. She was Invited Professor of the Organization of American States Scientific and Technological Program, Buenos Aires, in 1977, Invited Scholar of the Tokyo Metropolitan Institute of Medical Science, Tokyo, in 1982, and Invited Foreign Scholar of CNRS, Paris, from 1983 to 1984. She is a member of the American Society of Biological Chemistry and is presently the Chairperson of Bioenergetics Subgroup of the Biophysical Society.

She was the first to isolate tightly coupled, intact mitochondria from yeast and demonstrated that they are different from bovine heart mitochondria, because they oxidize exogenous NADH in an ADP-controlled manner. She has applied liquid helium temperature EPR to the study of the mitochondrial respiratory chain. She characterized basic thermodynamic and EPR properties of iron-sulfer clusters as well as bound forms of semiquineone species and flavin free radicals. She pioneered the discovery that mitochondrial genetic diseases can be caused by the deficiency of iron-sulfur clusters in the NADH-ubiquinone oxidoreductase. She also developed a paramagnetic probe technique to determine spatial organization of intrinsic redox components within the energy transducing membranes.

She has given over 20 invited lectures and 50 presentations in national and international meetings. She has published 170 papers and has been a recipient of consecutive grants from the National Institutes of Health and the National Science Foundation. In addition, she recently received a NIH Fogarty International Research Collaboration Award to work with scientists at the Moscow State University. She has served as a regular member of the Scientific Review Group of the National Institutes of Health.

CONTRIBUTORS

John R. Arthur
Principal Scientific Officer
Rowett Research Institute
Aberdeen, Scotland

Beverley A. Britt, M.D.
Professor, Department of
  Anaesthesia and Pharmacology
University of Toronto, and
Senior Staff Anaesthetist
Toronto General Hospital
Toronto, Ontario

Stanley N. Caroff, M.D.
Department of Psychiatry
University of Pennsylvania, and
Philadelphia Veterans Affairs
  Medical Center
Philadelphia, Pennsylvania

A. M. Cheah, Ph.D.
Department of Anesthesiology
The Laboratory for the Study of
  Malignant Hyperthermia
Hahnemann University
Philadelphia, Pennsylvania

Khay S. Cheah, Ph.D.
Department of Anesthesiology
The Laboratory for the Study of
  Malignant Hyperthermia
Hahnemann University
Philadelphia, Pennsylvania

C. Robert Cory
Department of Pathology
Ontario Veterinary College
University of Guelph
Guelph, Ontario

Garry G. Duthie, Ph.D.
Senior Scientific Officer
Rowett Research Institute
Aberdeen, Scotland

Makoto Endo, M.D., Ph.D.
Department of Pharmacology
Faculty of Medicine
University of Tokyo
Tokyo, Japan

J. E. Fletcher, Ph.D.
Department of Anesthesiology
The Laboratory for the Study of
  Malignant Hyperthermia
Hahnemann University
Philadelphia, Pennsylvania

Suellen L. Gallamore
MHAUS
Omaha, Nebraska

Gerald A. Gronert, M.D.
Department of Anesthesia
University of California at Davis
Davis, California

Gaisford G. Harrison, M.D., D.Sc.
Emeritus Professor of Anaesthetics
University of Cape Town
Cape Town, South Africa

Kirk Hogan, M. D.
Associate Professor of Anesthesiology
University of Wisconsin
  Medical School, and
William S. Middleton Veteran's
  Administration Hospital
Madison, Wisconsin

Barbara I. Kalow, D.V.M.
Department of Pathology
Ontario Veterinary College
University of Guelph
Guelph, Ontario

Werner Kalow, M.D.
Department of Pharmacology
University of Toronto
Toronto, Ontario

Amira Klip, Ph.D.
Department of Cell Biology
The Hospital for Sick Children
Toronto, Ontario

Jose Rafael Lopez-Padrino, M.D., Ph.D.
Centro de Biofisica y Bioquimica
Instituto Venezolano de
  Investigaciones Cientificas
Caracas, Venezuela, *and*
Department of Anesthesia
Brigham and Women's Hospital
Boston, Massachusetts

Wayne Macfadden, M.D.
Department of Psychiatry
University of Pennsylvania, *and*
Philadelphia Veterans Affairs
  Medical Center
Philadelphia, Pennsylvania

David H. MacLennan, Ph.D.
The Banting and Best Department
  of Medical Research
University of Toronto
Toronto, Ontario

Stephan C. Mann, M.D.
Department of Psychiatry
University of Pennsylvania, *and*
Philadelphia Veterans Affairs
  Medical Center
Philadelphia, Pennsylvania

Betty Martin
Sheffield, Alabama

George Massik
MHAUS Founder
Amherst, New York

**Peter J. O'Brien, D.V.M., D.V.Sc.,
  Ph.D.**
Associate Professor
Pathology Department
Ontario Veterinary College
University of Guelph
Guelph, Ontario

S. Tsuyoshi Ohnishi, Ph.D.
Director
Philadelphia Biomedical
  Research Institute
King of Prussia, Pennsylvania

Michael S. Phillips
The Banting and Best Department
  of Medical Research
University of Toronto
Toronto, Ontario

H. Rosenberg, M.D.
Department of Anesthesiology
The Laboratory for the Study of
  Malignant Hyperthermia
Hahnemann University
Philadelphia, Pennsylvania

Kenneth K. Sadanaga, D.V.M.
Philadelphia Biomedical
  Research Institute
King of Prussia, Pennsylvania

Scott R. Schulman, M.D.
Departments of Anesthesia and
  Pediatrics
University of California,
  Davis Medical Center
Sacramento, California

Hua Shen
Department of Pathology
Ontario Veterinary College
University of Guelph
Guelph, Ontario

Kenneth Sullivan, Ph.D.
Department of Psychiatry
University of Pennsylvania, *and*
Philadelphia Veterans Affairs
  Medical Center
Philadelphia, Pennsylvania

Alison Winks
British Malignant Hyperthermia
  Association
Nottingham, England

Xia Zhang
Department of Pathology
Ontario Veterinary College
University of Guelph
Guelph, Ontario

Yilin Zhang, M.D., Ph.D.
The Banting and Best Department
  of Medical Research
University of Toronto
Toronto, Ontario

INTRODUCTION
Contraction of the Skeletal Muscle

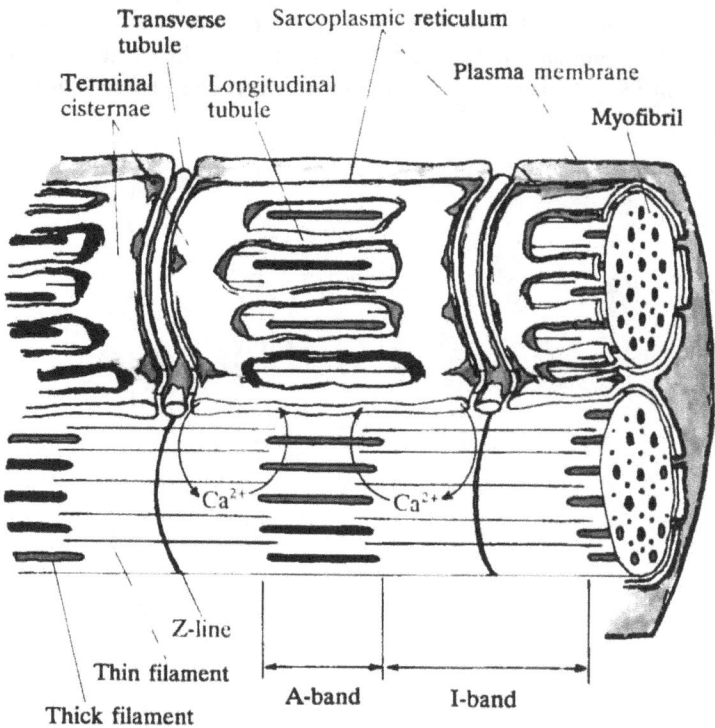

Shown above is a schematic illustration of the triggering of the contraction of skeletal muscle. When the impulse signal arrives at the muscle from the brain, the cell membrane of the muscle (called the *plasma membrane* or *sarcolemma*) is electrically depolarized, making the inside of the muscle cell positive. This depolarization also occurs at the membrane of the transverse tubules (which are the invaginations of the plasma membrane at the position of Z-line), triggering the release of calcium ions from within the sarcoplasmic reticulum at the terminal cisternae. The released calcium ions interact with troponin molecules on thin filaments (actin-tropomyosin complex which forms the I-band) of myofibrils. This induces the sliding movement of the thin filaments in reference to the thick filaments (myosin, which is the major protein in the A-band), thereby eliciting the muscle contraction. Subsequently, calcium ions are re-sequestered by the longitudinal tubule section of the sarcoplasmic reticulum via the Ca-ion pump, causing the relaxation of the muscle. In some mammalian muscles, there are transverse tubules near the intersection of the I-band and the A-band, which could improve the efficiency of calcium ion movement for the contraction.

After homogenization of the muscle tissue, the sarcoplasmic reticulum can be collected by differential centrifugation or density gradient centrifugation. The terminal cisternae can be collected in a higher density fraction (called *heavy SR*, which demonstrates both Ca-release and Ca-pump activities). The longitudinal tubule portion is collected in a lower density fraction (called *light SR*, which has only Ca-pump activity). See Chapter 6 for further details.

Part I
Prologue

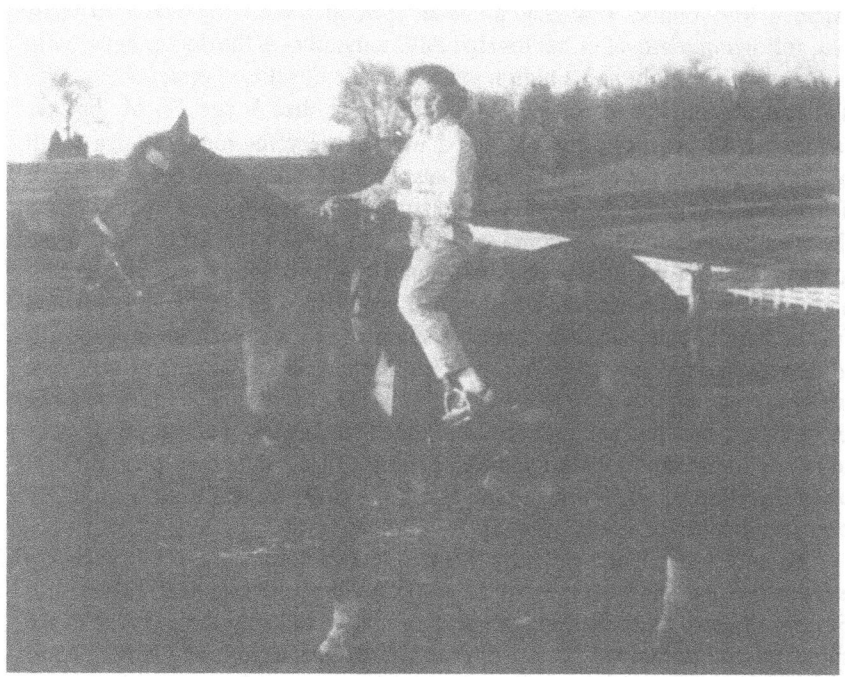

Francie Martin

Chapter 1

"IF ONLY DANTROLENE HAD
BEEN AVAILABLE THEN . . . "

Betty L. Martin

Dear Dr. Ohnishi:

I am so glad to hear that you are editing a book on MH. Every bit of information helps, as you know! I've spent several hours searching for a piece I wrote about the death of our daughter for a magazine several years ago (it was not published), but since I cannot find it I'll do the best I can, with my failing 72-year-old memory. As to family background — I am of German ancestry, with both maternal grandparents born in Germany. They were first cousins, which I think might be an important factor. Besides the two cases mentioned in my article, there have been three other items that might be of interest. My younger sister had an acute episode when I was about 10 years old, following removal of her tonsils. All I remember is the doctor being with her most of the night and a high fever. Later she developed epileptic seizures and spastic paralysis of her left leg and arm. She died at age 22. My brother fathered twin girls; one died at age 1 after surgery for removal of a small object she had swallowed. They now suspect MH might have been involved. The other twin developed epileptic seizures in her early teens, but outgrew them and now is a Ph.D. computer whiz. Other than that, the dozen or so grandchildren of the Frederick Post–Anna Bruning union have been healthy, active individuals. There have been minor problems with spinal curvature and foot deformity and pain due to muscle spasm. My own worst problem seems to be weakness in my upper leg muscles that makes me bend forward while walking, making me look like 92 instead of 72. My mother and two of her three sisters had this same problem. Other than fleeting pain in all parts of my body — no doubt due to muscle spasm — I lead an active, pleasant life, often traveling to visit two children and grandchildren. The following is my best recollection of Francie's story.

Though it happened so many years ago, I can still remember the happy expectation Jack and I felt as we flew to Chicago with our dear 13-year-old Francie. At last we were doing something that would stop the increase in the spinal curvature that was threatening to change her happy, active life. After talking with the specialists who would insert a spinal rod at the famous Children's Memorial Hospital in Chicago, they assured us that "this little tinkering" would not interfere with riding her beloved horse, and promised a quick recovery to normal activity after a few weeks in a body cast. We were so sure everything would go well we even left the hospital for an hour or so during surgery hoping to buy some special glasses so that Francie could read more easily while flat on her back.

On our return, we found we were being paged to go immediately to the operating room. Frightened beyond belief, and cursing ourselves for having been so foolish in leaving the waiting room, we learned from the assistant surgeon that Francie had developed an extremely high temperature (110°F.) and severe problems with heart rhythms. We waited for an interminable hour of anguish; I was praying only with hope for some medical miracle, my husband praying with his strong Christian faith. But the shattering blow came despite our prayers. Francie died on the operating table. I cry even 30 years later as I think of the anguish I felt at not even being able to hold her hand at the last, even though she was unconscious. The first years after her death would not have been livable had it not been for the loving kindness of friends and loved ones, and the knowledge that we could not let our grief flow over and smother the chance of a normal life for our two younger children.

Part of the dark hours was pervaded by the feeling that the doctors might be hiding some small accident in the operating room. Should we to try to investigate and bring the doctors to trial for taking the life of our daughter?

But that would not bring Francie back, and the doctors had been so kind and helpful: Would it be right to bring possible ruin to their reputations? So the sad years went by until about 5 years later, when a cousin called and said her brother's family was deep in grief over the death of their son during surgery. Would I call them? The situation was so like Francie's. There might be some connection. She gave me the number of the doctor at the university hospital where the surgery had been done. He expressed a deep interest in the case, as any anesthetist would, seeing a healthy young boy (age 13 again) die, perhaps as a result of his ministrations. In the course of the following year we exchanged many letters, and I found that the first writing in medical literature on the strange phenomenon called malignant hyperthermia had been published just about a year before Francie's death by an Australian pathologist, Dr. Michael Denborough.

In later years I contacted Dr. Claude Taylor at the University of Wisconsin Hospital, while vacationing nearby at the family cottage. He told me of the several incidents of MH in Wisconsin medical literature, and a year or two later he informed me that a national organization had been formed — MHAUS — headquartered in Darien, Connecticut. Since that time I have been in regular communication with MHAUS and have tried to "spread the word" to various hospitals in our area about the need to have dantrolene available in operating rooms and to have available the easily read charts MHAUS provides with a list of things that must be done in an MH emergency. Though I have attended only one yearly meeting of the group, I keep abreast of new developments by ordering tapes of the meetings and by reading their excellent newsletter. It's good to know that there is a number I can call if I need more information. I feel a real kinship with all the families who have lost loved ones to this mysterious, pernicious killer. I am amazed to hear about all the facts that have emerged by the many doctors and technicians involved in studying the disease, and I am sure that some day enough will be known and procedures perfected so that no patient will succumb during an episode which has come to be called "the anesthesiologist's nightmare".

Dear Dr. Ohnishi:

Thank you so very much for your letter that showed so much caring concern. I spent several hours yesterday trying to find a suitable picture of Francie, and was chagrined to find I had so few. I had an enlargement of the one I am sending, but it must be put away somewhere. All the other pictures I could find were when she was a little child. For several years we could not even look at pictures, it was just too painful. I hope you will return them, as I have so few.

Concerning the date, I believe the surgery was done on November 30, 1961, just about a month after Francie's 13th birthday. If only dantrolene had been available then, she probably would have lived, but of course the first writing on the MH syndrome had been published only a year before, so I doubt any of the surgical team had even heard of it.

I hope this information will be helpful to you, and I will hope to stay in touch with you and hear of results of your good work.

Sincerely,
Betty L. Martin

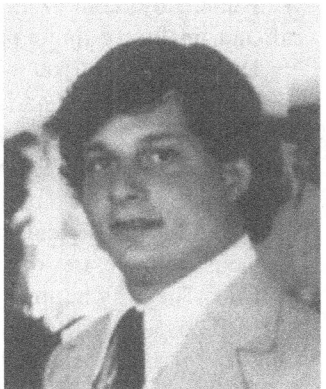

Daniel Massik

Chapter 2

Part 1
"I AM PUNCHING THE WALLS. MY HANDS ARE BLEEDING. I WANT DANIEL!"

George Massik

Daniel was 21 and finished with summer school. He needed organic chemistry credits, but had no time to squeeze them in during the biomedical engineering courses at Duke. So, summer school at home, then a week off, a family wedding, finish his medical school application, and start his trip back to school.

He had decided to ride his bicycle back to Duke. We live in Buffalo, NY, and decided that I would drive him into Pennsylvania and he would go on from there. We had a nice father and son drive for about 6 hours. We stopped for lunch, hugged and said our good-byes, and off he rode. Any parent knows the mixture of pride and dread one feels at such a moment, but still one has to let their children go.

He called the second morning. He had slept in a farm field and had bought a melon from the farmer for breakfast. Now he was off again. Had I heard hesitancy in his voice? I wasn't sure.

That night as I was talking with my sister by phone, the operator cut in with an emergency. Daniel had been hit by a car-carrier transport. The doctor told me he was stabilized, but needed to have his spleen removed and they could wait until I arrived.

0-8493-8093-6/94/$0.00 + $.50
© 1994 by CRC Press, Inc.

Panic, fury, cold hate, and finally the mind kicked into gear. Call after call and finally we find a private plane to take us to Gettysburg, PA.

During the flight you imagine that you are thinking. You aren't. You just think you are. Your mind is encased in an acrylic cube trying to break out.

Finally we got to the hospital, where we ran up the stairs. God, he's okay. He's talking, he's moving, he's alive.

Because Daniel is a pre-med student he is knowledgeable about medicine and the odds of a surgical accident. He knows how many unexplained deaths per thousand there are from anesthetics. I tell him I will talk to the doctors.

I do. They say he must have the surgery. I say I am not comfortable at a 48-bed hospital. They say he cannot be moved, and that they have adequate facilities for any emergency.

I tell him. He rebels. I yell at him, and he accepts.

We sit and wait. The chairs are near the surgery area. I notice people scurrying, and when they see me notice, they avoid my eyes. I'm sick. I'm really sick. What is it?

Finally they come out and tell me that something happened. They are in contact with people at Hershey Medical Center and will do all they can, but he is very, very sick.

I sit and wait. The anesthesiologist comes off the elevator with a thin book in his hand. He says he found the book in the library, and now he knows what happened.

I sit all night. People from the town come to offer help. There is one Jew in Gettysburg, a teacher and coach. He heard we were Jewish, and he came and brought me a prayer book. A young woman training to be a minister takes my hand. I feel them all giving so freely that I begin to believe. I force concentration. I connect with him and force him awake. The nurse came out to tell me I could see him for a while. I talk to him and tell him he must wake up. They tell me he can't hear, but I know better.

He does wake up. My God. I pound the floor with my fists. They think I've lost my mind and they want to sedate me. I talk to him, and he understands. He glances at the respirator, and I explain. I tell him he will have a semester off, and that I will take care of him. With his eyes he tells me he is in pain. I tell him I will let them know. I tell him to sleep. They ask me to leave, and I go out.

God, a miracle. He lives!

It's 2:30 a.m. and a doctor comes out and talks to me. What is he saying? Broken hip, broken arm, bed for months, kidneys are shut down, diuretics, but . . . ? He is very sick. I'm sick again.

During the night nurses and people of all kinds stop by. A held hand, a hope, a kind word, a smile. It all helps.

It's morning. It's sunny and beautiful. I go in. He is very quiet.

The doctors begin the assault. The orthopedist first. He is stern and matter of fact. He's originally from Buffalo. I know his family. Surgery, arm, restricted, hip, cast, pin, bed. Yes, I can take care of him. God, they're planning ahead. I feel better.

The surgeon comes out. He can't give him anything for the pain. He will try a little Valium. I must calm him, tell him not to get excited. He is talking to Hershey. They may move him by helicopter. Dangerous, but . . . We'll see. Trying new diuretics.

I go in. He blinks once for yes, twice for no. He's in pain. I calm him. He's angry and I know why. He knew about the anesthetics. I calm him. I go out. I'm sick.

Another long day and another long night. More people, some the same and all wonderful. He gets quieter. Last night's doctor again. Diuretics not working. Septicemia. Hershey. Fear. I'm sick again.

Morning. Yes, they will take him to Hershey by ambulance. We should start. They will meet us there. I'm in the back seat. Suddenly the car hisses and sputters, and then just goes on. I know. I feel it. My nephew Charles turns white at the wheel. He knows too.

We get to Hershey, and they tell us to go back. There has been a change in plans. We get back. His mother and brother are sitting on the front steps, and there doesn't seem to be a problem. Could I be wrong? I bound past them up the steps. There's the surgeon. Sorry. We did all we could. We waited for you to come back.

What am I doing? I'm punching the walls. My hands are bleeding. I control myself. I want to see him. There he is, quiet, bruised lips, bluish tint, fingernails blue. My God, it's Dan. Is this real? I want the comb. I want the head restraints. I want to remember. I want Dan.

Now it starts. Autopsy. Death certificate. Undertaker. Transportation. I want Dan!

It takes time. I am getting better. Then I hear the words malignant hyperthermia. Then I hear Dantrium. Then I hear Dr. Britt. Then it all comes out. He didn't need to die. I resolve not to let his life be wasted.

I became one of the four founders of MHAUS and originated the idea for the MHAUS Hotline. I see to it that every hospital in this area has posters about malignant hyperthermia.

Recently we went to Gettysburg and stopped at the hospital. There's a brand new one there, bigger and I hope better. They probably have Dantrium now.

POSTSCRIPT

Twenty five years ago when my nephew Charles was 6, he spiked an extremely high temperature during surgery. He recovered, and no one ever used the term malignant hyperthermia. Why? Doesn't any one ever go over old records to see who should be warned?

If there are others who would be interested in helping to raise funds to review old records to alert possible MH susceptibles, I would like them to contact me:

George Massik
94 Bondcroft
Amherst, NY 14226
716-832-9545

Part 2
THE HISTORY AND ACCOMPLISHMENTS OF THE MALIGNANT HYPERTHERMIA ASSOCIATION OF THE UNITED STATES (MHAUS)

Suellen Gallamore, George Massik

In October 1981, five people met as the founding board of the Malignant Hyperthermia Association of the United States (MHAUS) — Owen Davison, Suellen Long Gallamore, Robert T. Luckritz, George Massik, and Henry Rosenberg, M.D. All except Dr. Rosenberg had a personal interest in malignant hyperthermia (MH). Owen and George had lost young adult sons to MH, Bob had nearly lost an infant daughter, and Suellen had experienced numerous frightening encounters with physicians who were unconcerned and/ or unknowledgeable about MH. Dr. Rosenberg (an anesthesiologist with a special interest in MH) hosted the meeting at his office at Hahnemann University in Philadelphia.

The wheels had been set in motion several months earlier by Suellen, who perceived a need to educate the medical and lay communities about MH and serve as a resource to those families affected by it. She worked to recruit the board and professional advisory council to obtain the necessary legal and tax-exemption documents, and to define the need, goals and purposes of the group.

At its initial meeting, the MHAUS Board elected officers, agreed to the guiding principles set forth in the by-laws and articles of incorporation, adopted a logo, and agreed to make personal financial commitments to the fledgling organization and to establish an office in the home of its newly-elected president, Suellen Gallamore. As the Gallamores were in the process of moving from the Washington, D.C. area to the New York City area, they found a home in Darien, Connecticut, which then became the headquarters for MHAUS. The Gallamore family computer housed the MHAUS database; mailings were stuffed, labeled, sorted and bundled on the family room floor; and the MHAUS phone (red, for obvious reasons) rang at all hours of the night and day in the Gallamore kitchen.

The early months of MHAUS were spent establishing contact with all-important groups like Norwich Eaton Pharmaceuticals, the Medic-Alert Foundation, the Muscular Dystrophy Association (MDA), and the National Organization for Rare Disorders (NORD), among others. Owen Davison established contact with the World Health Organization (WHO), asking that they include MH among their list of recognized diseases and disorders.

Norwich Eaton invited MHAUS to share their booth space at the American Society of Anesthesiologists' meeting in Las Vegas during October 1982, and that exposure really put MHAUS "on the map". They also agreed to fund production of the MHAUS newsletter, *The Communicator*. Lastly, Norwich Eaton provided funds for MHAUS to purchase an exhibit which would travel to many scientific medical meetings during the next several years. Countless information was distributed in this manner.

The Communicator was first sent in the summer of 1982 to 288 names on the MHAUS mailing list, many of them friends and relatives of board members. With each subsequent issue, the mailing list nearly doubled as word of MHAUS began to spread in the medical and patient communities. Within a year or so, the mailing list contained the names of several thousand MH-affected families who yearned for information and support.

George Massik felt strongly that an information "hotline" was needed for physicians treating an MH emergency, and the board decided that he should make preliminary contacts with the Medic-Alert Foundation to see if MHAUS might tie into their 24-hour phone bank. After nearly a year of brainstorming, information-gathering, and negotiating. Medic-Alert agreed to accept MH-emergency calls and refer them to on-call MHAUS physician-consultants. To alleviate unnecessary calls to the Medic-Alert lines, MHAUS would publish an operating-room poster outlining the emergency treatment of MH (Figure 1). Less severe or problemmatic cases might be handled in this way. The poster also referred physicians to the MHAUS phone number to obtain information for their MH-susceptible patients. Tens of thousands of posters are now hanging in hospitals around the world. It is safe to say that the MHAUS/Medic-Alert Hotline has saved hundreds, if not thousands, of lives since its inception in 1983. The Hotline number is **(209) 634-4917**; the general information number is (203) 655-3007.

Dr. Rosenberg felt that MHAUS should sponsor opportunities for MH-susceptible families to come together for learning and sharing, and in 1983 Hahnemann University hosted the first annual MHAUS Family Conference. It brought participants from as far away as California, Arizona, and Georgia. MH experts from around the U.S. and Canada were there to lend their specialized knowledge and answer questions. A sense of "community" was emerging.

In 1985, the Gallamore basement could no longer contain the enormous stockpile of publications, files, and office equipment necessary to conduct business, so the office was moved into an empty classroom at a local church. Suellen Gallamore also stepped down as President during this time, becoming

Suggested Therapy for

Malignant Hyperthermia Emergency

1. All inhalation anesthetics should be discontinued and hyperventilation with 100% oxygen begun.
2. In the absence of blood gas analysis, bicarbonate 1-2 meq/kg should be administered
3. Dantrolene sodium should be obtained, mixed with sterile distilled water, and 2.5 mg/kg administered intravenously. At present dantrolene is packaged as a lyophilized preparation that contains 20 mg of dantrolene and 3 grams mannitol per vial.
4. Simultaneously, cooling should be started by all routes surface, nasogastric lavage, intravenous cold solutions, wound, and rectally
5. Change anesthetic tubing, and if possible, soda lime.
6. Arrhythmias will usually respond to treatment of acidosis and hyperkalemia. If they persist or are life threatening, 200 mg of procaineamide should be administered in repeated doses prn
7. Administer further doses of dantrolene as necessary titrated to the heart rate, muscle rigidity and temperature. Response to dantrolene should begin to occur in minutes; if not, more drug should be administered. Although the average successful dose of dantrolene is about 2.5 mg/kg, much higher doses may be needed (10 mg/kg and more) Fortunately dantrolene does not produce significant myocardial depression at these doses
8. Determine and monitor closely urine output, serum potassium, calcium, arterial blood gases, and clotting studies. Hyperkalemia is common in the acute phase of MH and should be treated with intravenous glucose and insulin.
9. Observe the patient in an ICU setting for at least 24 hours since recrudescence of MH may occur, particularly following a case that was difficult to treat.
10 Follow CPK, calcium and potassium until such time as they return to normal.
11 ECG should also be obtained and followed post operatively.
12 Monitor body temperature closely since overvigorous treatment of MH may lead to hypothermia. Temperature instability may persist for several days after the acute episode. Body temperatures of 41 to 42° are compatible with survival and normal brain function if treated promptly.
13. Insure urine output of greater than 1/ml/kg/hour. Consider CVP monitoring because of fluid shifts that may occur.
14. When the patient's condition has stabilized, convert from intravenous to oral dantrolene. Although data are not available regarding optimal doses and duration of treatment with dantrolene after an episode, the patient should probably receive a total dose of 4 mg/kg/day in divided doses for 48 hours post operatively.

CAUTION: This protocol may not apply to every patient and must of necessity be altered according to specific patient needs.

Names of on-call physicians available
to consult in MH emergencies may be
obtained 24 hours a day through:
**MEDIC ALERT
FOUNDATION INTERNATIONAL
(209) 634-4917**
Ask for: **INDEX ZERO**, Malignant
Hyperthermia Consultant List.

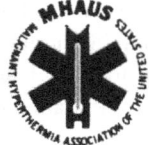

For Non-Emergency
or Patient Referral Calls:
MHAUS
(203) 655-3007

MHAUS P.O. Box 3231, Darien, CT 06820

FIGURE 1.   MHAUS poster.

a full-time paid Executive Director of MHAUS. She functioned in this capacity until 1988, when she moved to Omaha, Nebraska, as a result of her husband's job change.

MHAUS grew stronger and larger month-by-month and year-by-year, as it increased in visibility and program services. New board and advisory council members brought new talents and strengths to the organization, and new contacts with pharmaceutical and equipment manufacturers afforded new opportunities for financial independence. MHAUS had become a credible and respected provided in the anesthesia world and was truly making a difference.

John Larberg became president of MHAUS in 1985, and during his tenure the organization first began to find MH research. Two memorial funds, one established in the name of Jerry and Lila Lewis, the other in the name of Vincent Napolitano, were used for this purpose. Another significant achievement of John's presidency was that of assisting with the start-up of the North American MH Patient Registry. MHAUS also engineered and co-sponsored a North American Biopsy Standards Conference in the fall of 1987, bringing together MH investigators for the purpose of defining criteria for MH diagnosis using the caffeine/halothane muscle biopsy contracture test. The group agreed to cooperate by sharing information through the Registry, the goal being to standardize procedures and better understand results.

At this writing MHAUS is in its twelfth year of providing information, referral, and solace to the many families who had no where else to turn when MH was discovered in their lives. Those five who met in Philadelphia in 1981 could not begin to imagine the impact their efforts would have on so many.

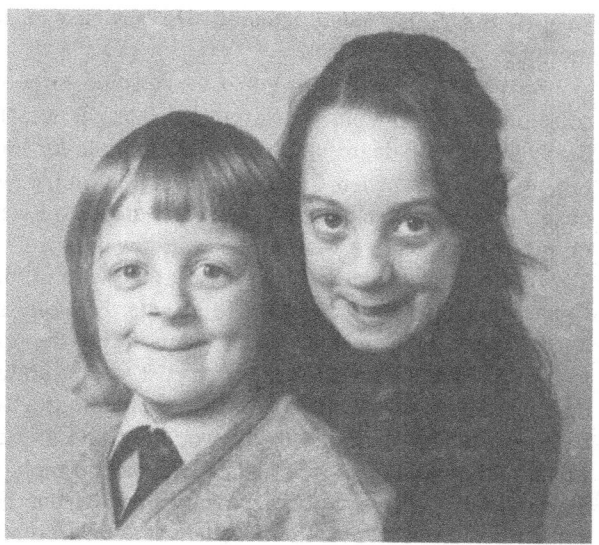

John and Tracey Winks

Chapter 3

Part 1
"WHY HIM? WHY US?"

Alison Winks

Looking back, I think I knew almost from the moment I entered the ward that I would not be taking John home again.

We had always said we wanted two children. Tracey and John were born 3 years and 4 months apart, both with cleft lip and palate. In a way I was glad they both were affected because neither would be able to say to the other, "Why me and not you." With a daughter and a son, both needing regular hospital admissions to repair and improve the lip and palate, we felt our family was complete.

By January 1982, Tracey had had three operations and John six. There was a dispute at the hospital and they were not calling adults for routine operations, so they started calling for as many children who were on waiting lists as possible. The letter came on the Friday and asked for John to be admitted the following Monday for another routine operation. These admissions had become a way of life. John was pleased to be going in to have a small fistula in his palate repaired. He was first on the list on Wednesday morning, January 13, 1982.

As usual, I intended to go to the hospital to be there when he arrived back on the ward from the surgical theater. It was intensely cold, a very heavy frost, −10 degrees, I think. Very unusual for England. The accelerator on my car stuck when I started the engine and it was racing. I rang my husband Geoff who explained what to do and then I was on my way. I picked up my mother and we went to the ward together.

As we entered the ward, we were asked who we had come to see. When I gave his name, they asked me to go into the Sister's office. They told me not to worry, there had been a problem during the operation, but it was all right now. The Sister said the anesthetist wanted to talk to me and got him on the telephone. He said there was a problem, they were still in the theater trying to stabilize him and then I would be able to see him. He had tried to get me on the phone at home but there was no reply. I had been there, but we discovered there had been problems on the line because of the extreme cold. Now that I was at the hospital, he would come up and talk to me. I phoned Geoff and said he had better get to the hospital as we had a problem. He raced over, breaking a few speed laws, I think, and praying there were no policemen around. We waited in stunned silence for the anesthetist to arrive.

After what seemed like hours he came into the office and explained. About two hours into the operation John had been overbreathing. This sometimes happened if the anesthetic was a little light, as they never want to give any more than necessary. He increased the anesthetic a little and the problem was corrected. A few minutes later, the surgeon also thought there was a problem with his breathing. The anesthetist checked his temperature (not routinely monitored during operations in this country) which was about 42°C (107°F). He stopped the operation.

John's heart stopped. They tried to resuscitate him. It took a long time. His kidneys stopped working and they put him on dialysis. They eventually got his heart started and put him on a ventilator. They had noticed the problems about 11:00 in the morning. It was about 1:00 in the afternoon when I got to the hospital. From then on time had no meaning, minutes were hours, hours seemed like days, and we waited to be allowed into Intensive Care. It was about 3:00 in the afternoon when we were able to go to him.

So many wires. The constant noise of the ventilator. His hands were icy cold from the cooling they had tried to do. Lots of people were around the bed, checking blood, emptying dialysis bags, giving injections, discussing in hushed whispers in the corner. We just sat there, helpless. How can two grown adults, parents, be so helpless?

Tracey! Someone had to get her from school, stay with her. But for how long? We phoned a neighbor who collected her and then told my sister who collected her after work. The hospital arranged a taxi to take my mother home. She phoned the hospital every hour for news. We just waited, helpless.

Out of the window there was a glorious red and orange sky. The kind you only get with intense cold. I remember thinking "red sky at night, shepherds delight" — it will be all right, it will. Ten minutes later, at 8:30 in the evening, his heart stopped again. They tried to revive him. They couldn't. They did not need to tell us. The doctor just stood in the doorway.

They removed all their equipment, and we went to see him. So tiny, so still. They had given him some flowers, freesias, to hold. I don't even re-member whether there were tears then. Just numbness, stunned helplessness.

The anger came later, as it does. If only. If only there had not been a dispute. If only he had not needed the operation. If only I hadn't signed the consent form. If only they had said the slight cold he had was a problem and sent him home. And the questions. Why did they not know earlier? Why did it take so long to revive him? Why him? Why us? They do such marvelous things these days. Why couldn't they save him?

His entire class came to his funeral. They played their recorders and sang his favorite hymn from school. So quickly he was gone, our gorgeous, cheeky, lively, blonde, and happy, 7-year-old son. Everyone said how happy a child he was. Why him?

Then the anesthetist sent one of his colleagues to our home to tell us about this malignant hyperpyrexia that had killed him. It's hereditary, and for him to be affected one of us must be, and Tracey might be too. All the family must not have anesthetics of any kind without telling the doctors of the problem, until testing could be arranged. Having been told we must avoid anesthetics, we were told we had to go to Leeds, the only unit in the country doing the tests, and have a general anesthetic so that they could do a muscle biopsy to test for this problem. They had to be joking! But they weren't. I was chosen to go first. It was only about 10 weeks since John had died and I was on my way to Leeds for this biopsy, April 1st, All Fools Day! I don't know how I decided to go, still numb I suppose. I do remember thinking I wasn't coming back. Perhaps I even wanted to die, to be with him. Geoff was banging on the door trying to find out if I was all right. When I came round, I sobbed. I was all right, he wasn't. I was also negative. This meant Geoff and maybe Tracey had this problem. They went for their biopsies together in June. Both are positive. They can have anesthetics, but only "safe" ones, and they must be properly monitored before, during, and after the operation. There is a specific procedure for giving anesthetics to someone with MH. There should be no problem getting operations done.

It was very difficult to get the family to take seriously the avoidance of certain anesthetics. If this can happen in a family where someone dies, how could you expect families where someone lives to take it seriously at all. Something had to be done. I contacted Leeds. Was there a group or association for this problem? Not yet. So, with their backing, I started one.

The problem is so rare that affected people are spread all over the country. Just knowing there is someone else who understands is very important, es-pecially for those of us who have lost someone through MH. Getting doctors to take us seriously is by far the biggest problem connected with MH. A lot of them are arrogant, unsympathetic, and dismissive about the effects of MH. It is these attitudes we hope to change.

On August 27, 1989, John had been gone for as long as he had lived. Today, we have now spent more of our married lives without him than with him. The only thing we have is our memories. They at least can never be taken away. January 13, 1982, was the worst day of our lives. It was the longest and shortest day I have ever lived. The details of every minute are etched on our memories. We can recall them as though they were yesterday and yet it seems such a long, long time since we were able to hold him, play with him, and see him smile. How tall would he be? Would he still be blonde? Still be clever with math? What would he want to be? We will never know and our only hope is that research into this problem never ends until what we have gone through can never, ever happen to anyone else again.

Part 2
HISTORY OF THE BRITISH MALIGNANT HYPERTHERMIA ASSOCIATION

The British Malignant Hyperthermia Association (BMHA) was started in 1983 by Alison Winks following the death of her son John the year before as a result of Malignant Hyperthermia. His death occurred during his seventh operation, and there had been no previous indication of problems. He was 7 years old.

Feeling isolated, frustrated, angry, and worried about future medical care for her daughter, Tracey, and her husband, Geoff (both affected by MH), Alison felt the need to make this problem better known and to help others affected by MH. With the support of the Leeds MH Investigation Unit, she contacted others susceptible to MH. Encouraged by the initial response, she began producing newsletters and organized members' meetings. A year later, she succeeded in convincing the BBC to feature the BMHA on one of their prime time news programs. Articles have appeared in anesthetic and nursing journals; representatives have been sent to international MH conferences to promote the work of the BMHA and to maintain links with MH professionals.

In 1989, an Executive Committee was formed, and regional representatives (or link families) were established. Member information is now held on a computer database, and the association is registered under the Data Protection Act. It is also a registered charity. There are ten members working actively for the BMHA, which has no employees; all work is voluntary. The BMHA exists solely on the subscriptions of its members and fund-raising activities; it receives no direct sponsorship.

The BMHA provides the following emergency aid for its members:

● A 24-hour Hot Line (**0345 333 111** — when asked for a number, **0525 420**) covered at all times by members of the Leeds Investigation Unit.

- Literature explaining MH and the drugs to be avoided. The materials are available in several languages for travelers to carry with them when traveling abroad.
- A Medical Emergency Medallion inscribed with Hot Line information.

The BMHA secretary is

> Alison Winks
> 11 Gorse Close
> Newthorpe
> Nottingham NG16 28Z
> England

Part II
History of Malignant
Hyperthermia Research

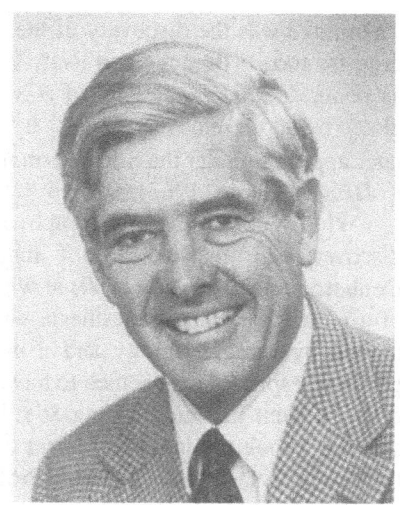

Dr. Michael A. Denborough (1984)

Chapter 4

THE EARLY HISTORY OF MALIGNANT HYPERTHERMIA — A PERSONAL PERSPECTIVE

Werner Kalow

This is a story of the beginnings of malignant hyperthermia (MH) observed by a witness or — if you prefer — by someone akin to a theater critic who by necessity has a different perspective than the leading actors. The narration of an observer may illuminate the discovery which has turned out to have lasting consequences. I accepted the invitation to write an account because I sometimes ponder the weave of coincidental factors that made me an early participant in the exploration of this syndrome.

Let me first present my credentials as a witness. In the mid-1950s I had observed a genetic variant of plasma cholinesterase which caused an abnormal response to the muscle relaxant succinylcholine (Kalow, 1956). This observation brought me, as a pharmacologist, in contact with geneticists, and it aroused my curiosity about other heritable changes that may alter the response to drugs. At that time, primaquine-induced hemolysis was still a relatively recent discovery, and the definition of its cause (Carson et al., 1956), as a deficiency of glucose-6-phosphate dehydrogenase, was an admired achievement.

Then there was the discovery of the slow elimination of the anti-tuberculous drug isoniazid (Bonicke and Reif, 1953; Hughes et al., 1954), later defined as being due to low activity of N-acetyltransferase. I was sufficiently stimulated by all these observations that I decided to compile a monograph, which later appeared under the title *Pharmacogenetics — Heredity and the Response to Drugs* (Kalow, 1962).

While writing this monograph, I was constantly looking out for further discoveries in this field. Thus I immediately noticed the letter in *Lancet* by Denborough and Lovell (1960) in which they described a frightening reaction of a patient to general anesthesia with halothane. This episode was characterized by muscle rigidity and a dramatic rise of body temperature. This peculiar response was deemed to have a genetic basis because several relatives of the patient had died during anesthesia, apparently under similar circumstances. I took the letter in *Lancet* to the Toronto General Hospital in order to show it to Dr. R. A. Gordon, Professor of Anesthesia, an influential man who eventually took a leading role in stimulating investigations into malignant hyperthermia (Gordon, Britt, and Kalow, 1973). He told me that reactions such as those of the patient described by Denborough and Lovell are uncommon but not unheard of in anesthesia. In other cases, the anesthetist did probably consider it to be a consequence of some inadvertently produced anoxic brain damage that must have occurred somehow during surgery and anesthesia. It is clear that such a despairing dead-end interpretation of the causes of a critical, perhaps fatal reaction was not particularly inducive to publication; the few pertinent reports were later summarized by Gordon (1973).

Denborough and his colleagues reinforced the impact of their letter with an article in the *British Journal of Anaesthesia* (1962) entitled *Anaesthetic Deaths in a Family*. This article contained a pedigree and more details than the original letter, and it was read by many anesthetists. At a meeting of interested investigators held in 1977 in Denver, CO (Aldrete and Britt, 1978), the proposal was made and formally discussed to honor Michael Denborough by calling this entity Denborough's myopathy (Kalow, 1978). All were in favor of the sentiment expressed by this motion, but marking a syndrome by a personal name was considered undesirable in principle. Among many proposals, malignant hyperpyrexia or malignant hyperthermia were the preferred terms. Considering the meaning of the Greek roots of the words hyperpyrexia and hyperthermia, the latter appears to be more appropriate.

In 1965, I took a year of sabbatical leave from the University of Toronto. When I returned in early 1966, there had been a case in Toronto such as described by Denborough. A child had died and the anesthetist, Dr. Beverley A. Britt, to whom this happened was devastated. Stimulated by this local case and by our previous discussions, Dr. Gordon had organized inquiries across Canada and thereby learned of 13 other cases that had occurred in recent times (Gordon, 1973). He became keen to stimulate research on this problem.

At a university, in contrast to industry, cross-departmental collaboration between willing but independently successful investigators cannot always be arranged unless special circumstances prevail. When Dr. Gordon called me and asked whether I would be willing to work on MH, I was in a position to accept his suggestion because the eloping of a student with his girlfriend had caused an unscheduled disruption of my plans for cholinesterase research. Dr. Gordon proposed that Dr. Britt should join me as a graduate student because she was highly motivated; she wanted to acquire research training to add to her medical qualifications in order to explore the syndrome. Thus Dr. Britt came to my laboratory, and as her supervisor I found myself cast in the role of an active player in the research on MH.

Two unforgettable events occurred during that time; one was the visit by a young English physician who had specialized to become a geneticist. He told me that during his internship in the west of England, a patient begged him not to give a general anesthetic because several of his relatives had died on the operating table. The anesthetist instructed the young intern to disregard such stories by patients because they are expressions of hysteria. The patient died. The attitude of many British anesthetists at that time was still that MH was a problem in North America or Australia but not in Britain. This story underlines the merits of Denborough, who had taken seriously the anxiety of his patient.

The second of these memorable events was closer to home. At a hospital in Ottawa, a child had died during minor surgery with muscle rigidity and fever. A year later, the brother of that child had a small injury that required some surgery. The parents fearfully reminded the anesthetist of the death of the first child and pleaded for special caution. The anesthetist assured them that a disaster like this may strike once in a million, but such a rare event would surely not happen to them twice. The anesthetist was obviously untrained in genetics. When this second child was on the operating table he became hot and extremely rigid with opisthotonos and developed cardiac irregularities. The surgeon in his desperation opened the child's chest to apply manual massage to his heart; he could feel the beats diminishing until the heart stopped in extreme systolic contraction. We knew from that time that MH represents an abnormality not only of the skeletal muscle, but sometimes also of the heart muscle.

In the laboratory, Dr. Britt and I tried to think of ways to study a syndrome as rare as MH. One obvious task was to get as many case reports as possible and to subject the information to statistical scrutiny (Britt and Kalow, 1970a, b). An observation by Satnik (1969) proved without doubt that the syndrome was caused by a primary defect in muscle and not in the nervous system: arm muscles temporarily excluded from circulation by a tourniquet remained flaccid while the rest of a patient's body became rigid during anesthesia. We therefore focused our attention specifically upon muscle, but our biochemical and histological scrutiny of muscle specimens from affected patients was of no avail (Britt and Kalow, 1968).

A considerable effort went into attempts to create animal models, for instance, by exposing rats to dinitrophenol, a poison that can cause fever and a muscle rigidity that turns into rigor mortis (Britt and Kalow, 1968). With my training in classical pharmacology, I had much experience measuring the contractile behavior of isolated muscle specimens *in vitro* (e.g., Kalow, 1954). We tested normal and dinitrophenol-exposed rat muscle. I knew that chicken biventer muscle is peculiar in responding to succinylcholine with contracture and not, as with most muscles, with relaxation; the biventer turned out not to have any other property of potential utility for us. A colleague in the department studied dog hearts so we could get some skeletal muscle from the same animals. We measured the responses to caffeine that were known to consist of contracture and enhanced twitch response by different mechanisms (Weber, 1968). I was excited when I found that dog muscle contracted on exposure to chloroform (we did not try halothane), something I had never seen with muscle from rats or guinea pigs.

It was these studies and frustrating experiences that made me think that the properties of human skeletal muscle might be better tested by pharmacological than by biochemical or histological means. Dr. Britt, through her clinical connections, was able to arrange for us to get muscle biopsy specimens for testing contractile properties.

None of the initially obtained specimens of human muscle contracted on exposure to halothane, neither those from survivors of MH nor the control specimens obtained during orthopedic surgery. However, the effects of halothane on skeletal muscle could be tested indirectly in the form of the potentiation of the contracture produced by caffeine. It was a crucial observation that both the responsiveness to caffeine contracture and the halothane potentiation could be used as semi-independent means to distinguish between subjects with and without predisposition to MH. We utilized these observations to arrange a pharmacologically sound, clinically useful test system to detect a person's predisposition to MH (Kalow et al., 1970).

After this discovery, Ellis et al. (1973) skillfully expanded the test system by showing that halothane itself could be used to recognize the predisposition. Several user-devised modifications of pharmacodiagnosis of MH have since been introduced (see Kalow et al., 1977; Britt, 1987; Ording, 1987). After Dr. Britt received her degree in pharmacology, she proceeded to use all of her skills and considerable energy to build a unique clinical testing laboratory for diagnosing and studying MH; in addition, she established a repository of information by collecting case reports from all over the world. She thereby created a model to show how a rare disease should be investigated, particularly if such a disease constitutes an experiment that will help us to understand human functions in health and disease.

I am satisfied that our development of a pharmacological assay — inadequate though it may be — has substantially helped the research on MH, both in humans and in pigs, by allowing a recognition of predisposition to this once dreaded pharmacogenetic disease.

REFERENCES

Aldrete, J. A. and Britt, B. A., Eds., *The Second Int. Symp. Malignant Hyperthermia*, Grune & Stratton, New York, 1978.

Britt, B. A., Muscle assessment of malignant hyperthermia susceptible patients, in *Malignant Hyperthermia*, Britt, B. A., Ed., Martinus Nijhoff, Boston, 1977, 193.

Britt, B. A. and Kalow, W., Hyperrigidity and hyperthermia associated with anesthesia, *Ann. N.Y. Acad. Sci.*, 151, 947, 1968.

Britt, B. A. and Kalow, W., Malignant hyperthermia: aetiology unknown!, *Can. Anaesth. Soc. J.*, 17, 316, 1970a.

Britt, B. A. and Kalow, W., Malignant hyperthermia: a statistical review, *Can. Anaesth. Soc. J.*, 17, 293, 1970b.

Bonicke, R. and Reif, W., Enzymatische inaktivierung von Isonicotinsaure hydrazide im menschlichen und tierschen organismus, *Arch. Exp. Pathol. Pharmakol.*, 220, 321, 1953.

Carson, P. E., Flanagan, C. L., Iokes, C. E., and Alving, A. S., Enzymatic deficiency in primaquine-sensitive erythrocytes, *Science*, 124, 484, 1956.

Denborough, M. A. and Lovell, R. R. H., Anaesthetic deaths in a family, *Lancet*, 2, 45, 1960.

Denborough, M. A., Forster, J. F. A., Lovell, R. R. H., Maplestone, P. A., and Villiers, J. D., Anaesthetic deaths in a family, *Br. J. Anaesth.*, 34, 395, 1962.

Ellis, F. R., and Harriman, D. G. F., A new screening test for susceptibility to malignant hyperpyrexia, *Br. J. Anaesth.*, 45, 638, 1973.

Gordon, R. A., History of the syndrome of malignant hyperthermia, in *Int. Symp. Malignant Hyperthermia*, Gordon, R. A., Britt, B. A., and Kalow, W., Eds., Charles C Thomas, Springfield, IL, 1973, p. 5.

Gordon, R. A., Britt, B. A., and Kalow, W., Eds., *Int. Symp. Malignant Hyperthermia*, Charles C Thomas, Springfield, IL, 1973.

Hughes, H. B., Biehl, J. P., Jones, A. P., and Schmidt, L. H., Metabolism of isoniazid in man as related to the occurrence of peripheral neuritis, *Am. Rev. Respir. Dis.*, 70, 266, 1954.

Kalow, W., The influence of pH on the ionization and biological activity of *d*-tubocurarine, *J. Pharmacol. Exp. Ther.*, 110, 433, 1954.

Kalow, W., Familial incidence of low pseudocholinesterase level, *Lancet*, 271, 576, 1956.

Kalow, W., *Pharmacogenetics. Heredity and the Response to Drugs*, W. B. Saunders, Philadelphia, 1962.

Kalow, W., Concluding remarks, in *The Second Int. Symp. Malignant Hyperthermia*, Aldrete, J. A. and Britt, B. A., Eds., Grune & Stratton, New York, 1978, p. 553.

Kalow, W., Britt, B. A., and Richter, A., The caffeine test of isolated human muscle in relation to malignant hyperthermia, *Can. Anaesth. Soc. J.*, 24, 678, 1977.

Kalow, W., Britt, B. A., Terreau, M. E., and Haist, C., Metabolic error of muscle metabolism after recovery from malignant hyperthermia, *Lancet*, Oct., 895, 1970.

Ording, H., The European MH group: protocol for in vitro diagnosis of susceptibility to MH and preliminary results, in *Malignant Hyperthermia*, B. A. Britt, Ed., Martinus Nijhoff, Boston, 1987, 269.

Satnik, J. H., Hyperthermia under anesthesia with regional muscle flaccidity, *Anesthesiology*, 30, 472, 1969.

Weber, A., The mechanism of the action of caffeine on sarcoplasmic reticulum, *J. Gen. Physiol.*, 52, 760, 1968.

Chapter 5

THE DISCOVERY OF MALIGNANT HYPERTHERMIA IN PIGS — SOME PERSONAL RECOLLECTIONS

Gaisford G. Harrison

TABLE OF CONTENTS

I.   Introduction 30

II.   The Discovery 30

III. The Genetic Aspect 35

IV.   Selection and Breeding 36

V.   Some Early Investigations 37

VI.   Conclusion 41

References 42

I. INTRODUCTION

It is ironic that although shock-like, stress-related syndromes had long been recognized in domestic swine and, because of their economic implications for the meat industry, they had been the subject of much veterinary research,[1,2] the identification of their manifestation of anesthetic-induced malignant hyperthermia (MH) was so entirely fortuitous. This discovery had to await the exposure of pigs to general anesthesia with halothane and succinylcholine occasioned by their use in medical research. Based, as it was, on observations by two independent groups of workers in places as far apart as Cambridge (Great Britain) and Cape Town (South Africa), the chance nature of this discovery that genetic strains of certain breeds of swine could serve as a valid experimental animal model of human MH can be judged from the fact that in the former instance the pigs were anesthetized for an investigation into atherogenesis, in the latter for experimental liver transplantation. Further at this time, about 1966, except for Denborough's original identification of this syndrome in a family in Australia,[3,4] published reports of MH in humans had been confined to the North American continent.[5,6] No cases had yet been documented as such in Great Britain or South Africa. Because so much of what we understand today of the pathogenesis of this pharmacogenetic, membrane-based myopathy MH, has come from experimental studies of malignant hyperthermia-susceptible (MHS) swine, a brief account of the circumstances surrounding the discovery of the "hot pig" is of interest and relevance to this volume.

II. THE DISCOVERY

The establishment of a program of liver transplantation in man was a primary objective of the Liver Research Group, an interdisciplinary group formed at the medical school of the University of Cape Town, South Africa in 1968.* To this end initial experience was sought in an animal experimental model. For this purpose we chose the domestic pig instead of the more usual surgical experimental animal, the dog. There were several reasons for this besides the very practical one that our research group's surgical leader already had considerable experience in experimental liver transplantation in swine, which he had acquired while working for a period at the medical school of the University of Bristol (Great Britain). First, the pig, in marked contrast to other animals, shows little evidence of rejection following liver homotransplantation, even of liver of nonrelated donors and in the absence of

---

* The original members of this group concerned with the "hot pig" discovery were J. Terblanche (surgeon), S. J. Saunders (physician), J. F. Biebuyck (anesthesiology resident), D. M. Dent (surgical resident), R. Hickman (surgical resident), and the author (anesthesiologist). In later years each of these attained professorial appointment in his/her particular discipline.

immunosuppression. This strange exception applies only to liver; kidneys, skin, and other organs being rejected, as usual, in these circumstances. Second, on surgical handling, pig liver does not develop venoconstriction with resultant venous outflow block as does that of dogs. Last, pigs were readily obtainable from local farm breeding lines in almost unlimited quantities and were cheap to maintain, and blood for transfusion during experimental surgery was readily obtainable from the local slaughterhouse.

The first animal models to be used in this project were locally bred Landrace piglets, 6 to 8 weeks old weighing 30 to 40 kg. These we anesthetized in the following manner. Having been starved for 16 h preoperatively (for surgical reasons), the unpremedicated pig was anesthetized in its transport pen by the inhalation of N_2O with O_2 (flow rates 6 and 3 l per minute, respectively) with halothane (concentration rapidly increased to 3%) delivered via a snout mask attached to a semi-open circuit, with the pig breathing spontaneously. When the pig lost consciousness, usually within 3 min, it was removed from its pen and placed supine on the operating table. Here, after anesthesia had been deepened for a further 3 to 5 min, orotracheal intubation was performed — a task considerably more difficult in the pig than in man — followed by the passage of a stomach tube and an esophageal thermistor for temperature monitoring. ECG monitoring was then instituted followed by femoral arterial and jugular venous catheterization for the measurement of arterial and venous pressure, arterial blood gas, acid/base and electrolyte monitoring, and to provide the conduit for blood and fluid replacement during surgery. For the surgery, anesthesia was maintained with N_2O/O_2 with halothane (1 to 2%) delivered via a nonreturn circuit by IPPV, powered by a standard automatic ventilator. Ventilatory volumes were adjusted to maintain normo- to mild hypocapnia and apnea. This method provided satisfactory operating conditions in the pig without the use of muscle relaxants. These we chose to avoid so as not to compound the difficulties in relaxant reversal and postoperative respiratory problems consequent to the inevitable early abdominal distension. Ambient temperature in the operating theater varied between 15 to 20°C. Thus the scene was set.

We had anesthetized but a few pigs in this manner without complication, when one reacted to anesthesia in the most bizzare and puzzling manner.[7] As the animal lost consciousness, instead of the usual quieting of respiration, it commenced panting, developing at the same time a blotchy skin cyanosis, despite good auscultated air entry and an FIO_2 of 0.3. Instead of the expected flaccidity, its legs became rigidly extended, so much so that once placed on the operating table, it had all the appearance of a pig in rigor mortis (Figure 1). Orotracheal intubation presented more than its usual difficulty because of masseter spasm and was no sooner successfully accomplished than the animal ceased breathing. IPPV was commenced and, as a good but fast pulse was palpable, we continued with our experimental protocol.

Commencement of ECG monitoring showed a sinus tachycardia of 200 beats per minute while the first blood sample from the femoral artery catheterization

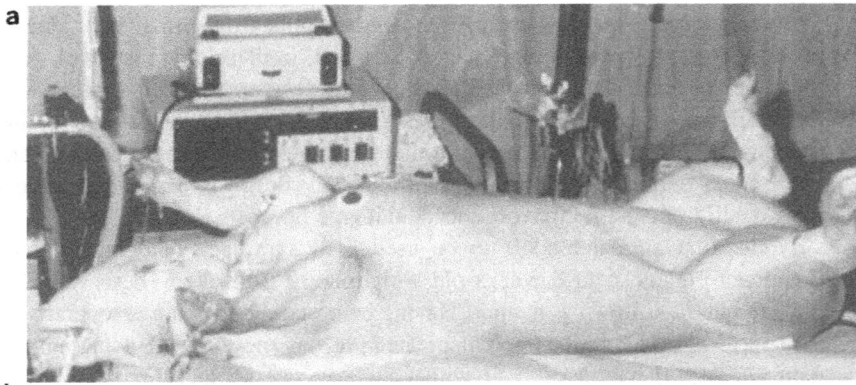

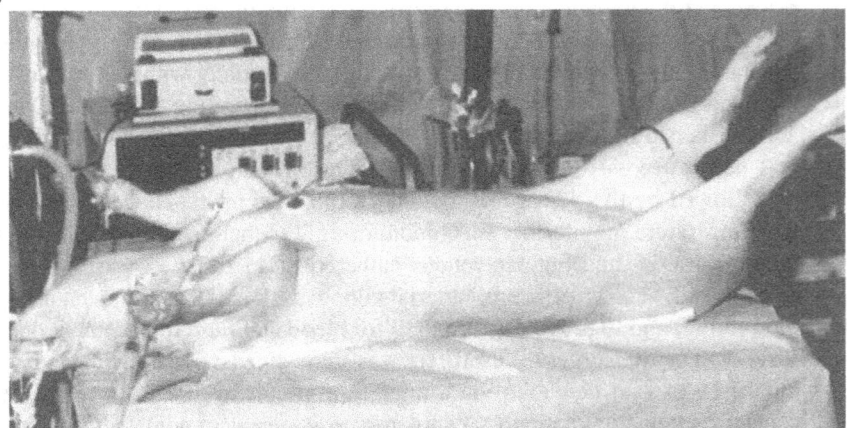

FIGURE 1. The characteristic ante mortem "rigor mortis" that first drew attention to PMH as an entity. (a) MHS pig anesthetized with thiopentone and (b) same pig after 10 min of inhalation of halothane.

revealed a metabolic acidosis so gross (pH 6.85) that we thought it had to be an artifact and immediately repeated it — with the same result. Afterwards, copious amounts of sodium bicarbonate made no impression at all on the acidosis. About 55 min had elapsed from the induction of anesthesia before the surgeon performed the laparotomy and immediately remarked on the extreme heat of the abdominal organs. (He insisted that steam arose from the peritoneal cavity.) The esophageal thermistor, just activated, registered the core temperature as an unbelievable 44°C! Blood pressure and circulation, which had been well maintained until this point, now commenced to fail. After several bursts of multifocal ventricular premature beats, the pig finally demised in ventricular fibrillation after 105 min of anesthesia.

Sporadically and quite unpredictably this same sequence of events was to be repeated exactly in 6 of the first 34 animals anesthetized in this manner. Therapeutic interventions proved fruitless and all died with the longest survival being 135 min, the shortest a mere 45 min from commencement of anesthesia.

At death, core temperatures, which during anesthesia had risen 1°C/5 to 10 min, ranged from 42.5 to 45°C (Figure 2) and all suffered severe metabolic acidosis — pH ≤ 6.85, PCO_2 ≥ 150 mmHg, base excess < −22 mEq/l — an acidosis seemingly uncorrectable by large amounts of sodium bicarbonate (Figure 3). We could discern no cause for all of this. Careful review of the clinical events of each death together with laboratory checks for such possible reasons as septicemia or pyrogens in infused fluids all proved negative.

Besides the unpredictability of its occurrence, the most ominous and frustrating aspect of what we were now coming to recognize as a specific syndrome was the fact that, although it was seemingly initiated in some way by the induction of anesthesia, once established discontinuance of all anesthetic agents and ventilation of the animals with O_2 alone made no difference whatsoever to its inexorably fatal progress. The anesthetic had, in some way, triggered a self-sustaining pathological process.[8]

The early random introduction of an alternate anesthetic technique omitting halothane and utilizing intermittent thiopentone with small doses of curare together with N_2O/O_2 by IPPV, soon demonstrated that when it did occur, the syndrome was only associated with the administration of halothane.

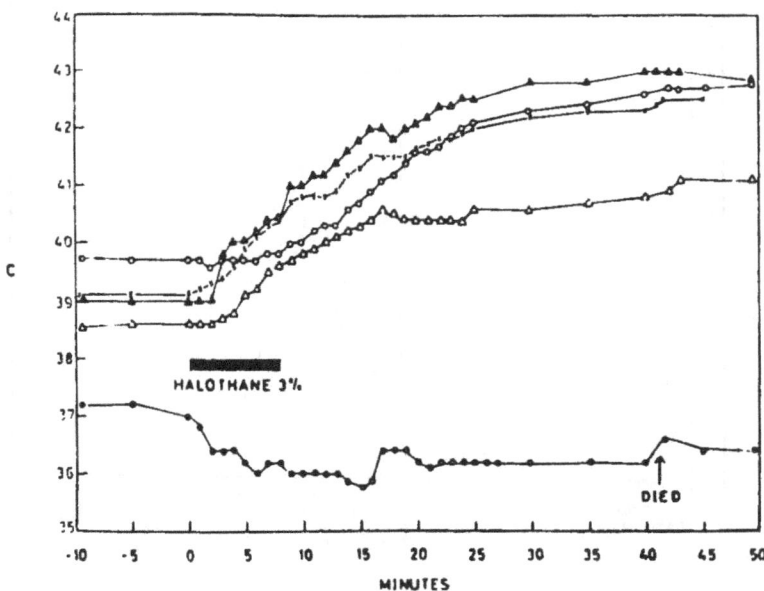

FIGURE 2. Multisite temperature changes recorded following halothane initiation of MH in an MHS pig following a control period of thiopentone anesthesia. Note extreme rapidity of MH onset and speed of temperature rise in internal organs. Skin vasoconstriction (blotchy cyanosis) has prevented a similar rise in skin surface temperature. X = esophagus; ○ = rectum; ▲ = liver; △ = muscle (gluteus); and ● = abdominal skin (surface). (From Berman et al. *Nature*, 225, 653, 1970. With permission.)

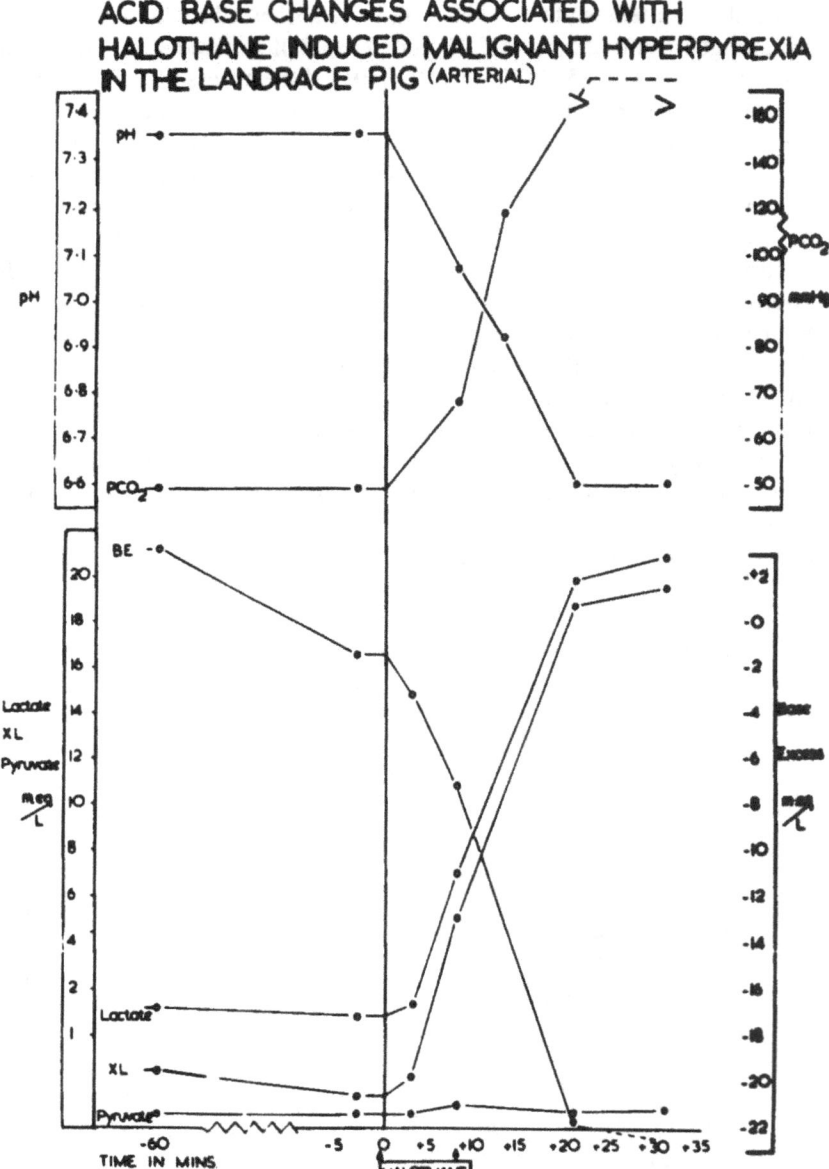

FIGURE 3. Arterial blood acid/base changes recorded in an MHS Landrace following initiation of MH after control period of thiopentone anesthesia. XL = excess lactate. Note speed and extremes of pH and related changes. (From Harrison, G. G., *Int. Symp. Malignant Hyperthermia*, R. A. Gordon, B. A. Britt, and W. Kalow, Eds., Charles C Thomas, Springfield, IL, 1971, 271. With permission.)

Addition of curare to the halothane technique did not prevent the onset, nor did it have any therapeutic effect.[8] Besides pointing the finger at halothane as the MH trigger in our original anesthetic protocol, this observation also identified an anesthetic technique that could be used safely on MHS swine — a technique we were to use subsequently for setting up *in vivo* the monitoring procedures and achieving control period steady states for investigations in such swine.

Clues as to the nature of this syndrome were given to us by two publications current at the time. The first was the 1966 September issue of the *Canadian Anaesthetic Society Journal* (now *Canadian Anaesthetic Journal*).[9] This carried reports by six groups of anesthesiologists — originally presented at a symposium organized by Dr. R. A. Gordon in Toronto — of 11 human fatalities following a syndrome induced by anesthesia, called then for the first time malignant hyperpyrexia. The second came from a preliminary communication by Hall and co-workers to the *British Medical Journal* the same year, which described an "unusual reaction to suxamethonium chloride" observed in three littermate pigs that had been anesthetized as experimental animals.[10] The component features and outcome of the syndromes described by these authors, in man and in swine, described exactly what we were observing; however, there was an important difference between the two groups of pigs. Whereas the "unusual reaction" in Hall's pigs at Cambridge (gross myotonia) was precipitated by the administration of suxamethonium chloride after a period of uncomplicated halothane anaesthesia, in our pigs halothane alone evoked the syndrome. In the human cases which, like Hall's pigs, had a genetic component both halothane and suxamethonium were incriminated. These findings led us to the conclusion that this bizzare hypercatabolic state, initiated in some swine by exposure to halothane, could well be a facsimile of the newly described lethal syndrome in humans of anesthetic-induced malignant hyperpyrexia. If they could be identified and salvaged in some way, we thought that such swine would serve as a valid and much needed experimental model of the syndrome.

III. THE GENETIC ASPECT

Establishing the genetic basis of this seemingly unpredictable susceptibility of our pigs to MH was made difficult for us by a local farming practice. The local pig breeders all corralled their post-weaned piglets in large groups according to weekly age. This made it impossible for us, at this stage, to identify accurately the pedigrees of the pigs supplied to us. Also, varying sources of supply resulted in our using Large White and Large White/Landrace Cross swine in addition to the original pure Landrace strain. As the number of pigs anesthetized increased, however, the genetic aspects of MH susceptibility become more obvious on a statistical basis. When this number had reached 160, we found MH had occurred in 25% of the pure Landrace, 3% of the Landrace/Large White Cross and not at all in the pure Large White breed.[8] This vulnerability of the Landrace was further borne out when an inquiry of Dr. Hall's group in Cambridge brought the reply that their "stiff" pigs that suffered this unusual reaction to suxamethonium were Landrace/ Wessex Cross breeds. (N. Woolf, personal communication).

Very soon reports of Porcine MH (PMH) from Europe,[11] America,[12,13] and Australia[14] showed that, far from being rare, this condition was widespread. In a genetic context, though, susceptibility to MH was limited, in that it was manifested by selected strains of but two major swine breeds other than Landrace. These were the Pietrain and Poland China breeds. All three are breeds genetically selected for the qualities of rapid growth, heavy muscling with high muscle/fat ratio, and high feed efficiency. These are the very breeds that manifest, in high incidence, the recognized stress-related syndromes, porcine stress syndrome (PSS), and pale, soft, exudative pork (PSEP). Indeed it was not long before subsequent research produced good evidence to support the hypothesis that PSS, PSEP, and PMH were all manifestations of the same covert genetic myopathy.[15]

MH-like syndromes have been documented but rarely in species other than swine, most notably the dog and the horse.[16] In these species, in contrast to MHS swine, evocation of the syndrome has needed much longer exposure of the animal to MH-triggering agents, progression of the syndrome has been slower, repeatability of the reaction in individual animals has not been established, and the role of genetic factors has not been as obvious as in swine or humans.

IV. SELECTION AND BREEDING

The association of PMH with stress syndromes and, once established, its rapid progress to a "malignant" irreversibility caused us much frustration in our early attempts to establish the MHS pig as the experimental model of the human condition. This required prospective diagnosis and thereafter inbreeding of the susceptible strain. Then, as now, observing the pig's response to the inhalation of halothane was the only reliable method of identifying MH-susceptible animals.[15] However, excitement from the stress of struggling while being manhandled profoundly enhances the sensitivity of the triggering and the speed of progression of the syndrome and may even be sufficient, of itself, to evoke it.

In these circumstances, MH may be fired by an inhalation of halothane for as short a time as 30 to 40 s. Muscle rigor with accompanying blotchy skin cyanosis occurs almost before the onset of anesthesia, so much so that it is often difficult to distinguish between the stiff leg of conscious induction struggling and the extended leg of MH rigor, so imperceptibly does one merge with the other. To compound these difficulties, the syndrome, having been aborted by very early discontinuation of halothane inhalation, may often recrudesce in highly reactive animals in the early period of recovery from anesthesia. Today, piglets that react so severely are salvaged easily and consistently by the i.v. administration of dantrolene,[17] but in those pre-dantrolene days we suffered the frustration of losing animals often in the diagnostic screening process.

Our first attempts at breeding the MHS strain were embarrassingly and laughably unsuccessful. In all innocence we had fed and pampered two MHS Landrace boars for 6 months before we discovered they had been castrated! Unbeknown to us, male pigs destined for the meat market are routinely castrated shortly after being weaned, in the interests of improving meat palatability and quality and, on superficial examination, signs of castration in young pigs are not that obvious to the uninitiated. Thereafter, having acquired a noncastrated young MHS boar and nurturing him to reproductive age, our next breeding attempt was frustrated by the syndrome of "purple porcine passion". Our boar was so highly stress-susceptible, that his excited attempts at procreation evoked fulminant MH that led to his becoming stiff, hot, and blue and his immediate and premature demise. Our breeding frustrations were not confined to boars. Of the first three MHS gilts that we carefully reared to reproductive age, one had a vaginal abnormality, one developed sway back, and the third refused to mate.

V. SOME EARLY INVESTIGATIONS

Fortunately, we were not dependent for our supply of MHS swine on our own initially futile attempts at breeding this strain. The random incidence of the MHS gene in the Landrace and Landrace/Large White Cross swine we acquired for the surgical research program — 25 and 3%, respectively — ensured a supply of MHS animals sufficient for our early MH investigational needs. Later, by efficient screening and elimination of stress-susceptible animals, the local pig breeders were to reduce this incidence greatly but, by then, we had established our own MHS breeding line.

The early investigations of MH using the MHS pig model were especially fruitful and cost effective. In this exciting and virgin field, fundamental conclusions could be and were made from relatively simple, unsophisticated, and inexpensive experiments. In a short time these led to the identification of skeletal muscle both as the site of the lesion and the primary source of the heat production.[18] In briefly recalling some of these early fundamental investigations using the MHS pig model to conclude this account, as these are personal recollections, I am confining my remarks to our own investigations of the "hot pig." Of course, as MHS swine were identified widely geographically, similar research was being undertaken contemporaneously in Europe, England, America, and Australia with results that were confirmatory and/or complementary to our own, but I do not have the space here to review these.

In pigs dying from MH, the only tissue to show histological abnormalities (conventional light microscopy) was skeletal muscle. These changes were consistent with fiber damage and destruction from severe rigor.[8] The character of this rigor, clinically so like that of rigor mortis (see Figure 1), which was then known to correlate with depletion of ATP from muscle, led us initially to investigate specifically ATP content of MHS muscle and the effects on this of exposure to halothane. This relatively simple investigation revealed the presence of a fundamental, identifiable functional lesion in the skeletal muscle of the MHS swine. The rate of depletion of ATP from biopsies incubated *in vitro* was double that of muscle from non-MH pigs, and this depletion rate was enhanced by exposure to halothane (Figure 4). Ironically, as we soon found, the depletion of ATP *in vivo* was **not** by itself the cause

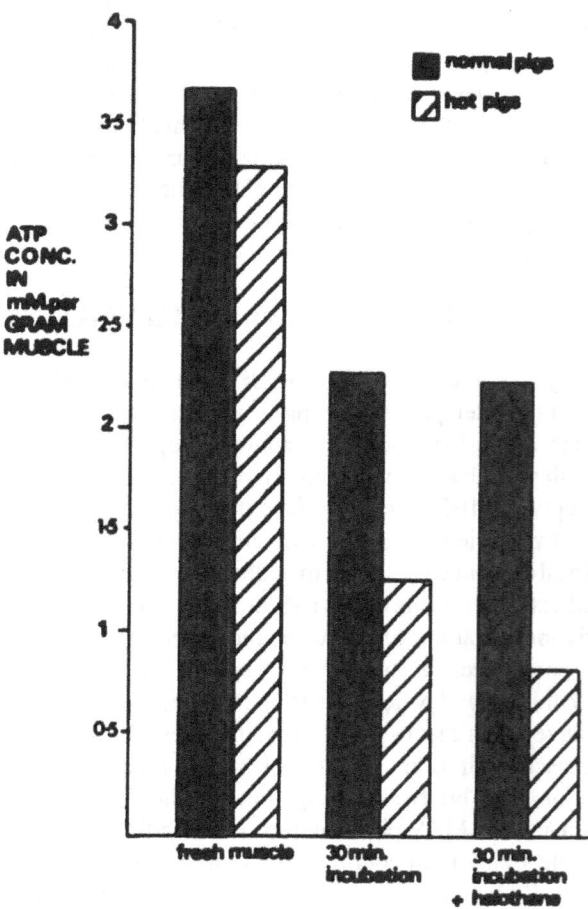

FIGURE 4. The effect *in vitro* on ATP content of muscle from normal and MHS swine of incubation in Krebs-Ringer solution and exposure to halothane. (From Harrison, G. G., *Porcine Malignant Hyperthermia in Malignant Hyperthermia*, B. A. Britt, Ed., International Anesthesiology Clinics, Vol. 17(4), Little, Brown, Boston, 1979, 25. With permission.)

of the muscle rigor. ATP levels in MHS muscle *in vivo* were well maintained early in the course of the MH syndrome initiated by halothane, at a time when muscle rigor was already well established. The levels of ATP fell only after there had been an appropriate depletion of creatine phosphate (Figure 5), which by itself correlated with a concomitant depletion of glycogen.[19]

This realization came from the subsequent, more sophisticated studies of the correlated dynamic *in vivo* biochemical changes in blood and serial muscle biopsies (liquid N_2 frozen) that accompanied progression of this syndrome to its fatal end.[18,19] The depletion of glycogen, which accompanied the concomitant development of gross acidosis (see Figure 3) with a stoichiometric increase in lactate (Figure 6), was the outcome of mass glycolysis that rapidly became anaerobic (Figure 7). Anaerobiasis was calculated as being responsible for at least 50% of the increased heat production. Anaerobic mechanisms had not previously been considered as a source of physiological or pathological heat. At the same time, no evidence was found of the uncoupling of oxidative phosphorylation that had been suggested by some as the source of the increased heat.[20]

The muscle rigor was fueled by the activation of the powerful myofibrillar ATPase and consequent hydrolysis of adenine nucleotides.

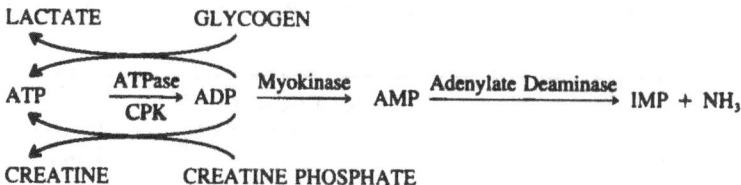

The originally observed depletion of ATP was the outcome of its rate of consumption in this system far exceeding its regeneration potential by anaerobiasis. Deprived of substrate by this reaction, various membrane ion pumps — in the sarcoplasmic reticulum (SR), mitochondria, and sarcolemma (SL) — progressively failed, leading to the a loss of membrane integrity, with the ultimate production of the biochemical conditions that characterize rigor mortis.

Both of these interrelated events: (1) activation of myofibrillar ATPase and rigor and (2) activation of glycolysis, were explainable, it was suggested, by the rapid release of calcium from intracellular sites. We provided pharmacological support for this contention that the release of calcium from intracellular binding sites was the primary event in the onset of the MH syndrome, by a demonstration *in vivo* that the triggering of the MH syndrome in MHS swine by halothane and succinylcholine was effectively blocked by the administration of procaine.[21] This drug was then well known to block caffeine-induced SR calcium release and so caffeine-induced muscle rigor *in vitro*, a reaction for which Kalow et al.[22] had shown the muscle of MH patients to have an abnormal sensitivity.[22] These observations provided the

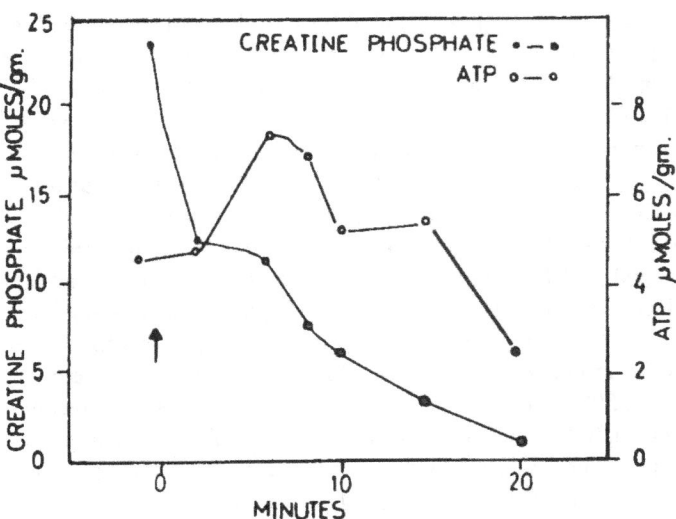

FIGURE 5. *In vivo* ATP and creatine phosphate content of serial muscle biopsies during progress of PMH provoked by inhalation of halothane. (From Berman, M. C. and Kench, J., *Int. Symp. Malignant Hyperthermia*, R. A. Gordon, B. A. Britt, and W. Kalow, Eds., Charles C Thomas, Springfield, IL, 1973, 287. With permission.)

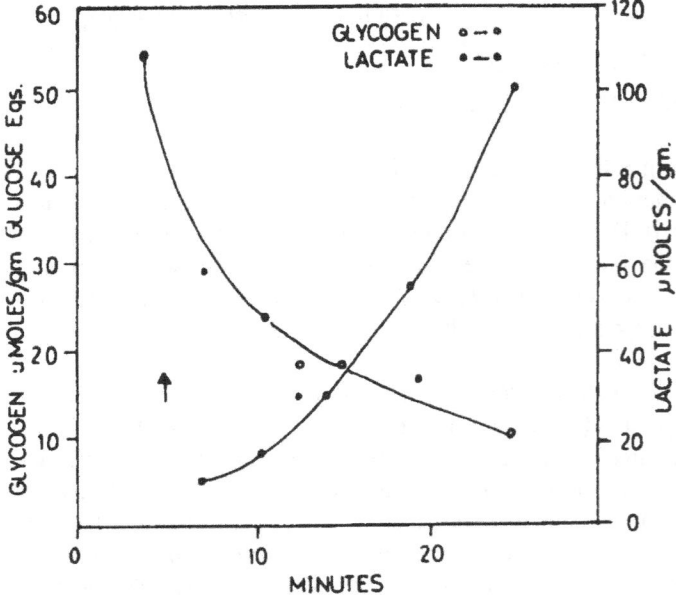

FIGURE 6. *In vivo* glycogen and lactate content of serial muscle biopsies during progress of PMH provoked by inhalation of halothane. (From Berman, M. C. and Kench, J., *Int. Symp. Malignant Hyperthermia*, R. A. Gordon, B. A. Britt, and W. Kalow, Eds., Charles C Thomas, Springfield, IL, 1973, 287. With permission.)

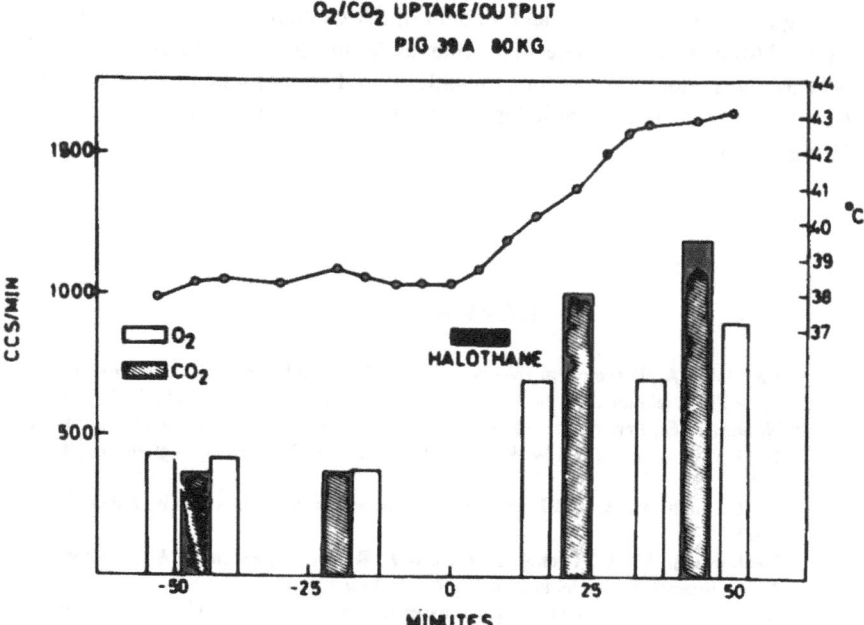

FIGURE 7. Oxygen uptake and CO_2 output with simultaneous esophageal temperature recorded during a course of PMH evoked by inhalation of halothane after a control period of thiopentone anesthesia. Note the disproportionate increase in CO_2 output compared to O_2 uptake indicating onset of anaerobiasis. (From Berman et al., *Nature*, 225, 653, 1970. With permission.)

rationale for the first and only specific therapy suggested for MH[23] before the introduction of dantrolene several years later.[17]

VI. CONCLUSION

Proposed in 1968 as an animal model for the study of the MH syndrome in man, the use of MHS swine has stood the test of time. Though the final minutiae of the pathogenesis of MH have still to be elucidated, knowledge that has come from worldwide extensive studies of PMH has shown it — and by inference the human syndrome — to be the functional result of a genetic membrane defect/dysfunction in the triadic SR/T-tubular junctional region of the myocyte.[24,25] In certain circumstances, this leads to a failure of the normal control of the calcium-release component of the excitation/contraction/coupling mechanism leading to the induction of an abrupt and sustained rise in myoplasmic free-calcium. This event initiates muscle contracture, activates glycolysis and mitochondrial activity, and sets in action a series of events that interact to form a vicious cycle.[26] Using the MHS pig as the pharmacological test bed, these insights into the pathogenesis of MH have been accompanied by the development of an effective therapy for the syndrome, a drug that reduces the rate and amount of SR calcium release, dantrolene.[17] This addition to the anesthetists' armamenterium has potentially eliminated MH as the major cause of unavoidable mortality attributable to anesthesia that it once was. Today, with correct management, survival from MH should be the norm.

REFERENCES

1. **Lawrie, R. A.**, Post mortem glycolysis in normal and exudative longissimus dorsi muscles of the Pig in relation to so-called white muscle disease, *J. Comp. Pathol.*, 70, 273, 1960.
2. **Nelson, T. E.**, Porcine stress syndromes, in *Int. Symp. Malignant Hyperthermia*, R. A. Gordon, B. A. Britt, and W. Kalow, Eds., Charles C Thomas, Springfield, IL, 1973, 191.
3. **Denborough, M. A. and Lovell, R. R.**, Anaesthetic death in a family, *Lancet* 2, 45, 1960.
4. **Denborough, M. A., Forster, J. A., Lovell, R. R., Mapleston, P. A., and Villiers, J. D.**, Anaesthetic deaths in a family, *Br. J. Anaesth.*, 34, 395, 1962.
5. **Britt, B. A.**, A history of malignant hyperthermia, in *Malignant Hyperthermia*, B. A. Britt, Ed., Martinus Nijhoff, Boston, 1987, xi.
6. **Gronert, G. A.**, Malignant hyperthermia, *Anesthesiology*, 53, 395, 1980.
7. **Harrison, G. G., Biebuyck, J. F., Terblanche, J., Dent, D. M., Hickman, R., and Saunders, S. J.**, Hyperpyrexia during anaesthesia, *Br. Med. J.*, 3, 594, 1968.
8. **Harrison, G. G., Saunders, S. J., Biebuyck, J. F., Hickman, R., Dent, D. M., Weaver, V., and Terblanche, J.**, Anaesthetic induced malignant hyperpyrexia and a method for its prediction, *Br. J. Anaesth.*, 41, 844, 1969.
9. **Cullen, W. G., Davies, L. E., Graves, H. B., Gordon, R. A., Hogg, S., Renwick, W., Lavoie, G., Relton, J. E. S., Creighton, R. E., Johnson, A. E., Pelton, D. A., Conn, A. W., Thut, W. H., and Davenport, H. T.**, Malignant hyperpyrexia: editorial and case reports, *Can. Anaesth. Soc. J.*, 13, 415, 1966.
10. **Hall, L. W., Woolf, M., Bradley, J. W., and Jolly, D. W.**, Unusual reaction to suxamethonium chloride, *Br. Med. J.*, 2, 1305, 1966.
11. **Sybesma, W. and Eikelenboom, G.**, Malignant hyperthermia syndrome in pigs, *Neth. J. Vet. Sci.*, 2, 155, 1969.
12. **Jones, E. W., Burnap, T. K., Nelson, T. E., Kerr, D. D., and Anderson, J. A.**, Preliminary Studies of Fulminant Hyperpyrexia in a Family of Swine, Ann. Meeting Am. Soc. Anesthesiologists, Abstracts of Scientific Papers, p. 47.
13. **Pollock, R. A., Standefer, J. C., Hildebrandt, P. K., Goodwin, B., and Li, T. K.**, Malignant hyperthermia in the American Landrace pig, in *Int. Symp. Malignant Hyperthermia*, R. A. Gordon, B. A. Britt, and W. Kalow, Eds., Charles C Thomas, Springfield, IL, 1973, 224.
14. **Denborough, M. A., Hird, F. J., King, J. O., Marginson, M. A. et al.**, Mitochondrial and other studies in Australian Landrace pigs affected with malignant hyperthermia, in *Int. Symp. Malignant Hyperthermia*, R. A. Gordon, B. A. Britt, and W. Kalow, Eds., Charles C Thomas, Springfield, IL, 1973, 229.
15. **Harrison, G. G.**, Porcine malignant hyperthermia — the saga of the "hot pig", in *Malignant Hyperthermia*, B. A. Britt, Ed., Martinus Nijhoff, Boston, 1987, 101.
16. **Klein, L. and Rosenberg, H.**, Malignant hyperthermia in animals other than swine, in *Malignant Hyperthermia*, B. A. Britt, Ed., Martinus Nijhoff, Boston, 1987, 137.

17. **Harrison, G. G.**, Dantrolene — dynamics and kinetics, *Br. J. Anaesth.*, 60, 279, 1988.
18. **Berman, M. C., Harrison, G. G., Bull, A. B., and Kench, J. E.**, Changes underlying halothane induced malignant hyperpyrexia in pigs, *Nature*, 225, 653, 1970.
19. **Berman, M. C. and Kench, J.**, Biochemical features of malignant hyperthermia in Landrace pigs, in *Int. Symp. Malignant Hyperthermia*, R. A. Gordon, B. A. Britt, and W. Kalow, Eds., Charles C Thomas, Springfield, IL, 1973, 287.
20. **Wilson, R. D., Nicols, R. J., Dent, T. E. and Allen, C. R.**, Disturbances of oxidative phosphorylation mechanism as a possible etiological factor in sudden unexplained hyperthermia occurring during anaesthesia, *Anesthesiology*, 27, 231, 1966.
21. **Harrison, G. G.**, The effect of procaine and curare on the initiation of malignant hyperpyrexia, in *Int. Symp. Malignant Hyperthermia*, R. A. Gordon, B. A. Britt, and W. Kalow, Eds., Charles C Thomas, Springfield, IL, 1971, 271.
22. **Kalow, W., Britt, B. A., Terreau, M. E., and Histe, C.**, Metabolic error of muscle metabolism after recovery from malignant hyperthermia, *Lancet*, 2, 895, 1970.
23. **Harrison, G. G.**, Anaesthetic induced malignant hyperpyrexia: a suggested method of treatment, *Br. Med. J.*, 3, 454, 1971.
24. **Kim, D. H., Sreter, F. A., and Ikemoto, M.**, Involvement of a 60 kDa phosphoprotein in the regulation of Ca^{2+} Release from SR of normal and malignant hyperthermia susceptible pig muscle, *Biochem. Biophys. Acta*, 945, 246, 1988.
25. **Mickelson, J. R., Gallant, E. M., Litterer, L. A., Johnson, K. M., Rempel, W. E., and Louis, C. F.**, Abnormal sarcoplasmic reticulum ryanodine receptor in malignant hyperthermia, *J. Biol. Chem.*, 263, 9310, 1988.
26. **Harrison, G. G.**, Malignant hyperthermia, in *General Anaesthesia*, J. F. Nunn, J. E. Utting, and B. R. Brown, Eds., 5th ed., Butterworths, London, 1989, 655.
27. **Harrison, G. G.**, *Porcine Malignant Hyperthermia in Malignant Hyperthermia*, B. A. Britt, Ed., International Anesthesiology Clinics, Vol. 17(4), Little, Brown, Boston, 1979, 25.

Chapter 6

HOW WAS THE ABNORMAL CALCIUM RELEASE CHANNEL FROM THE SARCOPLASMIC RETICULUM IDENTIFIED?

S. Tsuyoshi Ohnishi

TABLE OF CONTENTS

I.   Introduction 46

II.   Developing a Dual-Wavelength Spectrometer and the
        Murexide Method 46

III.   Struggling in a New Country 49

IV.   Starting from Scratch 50

V.   Success in Calcium-Induced Calcium Release from
        Isolated Skeletal SR 50

VI.   The Discovery that the Calcium-Release Channel of
        MH-SR is Abnormal 53

VII.   Again from Scratch 59

VIII.   Identifying the Difference between Skeletal and
        Cardiac Muscle 59

XI.   One More Time from Scratch 63

X.   Epilogue 64

References 65

I. INTRODUCTION

The previous two authors, who pioneered the research of malignant hyperthermia (MH), wrote their personal recollections, vividly describing historical events that led to the discovery of this disease. In comparison with their historical accomplishments, my experience in MH research is quite limited. However, I was able to participate in the quest to identify the true cause of MH and to make some critical contributions to its research.

What I did was to identify that the problem of this disease was in abnormal calcium-release channels of the sarcoplasmic reticulum (SR). To discover the secret at a time when no one knew the true mechanism was an endeavor that required courage, energy, and concentration. Once the mechanism was identified, it became much easier to confirm and extend the work. This discovery was the result of my lifelong pursuit of SR study.

II. DEVELOPING A DUAL-WAVELENGTH SPECTROMETER AND THE MUREXIDE METHOD

The story goes back approximately 30 years to Japan when I was a graduate student under Dr. Fumio Oosawa of the Department of Physics at Nagoya University. He was a pioneer in the field of biophysics in Japan. In the late 1950s, Dr. Oosawa began extracting the muscle protein, actin, from experimental animals and was studying its biophysical properties. Through him I learned the spirit of not being afraid to challenge a new field and the importance of observing experimental phenomena with one's own eyes. After I received my doctorate degree, Dr. Oosawa located a scholarship for me so that I could continue with my career. At his laboratory I discovered, in 1961, that the muscle protein actin could be found in cellular membranes, a finding that was ahead of other investigators.[1] Ten years later, the nonmuscular actin in the cytoskeleton became a popular area of research in cellular biology, but my earlier work was forgotten.

Around that time, Dr. Bunji Hagihara, who was the pioneer of the crystallization of soluble cytochromes, returned from the Johnson Foundation (JF) at the University of Pennsylvania and started his own laboratory in the Osaka University School of Medicine. He described to me a dual-wavelength spectrophotometer that Dr. Britton Chance had developed for measuring small absorbance changes in a turbid suspension, such as a mitochondrial suspension. He told me that no one else had succeeded in building such a machine outside of the JF, and asked me whether I could build it for him. Although I did not have any experience in building a spectrophotometer, I decided to try because I had some experience in electronics and optics. All I had were a few publications by Dr. Chance. Dr. Hagihara told me that the original machine used a mechanical vibrating mirror and a mechanical chopper with electric contacts that caused occasional instability.

It was at this time that semiconductors were being introduced to instrumentation, so I decided to try something new. I designed a rotating sector and semiconductor switching circuit which would eliminate the instability that was inherent to vibrating mirror-chopper systems. Fortunately, the new dual-wavelength spectrophotometer was completed in 1962 (Figure 1), and it worked very well.[2] I even built a three-wavelength spectrophotometer, because with this new design, the number of wavelengths at which we can simultaneously measure respective absorbance changes could be easily increased.[4] From Dr. Hagihara I learned the secrets of performing careful, patient experiments.

At that time, my scholarship funds ran out, but Dr. Oosawa found a visiting scientist scholarship for me. With this new scholarship, I started visiting Dr. Setsuro Ebashi's laboratory at the University of Tokyo School of Medicine. Dr. Ebashi had just found that the SR was an ATP-driven, calcium-sequestering organelle in skeletal muscle. He asked me whether I could develop a spectrophotometric technique to study the kinetics of calcium transport in the SR. I immediately decided to use the dual-wavelength spectrophotometer that I had just built, because the suspension of SR was quite turbid. With this spectrophotometer and using murexide, a metallochromic indicator, we were able to demonstrate ATP-induced calcium uptake by the SR (Figure 2).[3] I subsequently built myself a rapid flow apparatus (again by reading Dr. Chance's papers) and demonstrated that the speed of the calcium uptake was fast enough to account for the speed of muscle relaxation.[5] Murexide and tetramethyl murexide, which I used later,[9] were called the first generation calcium indicators.

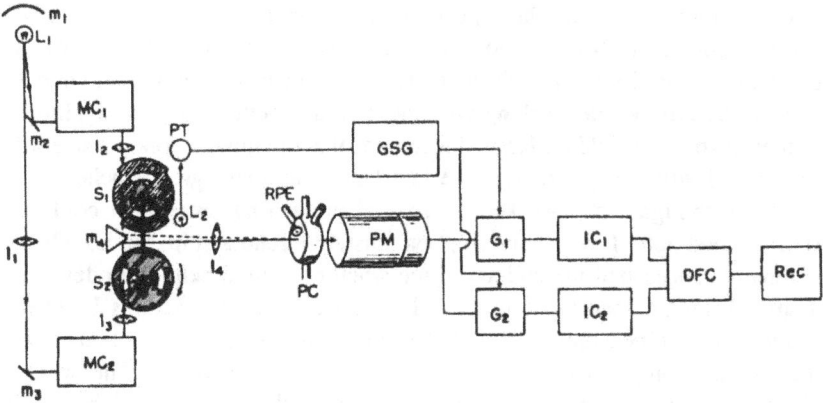

FIGURE 1. Outline of the apparatus. L_1, L_2, lamps; $l_{1,2,3,4}$, lenses; MC_1, MC_2, monochromators; $m_{1,2,3,4}$, mirrors; S_1, S_2, rotating sectors; PT, phototransistor; GSG, gate signal generator; G_1, G_2, gate circuits; PM, photomultiplier; IC_1, IC_2, integration circuits; DFC, difference circuit; Rec, recorder; PC, polarographic cell; and RPE, rotating platinum electrode. (From Ohnishi, S. T., Hagihara, B., and Okunuki, K., *J. Biochem.*, 54, 287, 1963. With permission.)

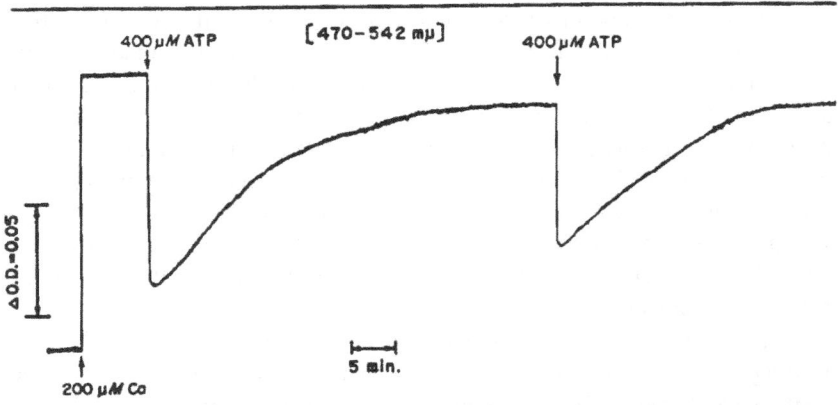

FIGURE 2. Instantaneous Ca binding of vesicles on addition of ATP. 30 μM murexide, 1.3 mg/ml vesicles, 0.1M KCl, 0.02M tris-maleate (pH 6.8), 2 mM MgCl$_2$, temperature 20°C. (From Ohnishi, S. T. and Ebashi, S., *J. Biochem.*, 54, 506, 1963. With permission.)

From Dr. Ebashi, I learned the principle of preparing good, active biological preparations. It was at this time that Dr. Ebashi discovered the mechanism of regulation of muscle contraction by isolating the calcium-binding protein troponin. Through his principle, he identified the role of SR and subsequently discovered troponin as an active component in tropomyosin. By that time, tropomyosin was regarded as a protein having no particular physiological functions. I also learned how important it was for a scientist to stay working at the laboratory bench. Dr. Ebashi had a motto that when he was working at the bench, the papers he wrote were of high quality, but if he was not working at the bench, the papers lost spirit and quality. Indeed, he worked every night at the bench, and his entire laboratory was full of spirit and excitement. Dr. Makoto Endo was also working in his laboratory, and we became friends. While working with these great teachers, who were pioneers in their respective fields, I learned a great deal about how to conduct scientific research. I will always treasure the fact that I met these great teachers.

Even though I had worked on several pioneering projects, I could not find a good job; I was surviving on unstable scholarship funds. Then a company approached me and asked me whether I could help them develop a dual-wavelength spectrophotometer. I taught them all the secrets I had discovered and helped them develop the optics and electronics. I thought that they would compensate my know-how, but I was too naive. The spectrophotometer became one of the company's best sellers and major laboratories in Japan had purchased it. The company had probably sold more than 1000 instruments, but I did not receive a penny. My name was not acknowledged anywhere in the company's pamphlet, although without my assistance it was impossible for the company to build this instrument. My concept of using a rotating sector and an electronic switching system has been widely accepted and today almost all spectrophotometers in the world use this system.

III. STRUGGLING IN A NEW COUNTRY

In 1967 I was a visiting scientist at the JF. There I taught Dr. Lena Mela about the murexide method, which she began to use for the measurement of calcium uptake by mitochondria. Dr. Antonio Scarpa, who joined the JF later, extended this method and screened various compounds. He found that arsenazo III and antipirazo III were more favorable, because they were more sensitive than murexide and because longer wavelengths were used for measurements (meaning less interference by turbidity). They were called the second generation calcium indicators. The method of measuring calcium concentration by dyes became suddenly very popular not only at the JF, but also throughout the world.

For myself, as an unknown scientist in the American scientific community, it was a long struggle to build my career. I lost my job twice and had to survive for many months by finding small consulting jobs for local companies. Around that time, I developed a simple, inexpensive dual-wavelength spectrometer that did not require any rotating sector-switching system. It used two interference filters for providing two wavelengths and DC amplifiers.[6,10] It had been a common belief that a DC amplifier was unstable, and therefore, we had to use a chopper amplifier to obtain high performance. However, I found that with certain precautions we could build a high-performance spectrophotometer with DC amplifiers, thanks to the availability of integrated circuits (IC). This spectrophotometer, which I built in 1971, has become the most popular instrument in my laboratory.[10] I have been using it, sometimes day and night, every day, for more than 20 years, and it still works without any problems.

Then a company wanted to commercialize this spectrophotometer. Because I had had a bad experience previously, we exchanged a document that stated that I would receive a commission if the company sold it. Again, I taught them how to build it. Unfortunately, it did not sell well, because no one was interested in a spectrophotometer that used interference filters. However, a few years later, someone else was developing a technology in an oxygen analyzer. My new dual-wavelength spectrophotometer was perfect for that application, because it was simple and inexpensive. Again I helped the company that had been trying to sell this spectrophotometer. The new instrument worked very well and was better than any other previous instrumentation. Although the market for this analyzer was not great, at least the company seemed to be selling the instrument occasionally. However, I did not receive a commission and was wondering why. Years later, I found that the instruments that the company was selling used the printed circuit boards that were copied from my original instrument. I did not give the company the design for the circuit boards, but they copied the boards from the first instrument I built and did not need my assistance. Then, another surprise came. Papers describing the development of this technology were published, but I did not find my name in these papers. Again, I did not receive any academic credit or financial benefit, although it was impossible for them to develop this new instrument without my participation.

IV. STARTING FROM SCRATCH

While I was struggling, it was Dr. C. Paul Bianchi (professor at the University of Pennsylvania in the early 1970s) who recommended me to Dr. Henry Price, an anesthesiologist. In 1973, I started working under Dr. Price to find out why halothane weakens heart contractions (negative inotropism). Dr. Price was a pioneer in this field, and he was the one who found that calcium antagonized the negative inotropic effect of halothane.[7,8]

I was given a small room equipped with only a pH meter and a classic triple-beam balance. I recalled the motto of Dr. Oosawa. He was always proud of having built his biophysics laboratory in a physics department where no instrumentation was available. It was his belief that a laboratory is something that one has to build by one's own effort. I started building instrumentation, doing experiments, and writing grant applications. I stayed in the laboratory until midnight almost every day. Finally, in 1975, we received an NIH grant. I started to study SR again after long years of interruption. I found that tetramethyl murexide was a better reagent, because it was pH insensitive.[9] I also found a problem with the arsenazo III dye. It strongly bound calcium ions so that the measurement of calcium concentration with this dye required correction.[10] I found a problem in the murexide method, too. The dye (especially tetramethyl murexide) was permeable to the SR membrane, a finding that could pose a problem under certain conditions;[11] however, this shortcoming was later changed into an asset. Using the permeability of this dye, I encapsulated the SR with both the tetramethyl murexide dye and 10-mM calcium ions. Then, I measured the rate of calcium release by measuring the absorbance changes of internally trapped dye.[17]

V. SUCCESS IN CALCIUM-INDUCED CALCIUM RELEASE FROM ISOLATED SKELETAL SR

After these experiences, I decided to change gears and to study calcium release instead of calcium uptake. Dr. Makoto Endo, with whom I established a friendship at Dr. Ebashi's laboratory, emphasized the importance of calcium release in the mechanism of muscle contraction.[12] At that time, techniques employed for the study of calcium release included using a single-skinned fiber (which Dr. Endo developed) or radioactive ^{45}calcium. I decided to develop a simpler method that used a dual-wavelength spectrophotometer and dye. This took years of hard work and staying every night after midnight. Finally, in 1979, I was able to develop methods that were easy to use: one was the depolarization-induced calcium release[13] and the other was the calcium-induced calcium release.[14-17] The secret to demonstrating the calcium-induced calcium release was very simple, once it was discovered: use a low magnesium concentration (0.5 mM) and pulse calcium until the SR is loaded to initiate calcium-induced calcium release (Figure 3A). I also found that the calcium-induced calcium release from the SR was triggered by halothane, enflurane, or caffeine (Figures 3B and Figure 4), but was inhibited by magnesium, tetracaine, or ruthenium red (Figure 5). After my first paper,[14] ruthenium red became a popular compound in the study of channel properties of SR all over the world.

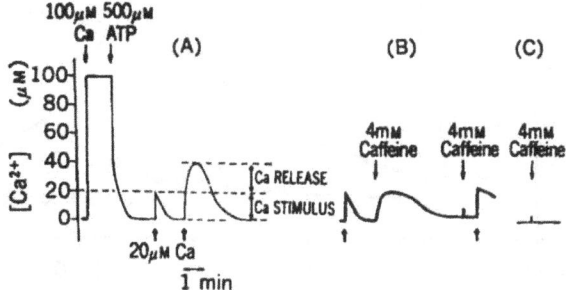

FIGURE 3. Preloading of the SR with Ca^{2+} is required before the demonstration of (A) Ca^{2+}-induced Ca^{2+} release and (B) caffeine-induced Ca^{2+} release. (C) Failure of caffeine-induced Ca^{2+} release before preloading was completed. Conditions are: 1.6 mg/ml protein, 75 mM KCl, 0.5 mM MgCl$_2$, 10 mM MES (pH 7.0), and 4 μM arsenazo III at 25°C. The arrows below the recordings indicate times of addition of CaCl$_2$ (to produce a Ca stimulus of 20 μM in the medium). In (B) and (C) the initial part of the recording showing the additions of 100-μM Ca and 500-μM ATP has been omitted for simplicity. The small spikes upon addition of 4 mM caffeine (20 μl of 100-mM solution) were optical noise caused by mixing. (From Ohnishi, S. T., *J. Biochem.*, 86, 1147, 1979. With permission.)

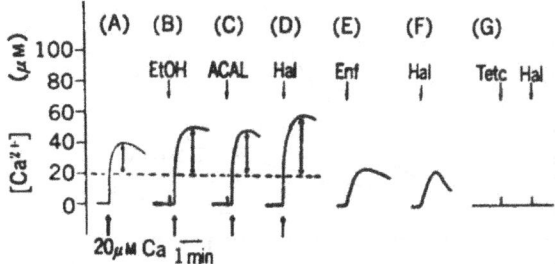

FIGURE 4. Effect of drugs on Ca^{2+}-triggered Ca^{2+} release. (A) Control, (B) 100-mM ethanol, and (C) 1-mM acetaldehyde. Ethanol and acetaldehyde were added 10 s before the addition of 20 μM Ca^{2+}. (D) Enhancement of Ca^{2+}-triggered Ca^{2+} release by the simultaneous addition of 0.6 mM halothane. (E) 1-mM enflurane- and (F) 0.6-mM halothane-triggered Ca^{2+} release. (G) Inhibition of the effect of halothane by 0.6 mM tetracaine. Conditions are: 1.6 mg/ml SR, 75 mM KCl, 0.4 mM MgCl$_2$, 10 mM MES (pH 7.0), 4 μM arsenaza III, 120 μM CaCl$_2$, and 0.5 mM ATP at 25°C. (For simplicity, the initial part of the recordings showing the addition of 120 μM CaCl$_2$ and 0.5 mM ATP prior to the start of each experiment has been omitted from the figures.) Arrows above the dotted line indicate the amounts of Ca^{2+}-triggered Ca^{2+} release. (From Ohnishi, S. T., *J. Biochem.*, 86, 1147, 1979. With permission.)

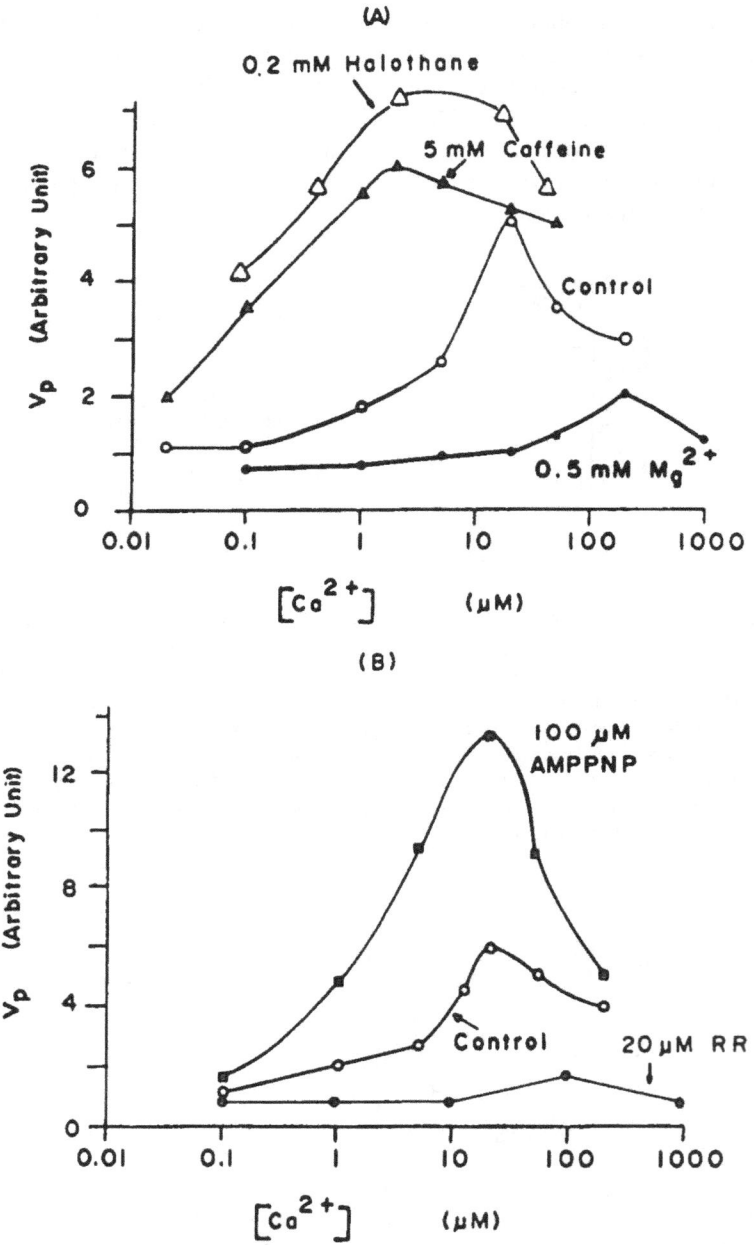

FIGURE 5. Effects of various agents on the passive calcium permeability of the heavy SR (from rabbit skeletal muscle). (A) 0.2 m*M* halothane, 5 m*M* caffeine, and 0.5 m*M* MgCl$_2$; (B) 0.1 m*M* AMPPMP (an ATP analog) and 20 μ*M* ruthenium red. (From Ohnishi, S. T., *Mechanism of Gated Calcium Transport Across Biological Membranes*, S. T. Ohnishi and M. Endo, Eds., Academic Press, New York, 1981, 275. With permission.)

With these accomplishments, Dr. Endo and I were able to receive a conference grant (jointly supported by the National Science Foundation and the Japan Society for the Promotion of Science) in 1981 to sponsor a U.S.-Japan international conference on calcium channels.[16,17] I reported the data that heavy SR has calcium-release channels that can be gated by calcium, halothane, or caffeine (Figure 6). I found that ethanol also increased the calcium-induced calcium release, but the mechanism was different from halothane in that ethanol did not trigger the release by itself (Figure 4B). I also found that ATP activated the release, but its energy was not needed, because nonhydrolyzable ATP analogs worked as well (Figure 5B). I presented a cartoon at the meeting that explained key mechanisms of calcium release from the SR (Figure 7). Although the scheme was a decade old, the ideas still seemed to be correct.

VI. THE DISCOVERY THAT THE CALCIUM-RELEASE CHANNEL OF MH-SR IS ABNORMAL

It was Dr. Price who informed me about a complication in the operating room called malignant hyperthermia (MH). I was interested in it and it was about this time that an excellent review on MH was written by Dr. Gerald Gronert.[18] According to his article, several investigators reported that MH-SR had more calcium uptake than normal SR, several other investigators reported that both MH-SR and SR had the same calcium uptake activity, and

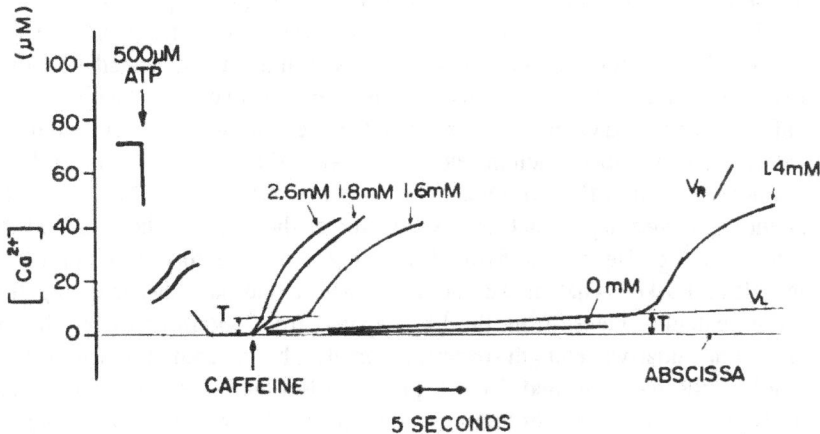

FIGURE 6. Effect of caffeine on the calcium-induced calcium release. Caffeine enhances the calcium leakage from SR, and thus slowly increases the external calcium concentration. When the external calcium concentration reaches the threshold value indicated by T, the gate is opened and the calcium-induced calcium release is triggered. (From Ohnishi, S. T., *Mechanism of Gated Calcium Transport Across Biological Membranes*, S. T. Ohnishi and M. Endo, Eds., Academic Press, New York, 1981, 275. With permission.)

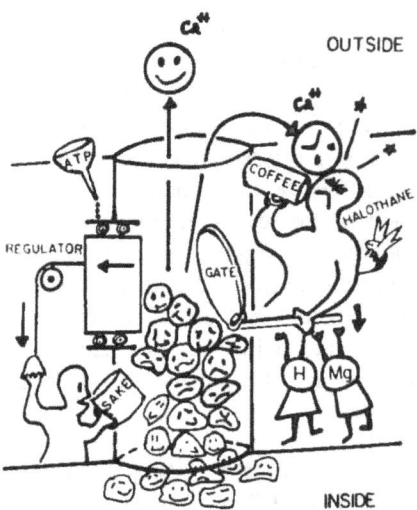

FIGURE 7. A cartoon showing the mechanism of the calcium release channel (proposed at the conference in 1981[17]). The calcium gate is opened by external calcium ions, which are leaked out from the inside of the SR. The gate opening is also accelerated by halothane and caffeine (coffee). The gate is inhibited by H^+ and Mg^{2+}. There is a regulator that changes the channel permeability, for example, ATP and alcohol (SAKE wine).

yet other investigators reported that MH-SR has less calcium uptake activity. These results led to the conclusion that SR may not be important in MH.

I knew instinctively that this confusion was derived from the fact that everybody was studying calcium uptake activity and felt that instead we should examine calcium-release activity. I knew already that both halothane and enflurane triggered calcium release from the skeletal SR.[14-16] I also found that caffeine could induce calcium release.[14-16] After this, it was only natural that I wanted to study MH and my chance came in 1981. On my way home after attending a meeting, I met an investigator at the airport who attended the same meeting. He was studying MH using a porcine model. I introduced myself and asked whether we could collaborate and publish papers together on the calcium release from the SR prepared from porcine muscle. He had an Aminco dual-wavelength spectrophotometer, but he could not demonstrate that MH-SR was abnormal. He accepted my offer and I flew to his laboratory in August 1981 and taught him how to prepare SR that was active enough to demonstrate calcium-induced calcium release. It was my training from Dr. Ebashi that "the active preparation" was the key. I also taught the investigator how to use the Aminco dual-wavelength spectrophotometer for calcium release study. The collaboration worked well. We were able to demonstrate that MH-SR released calcium in response to halothane, and that calcium-induced calcium release was abnormally high in MH-SR. We were excited, and I flew back to his laboratory again in October 1981 to finish the collaboration. However, things did not work well this time as we had a difference of opinion regarding which experiment should take priority. He decided that we should no longer work together. I was shocked as I had already made two trips and taught him all my techniques for preparing active SR and for applying dual-wavelength spectrophotometry for calcium release studies, especially the key technique for pulsing calcium to fill up the SR until the release takes place. Besides, we had already found that the calcium channels of the MH-SR were abnormal!

I had to look around again for someone who could collaborate with me. After many months of frustration, I recalled the review written by Dr. Gronert. I picked up the phone and called him. I introduced myself and asked whether we could collaborate on calcium release from porcine SR; fortunately, he accepted my offer. I flew to his laboratory in June 1982 (at that time, in Mayo University). I owe Dr. Gronert a great deal, because he gave me, a stranger, the key to his entire facility on the day I arrived. I worked around the clock. Because there was no dual-wavelength spectrophotometer available, I used an old Beckman single-wavelength spectrophotometer, which was located in another department. Still, I was able to reproduce the results that MH-SR has abnormal calcium-release channels and that halothane induces release in MH-SR. Because we did not study a large number of animals and because we did not use a dual-wavelength spectrophotometer, I had to come back again. I flew back to Mayo University in August, this time with Dr. Sadanaga (then a student of veterinary medicine at the University of Pennsylvania). I brought my home-built dual-wavelength spectrophotometer with me. We performed experiments with enough number of animals to confirm our findings (and most importantly, to convince Dr. Gronert). We even found that halothane-induced calcium release was inhibited by dantrolene, the only agent that was known to inhibit MH reaction (Figure 8). Another important finding was that the calcium uptake of MH-SR was the same as that of normal SR, but the release from MH-SR was abnormally higher than that from normal SR (Figure 9). Finally, after many years of sweat and tears, a historical paper describing the abnormality of MH-SR was published in 1983.[19] Dr. Endo also published a paper in 1983, describing that his skinned-fiber model using a biopsied specimens from a patient susceptible to MH demonstrated an abnormal calcium-induced calcium release.[20]

I then flew to Boston and collaborated with Dr. Noriaki Ikemoto. I taught him how to demonstrate calcium-induced calcium release, and he applied his expertise to the kinetic study. It was a pleasant collaboration. He acknowledged my contribution by making me a co-author.[21,22]

I started to purchase porcines susceptible to MH myself and finally was able to conduct SR studies at my own laboratory with the assistance of Dr. Sadanaga (then a resident of the University Pennsylvania Veterinary School). We furthered the understanding of calcium release channels of the MH-SR (Figures 10 through 12).[23-25] I found that another dye, calcein, could be used for the release study.[26] I also started studying the effects of ethanol on calcium release from SR.[27-28] We were full of hope and working hard, without the slightest idea of the problems that were waiting for us ahead.

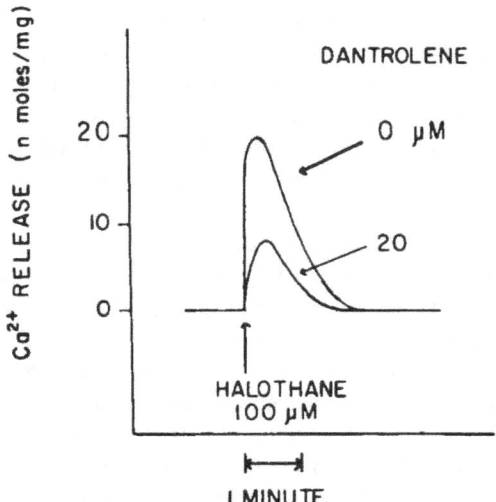

FIGURE 8. Inhibition of halothane-induced Ca^{2+} release by dantrolene. The concentration of halothane is 100 μM and concentrations of dantrolene are 20 μM. Other experimental conditions include: 150 mM KCl, 20 mM MES (pH 6.8), 2 mM MgCl₂, 1.5 mg SR protein/ml, 9 μM arsenazo III, 40 μM CaCl₂, and 1 mM ATP. (From Ohnishi, S. T., Taylor, S., and Gronert, G. A., *FEBS Lett.*, 161, 103, 1983. With permission.)

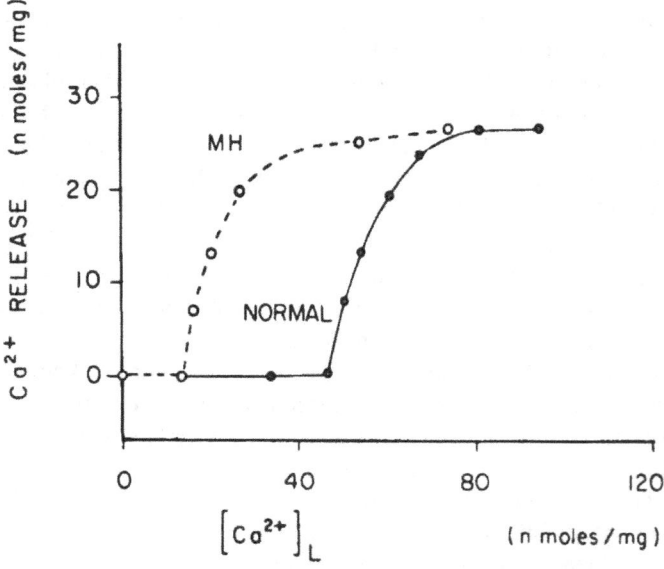

FIGURE 9. Relationship between the level of Ca^{2+} loading and the amount of halothane-induced Ca^{2+} release. Experimental conditions are the same as those in Figure 8, except for the Ca^{2+} concentration which was varied. The halothane concentration used to induce the Ca^{2+} release was 200 μM. (From Ohnishi, S. T., Taylor, S., and Gronert, G. A., *FEBS Lett.*, 161, 103, 1983. With permission.)

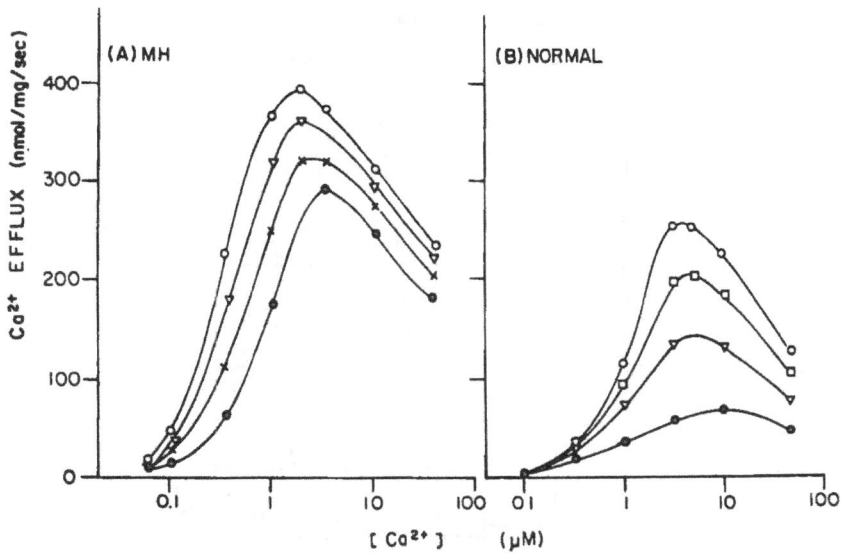

FIGURE 10. Effect of extravesicular calcium concentration on the calcium permeability of SR prepared from (A) malignant hyperthermic pig and (B) normal pig. Experimental conditions include: 120 m*M* KCl, 40 m*M* MES buffer (pH 6.8), 25°C. Halothane concentrations: ●, 0 μ*M*; ×, 25 μ*M*; ∇, 50 μ*M*; □, 100 μ*M* and ○, 200 μ*M*. (From Ohnishi, S. T., *Biochem. Biophys. Acta,* 897, 261, 1987. With permission.)

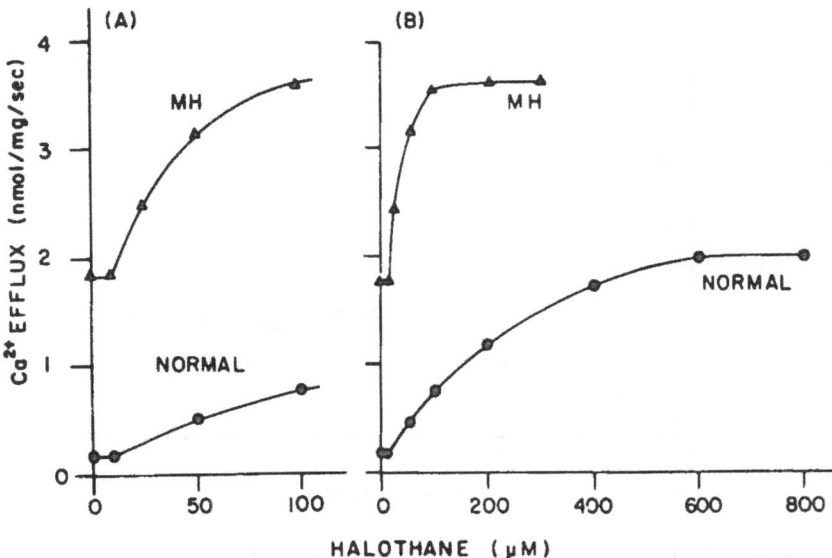

FIGURE 11. Effect of halothane concentration on the calcium permeability of MH and normal SR (A) at low halothane concentrations and (B) at higher halothane concentrations. The free Ca^{2+} concentration was 1 μM. Other conditions were the same as those in Figure 10. (From Ohnishi, S. T., *Biochem. Biophys. Acta,* 897, 261, 1987. With permission.)

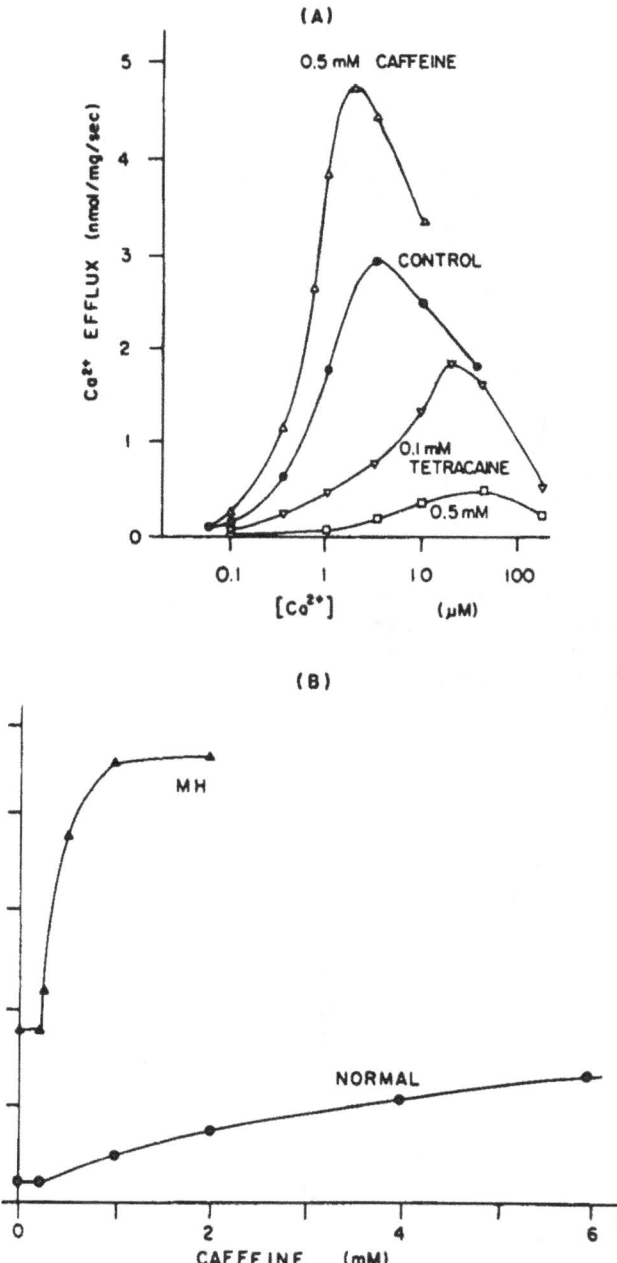

FIGURE 12.   (A) Effects of caffeine (0.5 mM) and tetracaine (0.1 and 0.5 mM) on the calcium permeability of MH-SR. (B) Effects of caffeine on the calcium permeability of MH and normal SR. Conditions were the same as those in Figure 10. (From Ohnishi, S. T., *Biochem. Biophys. Acta,* 897, 261, 1987. With permission.)

VII. AGAIN FROM SCRATCH

I was not working with Dr. Price anymore as he was on his way to retirement. He was a pioneer in his field and had done so much important work. I was working for other departments and became one of eight co-principal investigators on a 5-year-program project grant. A chairman of our school was the principal investigator. I performed experiments and wrote a segment of the project grant and it was funded. At that point, half of my salary was being paid by that project grant. I did some good work; however, in the second year, suddenly, the principal investigator eliminated my segment. When I lost half of my salary, my department chairman told me that I should leave in six months. When I was trying to find a job, another chairman, from whose department I had purchased all my equipment, told me that I could not take my equipment with me, because it was purchased from grants for which I was not the principal investigator. Although I was the only active investigator on these grants who performed all the experiments, wrote the grants, purchased all the equipment, and kept renewing the grants, I was still not the "principal investigator". How could I continue my research without that equipment? The employees I had hired were very unhappy and were complaining and nagging at me. What could I do? The stress mounted, and toward the end of 1984 I had a bleeding duodenal ulcer and was hospitalized in a room one floor above my laboratory. With the pressure of three chairmen, there was nothing I could do. In 1985 I left the laboratory that I had expanded from a room with a pH meter and a triple-beam balance to several well-equipped biophysics/biochemistry laboratory rooms with 13 years of hard work.

I then started working for a center. I rented a room from the center and decided to build a laboratory again, but what can a scientist do without equipment? It was a program director of NIGMS who saved my life. She knew that I had done some good work and that I was in limbo. She advised me that I should immediately write a supplementary grant to purchase the major equipment I had lost. I requested an ultracentrifuge, refrigerated centrifuge, dual-wavelength spectrophotometer, atomic absorption, and fluorescence spectrophotometer, worth more than $150,000. The grant was quickly approved and funded and I was able to purchase all the major equipment I had lost, this time as new equipment!

VIII. IDENTIFYING THE DIFFERENCE BETWEEN SKELETAL AND CARDIAC MUSCLE

With renewed determination, I started building a laboratory and doing experiments, even though the laboratory was not completely furnished. Although it took 2 years until the laboratory could fully function, we worked hard and the laboratory was growing again. A major breakthrough came when

I was able to answer the critical question: Why does halothane enhance contracture in MH muscle, while it weakens contraction in cardiac muscle? We measured calcium transients of isolated cardiac cells (myocytes) using Fura 2; one of the fluorescent calcium dyes which were developed by Dr. Richard Tsien and are called third generation calcium indicators. We also measured the total calcium content. Applying Dr. Endo's invention of measuring the calcium content of SR in muscle using the caffeine-purging method, we measured the calcium content of SR in myocytes in the presence and absence of halothane, enflurane, isoflurane, and caffeine. All of these compounds, which cause contracture of MH muscle, decrease the calcium transients (Figure 13) and concomitantly lower the calcium content in the cardiac

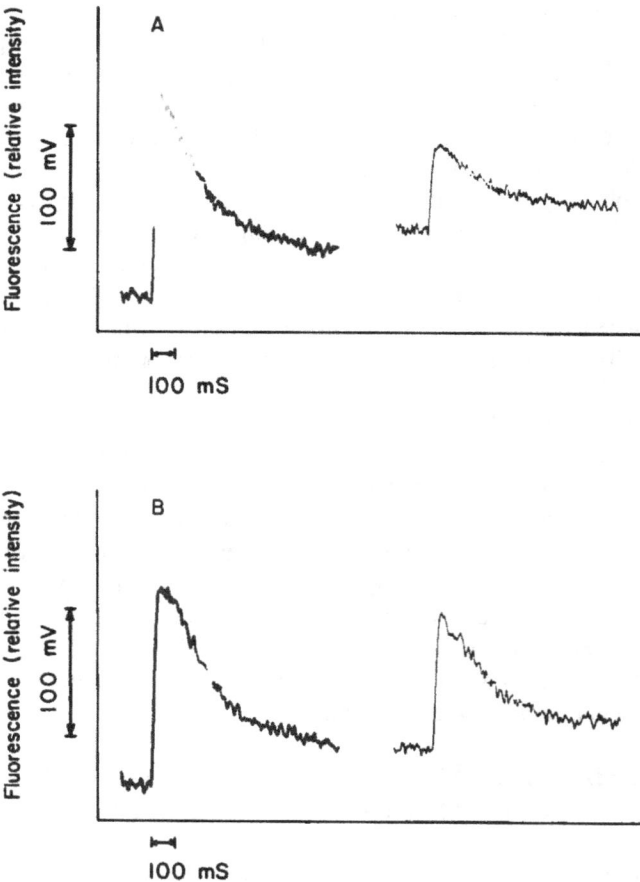

FIGURE 13. The calcium transient in myocytes. Left traces are the controls (no drugs), and the right traces are after the addition of a drug, (A) 4 m*M* caffeine and (B) 1 m*M* halothane. Myocytes were electrically stimulated every 5 s. Data from 20 traces were signal averaged.

myocytes (Figure 14), resulting in a decrease of the twitch contraction (negative inotropism).[29] We also used Langendorf's perfused heart model and obtained exactly the same results (Figures 15 and 16).[30] It is now clear that calcium channels of both skeletal and cardiac muscle behave similarly to inhalational anesthetics as well as to caffeine. All of these agents enhance calcium release. Then, why do these agents exert opposite effects in these two types of muscle? We found that it is because released calcium ions are recycled back into the SR in skeletal muscle, while calcium ions are pumped out of the cells when released from the SR in cardiac muscle.[31] There are at

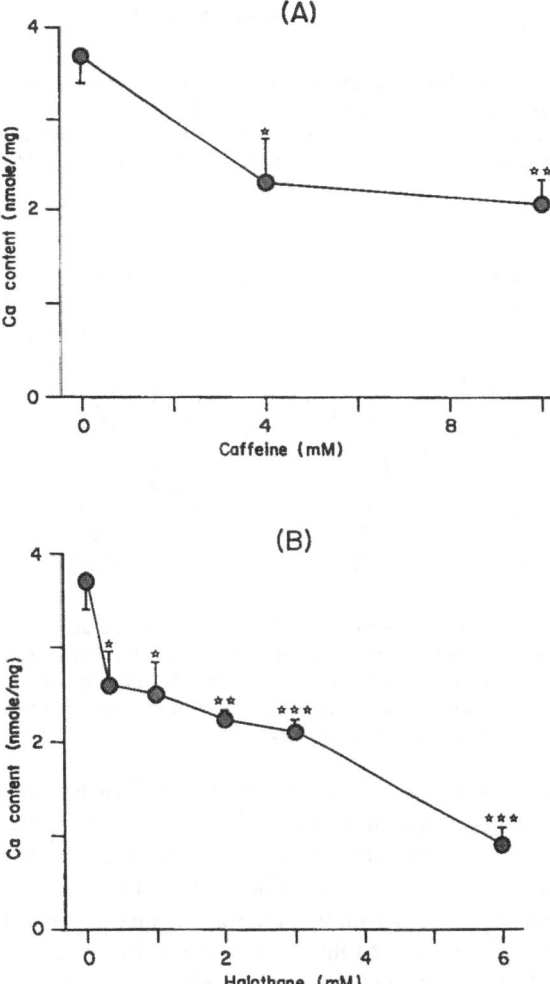

FIGURE 14. Effects of caffeine (A) and halothane (B) on calcium contents of myocytes as measured by atomic absorption.

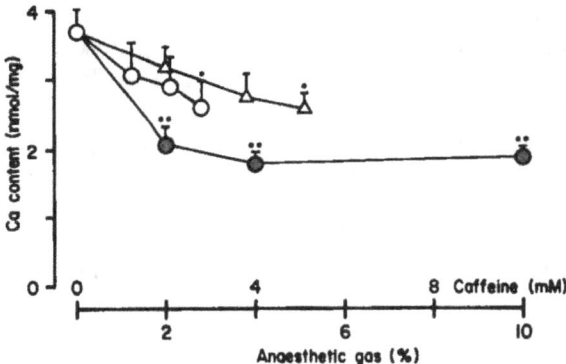

FIGURE 15. Effects of caffeine (●), halothane (○), and enflurane (△) on the calcium content of left ventricular muscle (mean and SEM); (*n* = 6). Calcium content was measured by atomic absorption spectrophotometry. Significant difference from normal perfusate: *, *p* <0.05; **, *p* <0.01. (From Katsuoka, M. and Ohnishi, S. T., *Br. J. Anaesth.*, 62, 669, 1989. With permission.)

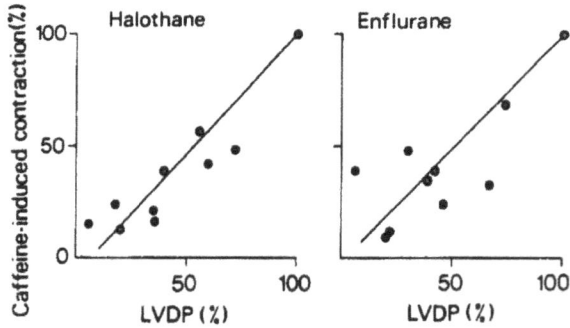

FIGURE 16. Effect of halothane (*r* = 0.95, *p* <0.001) and enflurane (*r* = 0.91, *p* <0.001) on the relationship between left ventricular developed pressure (LVDP = percentage of control) and calcium content in the SR. Calcium content in the SR was measured as a caffeine-induced contraction and expressed as a percentage of control. (From Katsuoka, M. and Ohnishi, S. T., *Br. J. Anaesth.*, 62, 669, 1989. With permission.)

least three reasons for this: (1) the cell membrane of cardiac cells (sarcolemma) has a well-developed calcium pump; (2) the sarcolemma has highly active calcium-sodium exchange; and (3) because cardiac muscle is about ten times smaller than skeletal muscle, the surface-to-volume ratio is ten times greater in cardiac muscle, favoring these pumping-out mechanisms (Figure 17).

This study finally solved the original query by Dr. Price of why inhalational anesthetics have negative inotropic effects. It took 20 years to answer this question and when I had an answer, he had already retired and I was no longer working in his laboratory. However, I was happy because I was able to finally answer his question.

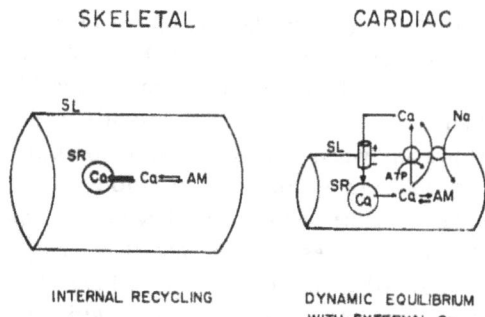

SKELETAL   CARDIAC

INTERNAL RECYCLING   DYNAMIC EQUILIBRIUM
WITH EXTERNAL Ca

FIGURE 17. Difference in calcium recycling between cardiac and skeletal muscle. AM stands for the actomyosin-troponin system and SL for the sarcolemma. On the SL of cardiac muscle there is a calcium channel, calcium pump, and Na-Ca exchange transport (from left to right). (From Ohnishi, S. T. and Katsuoka, M., *Adv. Exp. Med. Biol.*, 301, 73, 1991. With permission.)

If this scheme is correct, and if the calcium-release channels of both skeletal and cardiac SR are controlled by the same genes, the negative inotropic effect of inhalational anesthetics would be greater in the MH heart than in the normal heart. Someone should study this subject using the porcine heart, because it may be important.

IX. ONE MORE TIME FROM SCRATCH

When things are growing, obstacles always occur. It was when we were getting new grants, new personnel, and new discoveries that I was plagued with problems again. This time my employees started creating problems within the center. Due to the stress, I had another episode of bleeding from my duodenal ulcer. I did not need any more problems. What I needed was peace so that I could concentrate on my scientific experiments. I resigned in 1989 and again left a laboratory that I had built from scratch. Someone then found me a space in an old building in the suburbs that could be modified into a laboratory. I rented it and organized a nonprofit biomedical research institute. I thought I could transfer my equipment, because this time I was the principal investigator, but trouble occurred. The administrative office did not want to release the equipment and said that it was bought by the grants that were given to the center. I found that being the principal investigator did not protect me. It took long, tiring negotiations, but the office finally softened and started to release one piece of equipment at a time, once a week. I rented a truck and carried the equipment, one piece at a time, with the assistance of friends and my daughter. I started moving the laboratory on a hot summer day, when I finished it was going to snow.

I started doing experiments again, even though many boxes were still unpacked. I continued the experiments I had started when I was at the center. One experiment included an attempt to diagnose MH by measuring the membrane fluidity of human erythrocytes with electron spin resonance. I flew to Calgary and made a collaborative arrangement with Dr. A. K. W. Brownell (University of Calgary, Canada) whom I had previously met at the MH workshop held in England. Initially, we had promising results using blood sent from his laboratory.[32-34] However, when I started using blood sent from other laboratories, the results were not as consistent as before.

We also searched for other noninvasive diagnostic methods. I flew to the Department of Animal Sciences at Iowa State University and made an arrangement to purchase MH-susceptible and normal pigs that were littermates. Caging them at the University of Pennsylvania Veterinary School, we demonstrated the possibility of using intramascular temperature for diagnosis of MH (see Chapter 17). After two years, funds ran out. Some months I had to pay the institute's rent out of my own pocket, which had already hit rock bottom. All personal lines of credit had reached the limit. I had previously applied for several grants and one of them was approved with an extremely high priority. I was very happy for only a few months, until I was notified by the grant administrator that they could not fund the grant because my institute had no money. I needed money, but in order to receive money, I had to have money. After 6 months of negotiation with the feeling that my life was being cut short day by day, it was proposed that I might be considered for funding if I could raise $35,000 as an operating fund for the institute. I asked several banks for the loan; all turned me down. After 2 months of desperate trials, a bank agreed to a loan with the condition that I use my house as collateral. After another 2 months of walking on thin ice, the grant finally was funded. If it had been 1 month later, both the institute and I would have been bankrupt.

X. EPILOGUE

Why am I still working after all these hassles? It is because I believe that the ultimate goal of scientific research is to improve the welfare of mankind, and that I have a mission that only I can fulfill. It may be in my blood. My father was a family physician in a small Japanese town, using his home as a doctor's office. With the support of my mother he worked for 40 years for the welfare of the town. After he retired from his office, he volunteered to be the attending physician of an institute for seriously mentally retarded children. He visited there twice a week, staying overnight. He continued this until the age of 75 when he had a stroke at the institute and died (my brother is now the attending physician).

Although I became neither famous nor wealthy, I am satisfied because all aspects of my 30 years experience — instrumentation, indicator methods, SR preparation, and a never-give-up spirit — altogether led to the discovery of the abnormal calcium release channel in the MH-SR. Based upon my discovery, many capable investigators around the world have developed and expanded this field. Finally, the genetic mutation that causes MH was identified and noninvasive genetic diagnostic methods are being developed (please see Chapters 18 through 20).

I am happy because I have had great mentors and have some good friends including Drs. Endo, Ikemoto, and Sadanaga. I am happy because I have a wife and children who understand and support (or more or less gave up on) what I have been doing, and, more than anything else, because I was able to participate in the campaign to stop miseries caused by MH. So, until we can eliminate miseries from the world, *"Let's go back to the bench!"*

REFERENCES

1. **Ohnishi, T.**, Extraction of actin- and myosin-like proteins from erythrocyte membrane, *J. Biochem.*, 52, 307, 1962.
2. **Ohnishi, T., Hagihara, B., and Okunuki, K.**, A double-beam spectrophotometer without vibrating mirror-chopper system, *J. Biochem.*, 54, 287, 1963.
3. **Ohnishi, T. and Ebashi, S.**, Spectrophotometrical measurements of instantaneous Ca-binding of the relaxing factor of muscle, *J. Biochem.*, 54, 506, 1963.
4. **Ohnishi, T.**, Bau eines Dreistrahlenspektrophotometers, *J. Biochem.*, 55, 172, 1964.
5. **Ohnishi, T. and Ebashi, S.**, The velocity of calcium binding of isolated sarcoplasmic reticulum, *J. Biochem.*, 55, 599, 1964.
6. **Ohnishi, S. T., Masoro, E. J., Bertrand, H. A., and Yu, B. P.**, Analysis of a calcium ion binding system composed of two different sites, *Biophysical J.*, 12, 1251, 1972.
7. **Price, H. L.**, Calcium reverses myocardial depression caused by halothane: site of action, *Anesthesiology*, 218, 576, 1974.
8. **Price, H. L.**, Myocardial depression by nitrous oxide and its reversal by calcium ions, *Anesthesiology*, 44, 211, 1976.
9. **Ohnishi, S. T.**, Characterization of the murexide method: dual-wavelength spectrophotometry of cations under physiological conditions, *Anal. Biochem.*, 85, 165, 1978.
10. **Ohnishi, S. T.**, A method of estimating the amount of calcium bound to arsenazo III, *Biochem. Biophys. Acta*, 586, 217, 1979.
11. **Ohnishi, S. T.**, Interaction of metallochromic indicators with calcium sequestering organelles, *Biochem. Biophys. Acta*, 585, 315, 1979.
12. **Endo, M.**, Calcium release from the sarcoplasmic reticulum, *Physiol. Rev.*, 57, 71, 1977.
13. **Ohnishi, S. T.**, A method of studying the depolarization-induced calcium release from fragmented sarcoplasmic reticulum, *Biochem. Biophys. Acta*, 587, 217, 1979.
14. **Ohnishi, S. T.**, Calcium-induced calcium release from fragmented sarcoplasmic reticulum, *J. Biochem. (Tokyo)*, 86, 1147, 1979.
15. **Ohnishi, S. T.**, Calcium release from fragmented sarcoplasmic reticulum: development of an optical method for the rapid kinetic studies, in *Cation Flux Across Biological Membranes*, Y. Mukohata and L. Packer, Eds., Academic Press, San Francisco, 1979, 163.
16. **Ohnishi, S. T. and Endo, M., Eds.**, *Mechanism of Gated Calcium Transport Across Biological Membranes*, Academic Press, New York, 1981.
17. **Ohnishi, S. T.**, Calcium-induced calcium release as a gated calcium transport, in *Mechanism of Gated Calcium Transport Across Biological Membranes*, S. T. Ohnishi and M. Endo, Eds., Academic Press, New York, 1981, 275.
18. **Gronert, G. A.**, Malignant hyperthermia, *Anesthesiology*, 53, 395, 1980.

19. Ohnishi, S. T., Taylor, S., and Gronert, G. A., Calcium-induced calcium release from sarcoplasmic reticulum of pigs susceptible to malignant hyperthermia: the effect of halothane and dantrolene, *FEBS Lett.*, 161, 103, 1983.

20. Endo, M., Yagi, S., Ishizaka, T., Horiuti, K., Koga, Y., and Amaha, K., Changes in the calcium-induced calcium release mechanism in the sarcoplasmic reticulum of the muscle from a patient with malignant hyperthermia, *Biomed. Res.*, 4, 83, 1983.

21. Kim, D. H., Ohnishi, S. T., and Ikemoto, N., Kinetic studies of calcium release from sarcoplasmic reticulum *in vitro*, *J. Biol. Chem.*, 258, 9662, 1983.

22. Kim, D. H., Streter, F. A., Ohnishi, S. T., Ryan, J. F., Roberts, J., Allen, P. D., Meszaros, L. G., Antoniu, B., and Ikemoto, N., The kinetic studies of calcium release from sarcoplasmic reticulum of normal and malignant hyperthermia susceptible pig muscles, *Biochim. Biophys. Acta*, 775, 320, 1984.

23. Ohnishi, S. T., Flick, J. L., and Rubin, F., Ethanol increases calcium permeability of heavy sarcoplasmic reticulum of skeletal muscle, *Arch. Biochem. Biophys.*, 233, 588, 1984.

24. Ohnishi, S. T., Waring, A. J., Fang, S. G., Horiuchi, K., Flick, J. L., Sadanaga, K. K., and Ohnishi, T., Abnormal membrane properties of the sarcoplasmic reticulum of pigs susceptible to malignant hyperthermia: modes of action of halothane, caffeine, dantrolene and two other drugs, *Arch. Biochem. Biophys.*, 247, 294, 1986.

25. Ohnishi, S. T., Effects of alcohol and halothane on the structure and function of sarcoplasmic reticulum, *Ann. N.Y. Acad. Sci.*, 492, 138, 1987.

26. Ohnishi, S. T., Effects of halothane, caffeine, dantrolene and tetracaine on the calcium permeability of skeletal sarcoplasmic reticulum of malignant hyperthermic pigs, *Biochim. Biophys. Acta*, 897, 261, 1987.

27. Ohnishi, S. T., Chronic alcohol ingestion alters the passive calcium ion permeability of sarcoplasmic reticulum, *Membr. Biochem.*, 6, 33, 1985.

28. Ohnishi, S. T., Waring, A. J., Horiuchi, K., Fang, S. G., and Ohnishi, T., Sarcoplasmic reticulum membranes of rat skeletal muscle are disordered by chronic alcohol ingestion, *Membr. Biochem.*, 6, 49, 1985.

29. Katsuoka, M., Kobayashi, K., and Ohnishi, S., Volatile anesthetics decrease calcium content of isolated myocytes, *Anesthesiology*, 70, 954, 1989.

30. Katsuoka, M. and Ohnishi, S. T., Inhalational anesthetics decrease calcium content of cardiac sarcoplasmic reticulum, *Br. J. Anaesth.*, 62, 669, 1989.

31. Ohnishi, S. T. and Katsuoka, M., Why does halothane relax cardiac muscle but contract malignant hyperthermic skeletal muscle?, *Adv. Exp. Med. Biol.*, 301, 73, 1991.

32. Ohnishi, S. T., Membranes of sarcoplasmic reticulum and red blood cells may have a common gene: a new possibility of using blood for non-invasive screening for malignant hyperthermia, in *Calcium Binding Protein in Health and Disease*, A. W. Norman, T. C. Vanaman, and A. R. Means, Eds., Academic Press, New York, 1987, 119.

33. Ohnishi, S. T. and Ohnishi, T., Halothane disorders red cell membranes of malignant hyperthermia susceptible subjects, *Cell Biochem. Funct.*, 6, 257, 1988.

34. Ohnishi, S. T., Katagi, H., Ohnishi, T., and Brownell, A. K. W., Diagnosis of malignant hyperthermia using red blood cells and spin labeling technique, *Br. J. Anaesth.*, 61, 565, 1989.

Part III
Current Understanding
of the Mechanism of
Malignant Hyperthermia

Chapter 7

CLINICAL FEATURES OF MALIGNANT HYPERTHERMIA IN MAN

Scott R. Schulman and Gerald A. Gronert

TABLE OF CONTENTS

I.   Introduction 70

II.   History 70

III.   Clinical Manifestations of Malignant Hyperthermia 71
        A.   Elevated End-Tidal CO_2 72
        B.   Skeletal Muscle Rigidity and Trismus 73
        C.   Tachydysrhythmias 73
        D.   Combined Metabolic and Respiratory Acidosis 74
        E.   Cyanosis and Mottling 74
        F.   Hyperkalemia 75
        G.   Rhabdomyolysis 75
        H.   Recrudescence 75
        I.   Disseminated Intravascular Coagulation 76
        J.   CNS Manifestations 76
        K.   Renal Failure 77

IV.   Malignant Hyperthermia Outside the Operating Room 77
        A.   Awake Triggering of MH 78

V.   Conclusion 78

References 79

0-8493-8093-6/94/$0.00 + $.50

I. INTRODUCTION

Malignant hyperthermia (MH) is frequently referred to as "the anesthesiologist's nightmare". MH is a subclinical myopathy that is unmasked upon exposure to anesthetic trigger agents, namely, the depolarizing relaxant succinylcholine and the volatile anesthetics halothane, enflurane, and isoflurane. Unless stressed by general anesthesia, affected individuals may go through life completely unaware that they have MH. Even prior exposure may not be sufficient, as 50% of people susceptible to MH have undergone uneventful general anesthesia with trigger agents.

In an MH episode, skeletal muscle acutely and unexpectedly increases its oxygen consumption and lactate production, resulting in greater heat production, respiratory and metabolic acidosis, muscle rigidity, sympathetic stimulation, and increased cellular permeability.

II. HISTORY

In 1929, Ombrédanne first noted an association between anesthesia and postoperative pallor and hyperthermia with significant mortality in children.[1] It was not until 31 years later that Denborough and Lovell published the first case report of MH.[2] They described a 21-year-old male with a compound fracture of the right leg who was more concerned about anesthesia than about surgery because 10 of his relatives had died after ether anesthesia. At about the same time, Locher in Wisconsin participated in the care of a family in which 30 members had died in conjunction with general anesthesia.[3] These reports marked the first recognition of a genetic susceptibility to the stress of certain anesthetic agents.

Subsequent to Denborough's original description there appeared several reports describing hyperthermia during general anesthesia. Much of our current understanding of the clinical manifestations of MH in humans stems from these reports.

Case 4: A 35-year-old woman was admitted on May 18, 1968, for tonsillectomy after recurrent bouts of tonsillitis. The past history was unremarkable except for a 2-month history of leg cramps and muscle weakness. The patient had no abnormal neurologic or orthopedic findings, but had responded dramatically to psychiatric therapy with complete relief of muscle symptoms 6 weeks prior to admission. The diagnosis at that time had been anxiety reaction. Physical examination revealed a robust 5 ft, 10 in., 185-lb. woman who was normal except for obesity. Results of routine laboratory studies of blood and urine were normal. On the afternoon of May 19, after premedication with secobarbital, 100 mg, and atropine, 0.4 mg, anesthesia was induced with thiopental, 275 mg, i.v. After the i.v. injection of succinylcholine, 100 mg, the jaw was noted to be rigid; no fasciculations occurred. An additional 80 mg of succinylcholine was then injected, and the mandible could be opened to permit intubation. Anesthesia proceeded with halothane (0.7 to 1.5%), nitrous oxide (3 l), and oxygen (2 l). An additional 60 mg of succinylcholine was required for the insertion of the mouth gag. Respirations were controlled and the level of anesthesia appeared adequate. At the end of the 35-min procedure, with spontaneous respirations present, a Kussmaul type of respiration was observed. After about 10 min, while the patient was still intubated and in the operating room, the skin was noted to be warmer than before. She was taken to the recovery room. The rectal temperature was 101°F. A thermistor probe was inserted rectally, and a Block-Aid Monitor showed no evidence of neuromuscular blockade, i.e., there was a strong twitch response with no post-tetanic facilitation and no fade of tetanus. The EKG revealed normal sinus rhythm with peaked T-waves. The patient, still unconscious, was placed on a cooling blanket, blood was drawn for electrolyte and blood gas determinations, and oxygen was given via the endotracheal tube. After these procedures, which took approximately 5 to 7 min, the temperature was 103°F. On admission to the recovery room, the blood pressure was 120/80 mmHg, and the pulse rate 140 beats/min. After 10 min the blood pressure was 180/110 mmHg and the pulse rate 190 beats/min. External cooling was continued and *d*-tubocurarine, 12 mg, and chlorpromazine, 25 mg, i.v. were given; controlled ventilation was begun with 100% oxygen. The temperature climbed rapidly to above 108.8°F in approximately 20 min. Ventricular arrhythmias appeared and the blood pressure fell to 40 mmHg systolic, then became unobtainable. Closed-chest massage was begun and iced sodium chloride and water were instilled through gastric and rectal catheters, together with surface cooling, with no effect on the hyperthermia. At this point reports of the results of blood studies were obtained. Serum potassium was 8.5 mEq/l; the pH of arterial blood was 7.15, with a base excess of -16.5 mEq/l. Sodium bicarbonate, 150 mEq, was administered i.v. The Wangensteen gastric hypothermia unit was then inserted via direct esophagoscopy. Inflow temperature was 2°C. The rate of flow was approximately 1.0 l/min. For almost 10 min the fluid returning from the stomach remained at 20°C, then began to fall, as did the patient's rectal temperature. When the rectal temperature reached 106.2°F, normal sinus rhythm returned and the blood pressure was 40 mmHg systolic. Arterial blood had a pH of 7.35 and a base excess of -3.2 mEq/l. Serum potassium was 6.2 mEq/l just after return of the patient's circulation. A second dose of *d*-tubocurarine, 6 mg, was given i.v., and assisted ventilation continued with a pressure-limited respirator. Over the next half hour the rectal temperature fell to 103°F and blood pressure rose to 80 to 90 mmHg, with normal sinus rhythm on the EKG. Arterial blood had a pH of 7.45. The serum potassium 3 h later had fallen to 2.3 mEq/l. Approximately 6.5 h after admission to the recovery room, the patient responded to commands. The trachea was extubated 4 h later. The patient was given morphine sulfate, 6 mg, i.v. in three divided doses over the next 3 h to alleviate severe muscle pains in the legs and arms. Urinary output was never less than 100 ml/h. The urine was red and analysis disclosed that it contained myoglobin. Serum potassium levels remained low during the evening, but rebounded to a level of 6.1 mEq/l at 9:00 a.m. the next morning. There was a slight metabolic and respiratory alkalosis from bicarbonate administration and controlled ventilation. The leukocyte count the following day was 33,000 with 93% neutrophils. Creatine phosphokinase was elevated and myoglobinuria persisted for 3 days. SGOT levels reached a peak of 940 units and remained elevated for 7 days. Anteroseptal T-wave changes in V_2 and V_3 persisted for 8 weeks. An electromyogram 1 week postoperatively revealed acute myopathic changes compatible with muscular destruction. Biopsy of the left gastrocnemius muscle revealed acute myopathic changes scattered randomly in the muscle fibers, with degeneration, vacuolation, and some fibrocytic activity with disintegration of muscle fibers. Following discharge the patient returned to her previous activity.[4]

The preceding case highlights many features that we now recognize as acute MH. Let us examine these in more detail.

III. CLINICAL MANIFESTATIONS OF MALIGNANT HYPERTHERMIA

MH is a clinical diagnosis. Affected individuals exhibit some combination of the following: (1) elevated end-tidal CO_2, (2) skeletal muscle rigidity, (3) tachyarrythmias, (4) combined metabolic and respiratory acidosis, (5) cyanosis and mottling of the skin, (6) hyperkalemia, (7) rhabdomyolysis, and (8) disseminated intravascular coagulation.

A. ELEVATED END-TIDAL CO_2

In 1984, Baudendistel et al. noted the importance of end-tidal CO_2 monitoring in the diagnosis and treatment of acute MH.[5]

Case 2: A 6-month-old male infant with a distal type of arthrogryposis multiplex congenita presented for open reduction of congenital hip dislocation. No other abnormality was disclosed by physical or laboratory examination, and the preoperative evaluation revealed no contraindication to general anesthesia. The patient was not receiving any medication. Anesthesia was induced by inhalation of oxygen, nitrous oxide, and increasing concentrations of halothane. The trachea was intubated with a 3.5-mm uncuffed tube, and the child's lungs were mechanically ventilated with 60% nitrous oxide in oxygen and 1% halothane. Monitoring consisted of arterial blood pressure by cuff, EKG, esophageal stethoscope and temperature probe, urinary catheter, and end-tidal $PetCO_2$ monitor (Datex). Minute ventilation was set to maintain the $PetCO_2$ between 34 to 40 mmHg.

A transient, moderate elevation in heart rate, concomitant with surgical incision, responded to an increase of the halothane concentration to 1.5%. Within minutes the initial small rise in $PetCO_2$ accelerated dramatically to 61 mmHg. Other monitored variables remained stable. Proper calibration and function of the CO_2 monitor was quickly established and the conventional causes of impaired CO_2 elimination were investigated. These considerations ruled out, increased CO_2 production appeared the viable explanation and a tentative diagnosis of MH was considered. Halothane administration was stopped, a radial arterial catheter inserted, and arterial blood sent for analysis. Mechanical ventilation of the lungs was discontinued and controlled manual ventilation started. The initial blood gas values PaO_2 235, $PaCO_2$ 57, pH 7.17, and base excess −7 mmol/l were consistent with the diagnosis of MH. Anesthesia was continued with tubocurarine, fentanyl, nitrous oxide, and oxygen, and the anesthetic system was replaced with an open high gas flow system. Although the measured temperature had only increased approximately 0.5°C (to 38°C) at this time, active cooling measures were begun. Within 30 min of initial concern, the $PetCO_2$ had risen to 69.8 despite a fourfold increase in minute ventilation, while esophageal temperature had risen approximately 1.5°C (to 39°C). Other monitored variables were not significantly changed from initial postinduction values. Dantrolene sodium (3 mg/kg) was infused over a period of 2 to 3 min. Within 10 min a decreasing $PetCO_2$ foretold the effectiveness of treatment which was confirmed by arterial blood gas analysis (PaO_2 159, $PaCO_2$ 47.3, pH 7.23, base excess −8 mmol/l). Throughout the period in question changes in temperature lagged relative to changes in $PetCO_2$.

With continuing improvement in the patient's clinical condition, mechanical ventilation was reinstituted. Surgery was completed without further incident. Following adequate reversal of neuromuscular blockade, the trachea was extubated and the patient was transported to the pediatric intensive care unit. Dantrolene sodium (2 mg/kg) i.v. every 6 h was continued for 48 h. The remaining hospital course was uneventful, and the patient was discharged on the fifth postoperative day.

As this case aptly illustrates, elevated end-tidal CO_2 during constant ventilation is one of the earliest, most sensitive signs of MH. Spontaneously breathing patients will become markedly tachypneic. Ventilation must increase not only to excrete the CO_2 produced by accelerated aerobic metabolism, but also to remove that which is produced by the bicarbonate buffering of organic acids of anaerobic glycolysis. If the anesthetic system includes a CO_2 absorber, the canister will heat rapidly and the soda-lime will be depleted. Increased ventilation may not be sufficient to prevent CO_2 from rising.

B. SKELETAL MUSCLE RIGIDITY AND TRISMUS

Approximately 75% of patients with MH exhibit rigidity. Historically it was felt that there were two distinct types of MH: rigid and nonrigid. This nosology has since been abandoned.[6] It is currently felt that the occurrence of rigidity is proportional to the magnitude of the rise in intracellular calcium concentration. If this rise is sufficiently large, rigidity occurs, because calcium levels have reached mechanical threshold.

Masseter muscle spasm, or trismus, is jaw muscle rigidity following succinylcholine. Historically, its occurrence was felt to herald an MH crisis approximately 50% of the time. However, two recent retrospective studies show that the incidence of trismus in children undergoing mask inductions with halothane followed by succinylcholine is 1%.[7,8] This high incidence of trismus contrasts with the 0.01% incidence reported by others.[9,10] Nonetheless, it has caused experts to reevaluate the role of trismus in MH. If one accepts the 1% incidence figure, this would suggest an overall incidence of MH of 50% of 1%, or 0.5%. The actual incidence of MH, when one considers anesthetic techniques utilizing the potent agents and succinylcholine, is 1/62,000 or 0.002%. Indeed, none of the patients who developed trismus in these two studies went on to show signs of MH.

Thus, trismus may be a physiologic rather than a pathologic response. Van der Spek et al. have shown that masseter muscle tone increases after succinylcholine administration in normal children under deep inhalation anesthesia with either halothane or enflurane.[11] Some instances, however rare, will mark the beginning of an MH episode, and the clinician must be prepared. Therefore, management of patients who exhibit trismus has become a topic of debate. Some experts advocate discontinuing the anesthetic; others believe it can be continued with or without triggering agents as long as there is careful monitoring for other signs of MH, i.e., elevated end-tidal CO_2 production, muscle tone, urine color, temperature, and acid/base status. Regardless of the decision made, all patients exhibiting trismus should be referred for muscle biopsy so that accurate epidemiologic data can be generated.

Masseter muscle spasm often makes endotracheal intubation difficult. Bag-and-mask ventilation is usually adequate until the spasm subsides. Neither an additional dose of succinylcholine nor a depolarizing relaxant relieves trismus. It usually subsides in 5 to 15 min without any intervention. If necessary, it may be combated with dantrolene 2 mg/kg i.v.

C. TACHYDYSRHYTHMIAS

Tachydysrhythmias are an early and reliable sign of MH. The heart rate is often elevated well beyond that which could be accounted for by the elevated metabolic rate due to temperature alone. (Heart rate increases by 10% of its resting value for each degree centigrade rise in body temperature.) Tachycardia in acute MH is likely a nonspecific response to stress and is mediated by serum catecholamines. Dysrhythmias may be ventricular or supraventricular and can be due to elevated serum potassium levels. Tachycardia is often initially dismissed as being due to a light plane of anesthesia. Other causes of tachycardia, such as administration of anticholinergic drugs, hypovolemia, and hypercarbia, should be ruled out before the diagnosis of MH is considered.

While most evidence suggests that the heart is not primarily involved in MH, myocardial failure frequently occurs. The tachydysrhythmias seen initially are often followed by hypotension, a low cardiac output state, and finally, cardiac arrest. This raises an important point. If the cardiac output falls early in the course of a fulminant MH episode, the patient's temperature may never rise. If there is no flow to muscle, the heat produced therein will never be carried away by the venous blood. This also has implications for treatment, for in order for dantrolene to effectively halt a hypermetabolic crisis, it must be given while there is still blood flow to muscle. Therefore, one must suspect MH anytime there is an unexplained, unusual response to an induction utilizing the halogenated agents and/or succinylcholine. Fever need not be a predominant feature.

D. COMBINED METABOLIC AND RESPIRATORY ACIDOSIS

When the clinical picture suggests MH, arterial blood gas analysis can confirm the diagnosis. A metabolic acidosis is present due to increased lactate production. The base deficit is frequently -5 to -10 mEq/l. If the patient is unable to increase ventilation as metabolism increases, respiratory acidosis ensues. If the $PaCO_2$ is greater than 60 mmHg and the base deficit is at least -5 to -7 mEq/l, the diagnosis is usually MH. Recall, however, that the arterial partial pressure of CO_2 does not always reflect the true severity of hypercarbia in MH. Normally the venous partial pressure of carbon dioxide is about 5 mmHg greater than arterial partial pressure. In acute MH, however, both arterial and venous CO_2 will be elevated, but the difference between them will also be greater. Thus, some investigators have suggested venous blood gases for more accurate assessment of the severity of an acute MH crisis.

E. CYANOSIS AND MOTTLING

"At the end of surgery, it was observed that the patient's skin was hot and mottled, and that he was peripherally cyanosed."[12] The skin change of an acute episode of MH is an erythematous macular eruption that rapidly develops into cyanotic mottling. The venous blood will appear quite dark due to maximal tissue extraction or a low cardiac output state. Many experts feel that cyanotic mottling and tachycardia in a previously well-oxygenated and -ventilated patient almost always means MH.

F. HYPERKALEMIA

Serum potassium levels greater than 8.5 mEq/l have been reported during acute MH. ATP depletion, fever, and acidosis destroy the integrity of the myofibril membrane and potassium leaks from the muscle cell into the systemic circulation. Data from muscle biopsy specimens taken during acute MH in a 12-year-old boy show significantly less potassium compared to normal controls.[12]

Hyperkalemia can exaggerate pre-existing cardiac arrhythmias. It can also occur when patients receiving calcium entry blockers are treated with dantrolene.[13,14] This hyperkalemia may then retrigger an episode of MH.[15]

The systemic acidosis in MH will drive potassium into the cells. Serum potassium determinations will then falsely underestimate elevated total body potassium. Later in the course of an MH crisis, marked and prolonged hypokalemia may ensue.

G. RHABDOMYOLYSIS

Muscle breakdown in fulminant MH leads to marked increases in serum myoglobin and creatine phosphokinase (CK). Normal CK levels are 0 to 225 U/l. Levels as high as 100,000 U/l occur in MH. Peak values are noted 12 to 24 h after the initial episode of muscle cell lysis. Serial CK determinations are mandatory in acute MH, as the disease may recrudesce. Immediate treatment of "port wine" urine is essential in order to prevent renal failure.

Once an acute MH crisis subsides, patients often complain of severe myalgias that last for days to weeks. The muscles are usually swollen and tender. Muscle weakness and atrophy can set in for a period of months when the swelling subsides.

H. RECRUDESCENCE

Mathieu et al. in 1979 described two cases of treated MH that recurred 16 to 24 h after the initial episode.[16]

Patient 1: A muscular, 20-year-old, 104-kg, 190-cm man had a closed, comminuted fracture of the left tibia and fibula. There was no significant past medical history, and the results of physical examination were unremarkable. The family anesthetic history was negative. Anesthesia was induced with thiopental, 300 mg, i.v. with use of succinylcholine, 160 mg, i.v. to facilitate endotracheal intubation. Endoscopy was performed with some difficulty due to insufficient relaxation. Anesthesia was maintained with nitrous oxide, 3 l/min, oxygen, 2 l/min, and halothane, 2%. Relaxation was obtained with pancuronium, 6 mg i.v. Within 10 min, the hyperpyrexia syndrome started, with an increase in esophageal temperature to 42°C, hypotension, and cutaneous signs of hypoxia. At their worst values, arterial blood gas values (FIO_2 1.0) were pH 6.96, PCO_2 73 mmHg, and PO_2 320 mmHg. The patient was immediately given gastric lavage with cold saline solution and packed in ice. Treatment also included bolus intravenous injections of sodium bicarbonate 200 mEq, procainamide, 300 mg, and lidocaine, 100 mg, for ectopic ventricular beats, and continuous infusion of dopamine, 10 to 20 µg/kg/min. Furosemide, 100 mg, and mannitol, 5 g, i.v. were also administered. These drugs were administered intermittently until blood gases were restored to normal values.

After active treatment for the initial episode of MH, the patient was successfully treated for diffuse intravascular coagulation. Twelve hours after the initial episode the patient was awake and asking for food. At this point, cardiovascular dynamics were stable, respiratory function was good, and the patient was no longer acidotic. His condition remained stable for the first 20 h except for continued slight muscle rigidity, increased fluid volume requirement to maintain an adequate central venous pressure (CVP), and inadequate urinary output. Leg abduction and arm flexion produced moderate resistance throughout the postoperative period. Thirty hours after the initial episode the patient suddenly became apprehensive, had masseter spasm, and became cyanotic, dyspneic, and tachypneic. Despite hyperventilation with oxygen, within 20 min he had a cardiac arrest. The presumptive diagnosis of cardiac arrest due to hyperkalemia and recrudescence of MH was made, and cardiopulmonary bypass and renal dialysis were rapidly instituted. The patient's temperature at this point was 36°C, and he remained afebrile until death. The first serum potassium value obtained after establishment of bypass was 14.2 mEq/l. Arterial blood gas values were pH 6.94, PO_2 400 mmHg and PCO_2 54 mmHg. A regimen of procainamide, 15 mg/kg, dantrolene 1.5 g, i.v., mannitol, glucose, sodium bicarbonate, insulin, and cooling was instituted. When the serum potassium fell below 7.8 mEq/l, the heart spontaneously defibrillated. Despite vigorous dialysis, potassium could not be reduced to below 6.6 mEq/l. With vasopressor support, an unsuccessful attempt was made to wean the patient from bypass. He succumbed to pulmonary edema and heart failure.

I. DISSEMINATED INTRAVASCULAR COAGULATION

Disseminated intravascular coagulation (DIC) is a well-known complication of MH and it was first reported by Purkis.[17] In 1969, Daniels et al. reported a fatal case of MH with DIC:[18]

By 11:30, the patient was bleeding from all needle puncture sites, the surgical incision, and the gastrointestinal tract. Large hematomas had formed in both groins. Increasing brawny edema and abdominal distention were noted. At 2:00, coagulation studies revealed platelets, less than 20,000; fibrinogen, none; prothrombin time, 3 min 47 s. The diagnosis of DIC was made. He was given heparin, 50 mg, i.v. and an infusion of 3.25 g of fibrinogen. Transfusion of whole blood was started.

By 3:00, he had received 10 l of lactated Ringer's solution, 1500 ml of dextran, 1000 ml of whole blood, and an additional 500 mg of hydrocortisone. A unit of fresh whole blood was running. Venous pressure had risen to 12 cm of water, but intra-arterial blood pressure had fallen to 30 to 40 mmHg systolic. The pupils were widely dilated and fixed. There was still no urine output. The extreme muscle rigidity persisted. To provide a tidal volume of 1 l now required 40 cm of water inflation pressure. At 4:00, the electroencephalogram revealed complete absence of brain activity in all leads. Heart action stopped at 5:25, and the patient was pronounced dead at 5:30.

The occurrence of a consumptive coagulopathy in association with MH is a poor prognostic indicator. Postulated causes of DIC in fulminant MH include: hemolysis, release of tissue thromboplastins, cardiogenic shock, or a generalized increase in permeability leading to release of humoral factors capable of activating the coagulation cascade.

J. CNS MANIFESTATIONS

Some patients will survive an acute MH crisis only to be left with permanent neurologic sequelae. Although there are no incidence data, patients exhibiting the most fulminant symptoms of MH are the ones who sustain the worst CNS damage. In 1982 Fletcher et al. reported the case of an 18-month-old boy with congenital muscular dystrophy who exhibited signs of MH that persisted for 2 days postoperatively despite continued treatment with dantrolene.[19] After the third postoperative day a dense left hemiparesis was noted. CT scans demonstrated a right-sided cerebral infarction.

Other patients suffer more global neurologic damage. The cerebral insult is presumably secondary to acidosis, hypoxia, hyperkalemia, and hyperthermia. These interfere with oxidative metabolism and hence deplete energy stores necessary for neuronal electrical activity. The clinical picture is one of acute cerebral edema and intracranial hypertension. The symptoms are coma, areflexia, and fixed and dilated pupils. Some patients proceed to brain death.

K. RENAL FAILURE

Renal failure as a complication of MH was simultaneously noted in 1970 by Ryan and Papper[4] in the U.S. and by Britt and Kalow[20] in Canada. Oliguria or anuria occur and are associated with a high mortality rate. Lieberman et al. reported a case of nonoliguric renal failure complicating MH that necessitated hemodialysis for several months.[21] The patient subsequently recovered full renal function.

Renal failure in MH is due to plugging of the tubules with myoglobin, as well as the deleterious effects of shock, acidosis, hypoxia, and hypercarbia on the renal circulation. When DIC occurs, fibrin deposition in the renal microvasculature causes further damage.

IV. MALIGNANT HYPERTHERMIA OUTSIDE THE OPERATING ROOM

Several recent case reports suggest that human MH can occur without exposure to anesthetics in susceptible individuals. Feuerman et al. reported such a case in a head-injured patient.[22]

The 21-year-old black man was found unconscious, apparently having been assaulted. Upon arrival at the hospital his vital signs were normal. On neurological examination he was noted to have a Glasgow Coma Scale score of 9. Cranial nerve examination was unremarkable except for a right VI nerve palsy. He withdrew all extremities equally in response to painful stimuli. Deep tendon reflexes were symmetrical with hyperactive Achilles reflexes. Plantar responses were flexor bilaterally. A CT scan of the head was normal.

Approximately 36 h after his injury the patient became agitated and diaphoretic. His temperature rose to 39.5°C. Over the next hour he began to exhibit decerebrate posturing. Three hours later his temperature was 42.3°C. He was tachycardiac, hypotensive, and tachypneic. Arterial blood gas analysis revealed a metabolic acidosis. The patient was intubated and ventilatory support was begun. He was given i.v. fluids and started on a course of dopamine. At that time he did not respond to pain but retained pupillary responses to light and other brainstem reflexes. He was treated with mannitol and hyperventilation. A repeat CT scan of the head was again normal. An intracranial pressure monitor was placed and gave an initial reading of 28 mmHg.

Aggressive cooling measures were taken, and over the next 24 h the patient's temperature returned to normal. Multiple blood, sputum, urine, and cerebrospinal fluid cultures all failed to grow any organisms. The patient continued afebrile throughout the remainder of his hospital course. By the fourth hospital day he began to manifest laboratory evidence of rhabdomyolysis, renal failure, liver failure, and DIC. On the sixth day he underwent biopsy of his right vastus lateralis muscle to confirm the then suspected diagnosis of MH. He died on the 24th hospital day, having remained comatose throughout his course after the episode of hyperthermia. Muscle biopsy results were consistent with MH.

A. AWAKE TRIGGERING OF MH

Several recent case reports relate heatstroke, sudden death, unusual fatigue, and myalgias to possible awake MH episodes. Some of these may actually represent human MH independent of the anesthesia environment. Consider the following.[23]

We evaluated the condition of a 20-year-old black offensive lineman who played for a college football team. He was 6 ft, 2 in. tall and weighed 285 lbs. During his football career, he had had many muscle problems that indicated muscle dysfunction, including shin splints, anterior compartment syndrome, arch pain (probably because of extremely flat feet), and low back pain (because of lordotic lumbar spine). He had frequent muscle cramps during and after practice. Many of his muscle problems did not develop until after he had stopped exercising.

Two incidents led us to suspect that he might have a muscle disorder. First, during spring practice, he complained of dyspnea, dizziness, and chest pain. A cardiac workup including an EKG, a 24-h Holter monitor, and an echocardiogram revealed few significant findings. Cardiac stress testing showed only early tachycardia, which was attributed to decreased conditioning. The patient was allowed to return gradually to conditioning exercises in anticipation of the fall football season. He continued to have generalized muscle aches and pains that were again attributed to lack of conditioning.

The second incident occurred in July after the patient finished running on a particularly hot and humid afternoon. He returned to the locker room without difficulty and took a cold shower. Within 10 to 15 min, he began to have cramps in all extremities and became dizzy. He was transported to the student health service on campus. On arrival, he was conscious but dizzy, short of breath, and cramping severely. His initial rectal temperature was 106.1°F. Vigorous i.v. therapy and ice administration lowered his temperature to normal within 2h. He continued to have headaches and cramps for approximately 1 week.

Several factors indicated to us that he might have a condition such as MH: (1) He had an unusually high number of muscle-related complaints; (2) many of these symptoms did not occur until he had finished exercising; and (3) his rectal temperature was elevated 10 to 15 min following exercise, when he was resting after taking a cool shower. To confirm the diagnosis, the patient was sent to Hahnemann University Hospital for a possibly confirming test on biopsied muscle to diagnose MH.

Following a muscle biopsy that verified MH susceptibility, his 4-day resting CK level was 141 U/l (normal = 0 to 110 U/l). The patient chose to discontinue playing football at the urging of team physicians. He was cautioned about undergoing anesthesia and was issued a medical alert bracelet. Members of his family were informed that they might carry the trait for MH susceptibility.

Other case reports must be viewed with skepticism until thoroughly investigated. The incidence of awake MH episodes in humans is undoubtedly rare.

V. CONCLUSION

The clinical manifestations of human MH are protean. Because the disease is rare, much of our knowledge comes from case reports. Classically, MH presents as an elevated end-tidal CO_2, unexplained or undue tachycardia, rigidity, cyanosis, mottling, diaphoresis, and fever. Its onset can be immediate or delayed several hours after exposure to anesthetic triggering agents. Electrolyte and arterial blood gas analyses reveal hyperkalemia, hypercalcemia, and a combined metabolic and respiratory acidosis. DIC and renal failure due to rhabdomyolysis can occur, but these are poor prognostic signs. Neurologic sequelae range from hemiparesis to brain death. MH can occur in association with other diseases, and it may even occur in certain susceptible individuals without exposure to general anesthesia.

Untreated, the mortality of MH is greater than 70%. Because of a greater awareness among clinicians and better means of detecting the signs of an impending MH crisis, it is being diagnosed and treated with dantrolene earlier. This has reduced the mortality to less than 10%. The past generation has seen tremendous progress in our understanding of this perplexing disorder, but there is still much to discover.

REFERENCES

1. **Ombrédanne, L.**, De l'influence de l'anesthesique-employé dans la genése des accidents post-opératoires de paleur-hypertherme observés chez les nourrissons, *Rev. Med. Fr.*, 10, 617, 1929.
2. **Denborough, M. A. and Lovell, R. R. H.**, Anaesthetic deaths in a family, *Lancet*, 2, 45, 1960.
3. **Britt, B. A., Locher, W. G., and Kalow, W.**, Hereditary aspects of malignant hyperthermia, *Can. Anaesth. Soc. J.*, 16, 89, 1969.
4. **Ryan, J. F. and Papper, E. M.**, Malignant fever during and following anesthesia, *Anesthesiology*, 32, 196, 1970.
5. **Baudendistel, L., Goudsouzian, N., Coté, C., and Strafford, M.**, End-tidal CO_2 monitoring, *Anaesthesia*, 39, 1000, 1984.
6. **Gronert, G. A., Mott, J., and Lee, J.**, Aetiology of malignant hyperthermia, *Br. J. Anaesth.*, 60, 253, 1988.
7. **Schwartz, L., Rockoff, M. A., and Koka, B. V.**, Masseter spasm with anesthesia: incidence and implications, *Anesthesiology*, 61, 772, 1984.
8. **Carroll, J. B.**, Increased incidence of masseter spasm in children with strabismus anesthetized with halothane and succinylcholine, *Anesthesiology*, 67, 559, 1987.
9. **Ording, H.**, Incidence of malignant hyperthermia in Denmark, *Anesth. Analg.*, 64, 700, 1985.
10. **Berry, F. A. and Lynch, C.**, Succinylcholine and trismus, *Anesthesiology*, 70, 161, 1989.
11. **Van der Spek, A. F. L., Fang, W. B., Ashton-Miller, J. A., Stohler, C. S., Carlson, D. S., and Schork, M. A.**, The effects of succinylcholine on mouth opening, *Anesthesiology*, 67, 459, 1987.
12. **Rutberg, H., Henriksson, K.-G., Jorfeldt, L., Larsson, J., Martensson, J., and Schildt, B.**, Metabolic changes in a case of malignant hyperthermia, *Br. J. Anaesth.*, 55, 461, 1983.
13. **Yoganathan, T., Casthely, P. A., and Lamprou, M.**, Dantrolene-induced hyperkalemia in a patient treated with diltiazem and metoprolol, *J. Cardiothor. Anesth.*, 2, 363, 1988.

14. **Rubin, A. S. and Zablocki, A. D.**, Hyperkalemia, verapamil, and dantrolene, *Anesthesiology*, 66, 246, 1987.
15. **Gronert, G. A., Ahern, C. P., Milde, J. H., and White, R. D.**, Effect of CO_2, calcium, digoxin, and potassium on cardiac and skeletal muscle metabolism, *Anesthesiology*, 64, 24, 1986.
16. **Mathieu, A., Bogosian, A. J., Ryan, J. F., Crone, R. K., and Crocker, D.**, Recrudescence after survival of an initial episode of malignant hyperthermia, *Anesthesiology*, 51, 454, 1979.
17. **Purkis, I. E., Horrelt, O., DeYoung, C. G., Fleming, R. A. P., and Langley, G. R.**, Hyperpyrexia during anaesthesia in a second member of a family with associated coagulation defect due to increased intravascular coagulation, *Can. Anaesth. Soc. J.*, 13, 183, 1967.
18. **Daniels, J. C., Polayes, I. M., Villar, R., and Hehre, F. W.**, Malignant hyperthermia with disseminated intravascular coagulation during general anesthesia: a case report, *Anesth. Analg.*, 48, 877, 1969.
19. **Fletcher, R., Blennow, G., Olsson, A.-K., Rankley, E., and Törnebrandt, K.**, Malignant hyperthermia in a myopathic child. Prolonged postoperative course requiring dantrolene, *Acta Anaesth. Scand.*, 26, 435, 1982.
20. **Britt, B. A. and Kalow, W.**, Malignant hyperthermia. A statistical review, *Can. Anaesth. Soc. J.*, 17, 293, 1970.
21. **Lieberman, P., Iaina, A., David, R., Agranat, O., Ohry, A., Ramon, I., and Eliahou, H.**, Non-oliguric acute renal failure following malignant hyperthermia, in *Malignant Hyperthermia*, J. A. Aldrete and B. A. Britt, Eds., Grune & Stratton, New York, 1977, 451.
22. **Feurman, T., Gade, G. F., and Reynolds, R.**, Stress-induced malignant hyperthermia in a head-injured patient, *J. Neurosurg.*, 68, 297, 1988.
23. **Hunter, S. L., Rosenberg, H., Tuttle, G. H., DeWalt, J. L., Smodic, R., and Martin, J.**, Malignant hyperthermia in a college football player, *Physician Sportsmed.*, 15, 77, 1987.

Chapter 8

THE PORCINE HYPERTHERMIA AND STRESS SYNDROMES

Gaisford G. Harrison

TABLE OF CONTENTS

I.   Introduction 82

II.   Stress Syndromes in Swine 82

III. Inheritance and Identification 82

IV.   The Clinical Syndrome 84
      A.   Modifications of the Syndrome 85

V.   The Biochemical Accompaniments 86

VI.   Pathogenesis 87
      A.   Myoplasmic Free Ca^{2+} 91
      B.   Sarcoplasmic Reticulum 91
      C.   The Vicious Cycle 92
      D.   The Milieu of Irreversibility 93
      E.   Mitochondria 94
      F.   Sarcolemma 94
      G.   Contractile Proteins 94
      H.   Other Membranes 95

VII. The Role of the Sympathetic Nervous System 95

VIII. Capture Myopathy 96

IX.   The Triggering of PMH 96

X.   Drug Screening in MHS Swine 97

XI.   Future Directions 99

Acknowledgments 99

References 99

I. INTRODUCTION

Malignant hyperthermia in swine (PMH) is the specific drug-induced syndrome of hypercatabolism and muscle rigor exhibited by swine, the subjects of a covert pharmacogenetic myopathy known as malignant hyperthermia susceptibility (MHS) or more generally, stress susceptibility (SS). The discovery of this lethal syndrome in swine was serendipitous and, as with man, it had to await the chance exposure of genetically susceptible animals to the classic MH-triggering agents, halothane and/or succinylcholine, occasioned by their use in medical research (see Chapter 5).

Evoked in these swine, the MH syndrome displays all the features of its counterpart in man, validating the use of MHS swine as the animal experimental model of this life-threatening syndrome in man.[1,2] There may be some differences but, being quantitative rather than qualitative, they do not appear to be fundamental.[3] MH-like syndromes have been observed in species other than swine and man, but with a rarity that renders them but biological curiosities. Only in MHS swine does the syndrome occur predictably and reproducibly. Most of our knowledge of the acute biochemical changes that characterize the human syndrome and hypotheses of its pathogenesis in this volume will have been derived by extrapolation from controlled experiments conducted on MHS swine.

II. STRESS SYNDROMES IN SWINE

Whereas in man MH has been documented in most broad racial groups, in swine affliction with the MHS genes is confined, strangely, to selected strains only of five major pig breeds, the Landrace, Pietrain, Poland China, Yorkshire, and Duroc.[4] These are the selfsame breeds that are subject to the long recognized porcine (sudden death) stress syndrome (PSS) and its resultant postslaughter carcass condition of pale, soft, exudative pork (PSEP) — pork that exhibits unfavorable meat quality, being pale, soft, and watery.[1]

Documented separately chronologically, PSS, PMH, and PSEP are now accepted as manifestations of the same covert myopathy. PSS and PMH both present as the florid MH syndrome, in the former instance evoked naturally by severe stress such as engendered by social order fighting, exercise, manhandling, hot environment, etc. and in the latter, artificially by exposure to certain drugs. PSEP follows from the accelerated postmortem glycolysis, concomitant myolactosis, and abnormally rapid postmortem fall in muscle pH peculiar to this myopathy. This, it is proposed, alters the muscle water-holding capacity and texture by denaturation of the sarcoplasmic protein.[5,6]

III. INHERITANCE AND IDENTIFICATION

Considering the economic losses sustained by pig breeders around the world from the effects of PSS,[7] losses preslaughter in transport and postslaughter from PSEP, it is strange how inconclusive our knowledge is of the inheritance patterns of this myopathy. These patterns have turned out to be considerably more complex than appeared at first sight. There are good data to support hypotheses of both autosomal dominant and recessive modes of inheritance.[1,8]

A major difficulty that arises in the conduct of breeding experiments is the manner in which SS is identified. In many studies, especially in the past, animals were identified as SS retrospectively postslaughter by the presence of PSEP.[9] Since the discovery of PMH, this method has been superseded by the more objective *in vivo* barnyard halothane test; the observance of the animal's response to brief mask inhalation of halothane.[1] However, the correlation between genotype and phenotype is not absolute.[4] For this reason some investigators only consider an animal completely MHS/SS negative when response to succinylcholine in addition to that to halothane is negative.[10] To these criteria Williams adds the requirement of an unraised basal metabolic rate.[11]

Of simple blood sample tests, none have proved to be specifically diagnostic. The variability observed in the serum levels of the muscle enzyme markers of this myopathy is such that the levels recorded in an individual pig are of little diagnostic significance.[12-14] As in humans, the only diagnostic screening test with any pretensions to sensitivity and specificity of a high order involves *in vitro* contracture testing (IVCT) of muscle biopsy material.[15] While these have been used to evaluate some breeding experiments,[10,16] logistic difficulties obviate its widespread use in this sphere.

In terms of autosomal dominant inheritance, current data of graded genotype response support the view that this is multigenic (at least two gene alleles), the genes involved being codominant. The likelihood of a multifactorial pattern of inheritance is further suggested by evidence of the cross-linkage of this myopathic trait with other characteristics, e.g., blood group.[17] On the other hand, workers, especially in Europe, report data from breeding programs in the Dutch Landrace and Pietrain breeds that strongly support the existence of a recessive inheritance pattern in these swine involving a single major recessive gene exhibiting complete penetrance. In these studies, identification of MHS/SS was not corroborated with IVCT.[8,18]

Although all the reported studies in Poland China swine have evidenced a dominant inheritance pattern, both dominant and recessive patterns have been documented in the Landrace, Pietrain, and crossbreeds of these. The present data seem to support the hypothesis that swine, as do humans, suffer covert subclinical myopathic states both dominantly and recessively transmitted that manifest the MH syndrome as the functional final common pathway.

The recent localization of the functional defect responsible for the MH reaction to the ryanodine receptor calcium release channel of the sarcoplasmic reticulum (see Section VI.B.) has afforded us a rational and more accurate insight into the transmission of the PMH/SS trait. In the human, the gene for the ryanodine receptor (ryr 1) has been localized to chromosome 19q 13.1 and susceptibility to MH has been linked to mutations of this gene.[4a] In the pig, the ryr 1 gene and the PMH (hal) locus have been localized to chromosome 6p11-q21. Fujii et al[4] have demonstrated a single point mutation in this gene to be correlated with the PMH/SS phenotype in the five major breeds which manifest the condition — knowledge which has allowed the development of a simple, accurate, and noninvasive diagnostic test that can provide the basis for elimination of this mutation if desired or, in view of its association with leanness and muscularity, its controlled retention as the N/n genotype.

IV. THE CLINICAL SYNDROME

Evoked in highly reactive MHS/SS swine by stress alone, or *ab initio* by the inhalation of halothane alone, the PMH syndrome is manifested by the following clinical signs that progress simultaneously and worsen rapidly:

1. Generalized blotchy cyanosis of the skin with well-marked cyanosis of the snout
2. The onset of sinus tachycardia often to extreme rates of 200 beats/min; untreated, this progresses through multifocal ventricular premature systoles to ventricular fibrilation
3. Distressed open mouth breathing with increasing hyperventilation that progresses to apnea in 15 to 20 min
4. Tail twitching and sporadic fasciculation of muscle, most obvious in the thighs; this progresses inexorably to generalized muscle rigor that causes a characteristic rigid extension of the hind legs (see Figure 1 in Chapter 5). So rigid do the legs become that they are impossible to flex passively. In the absence of endotracheal intubation, this generalized rigor may be accompanied by laryngospasm.
5. An explosive sustained rise in muscle and core temperature at rates as extreme as 1°C per 5 to 10 min, reaching 43 to 45°C antemortem (see Figure 1).

Left untreated, other than for the provision of IPPV when apnea supervenes, death usually follows 45 to 100 min from initiation of the syndrome.

If exposure to halothane is discontinued within minutes of the first appearance of any of the major clinical signs, the syndrome is spontaneously reversible. This maneuver is the basis of the simplest diagnostic screening test for MHS already referred to, the so-called "barnyard test" (see Section III). If, however, exposure to the triggering agent is continued for more than several minutes thereafter, the syndrome rapidly becomes irreversible and will continue independent of the stressor drug. This can now be seen to have acted as a trigger.

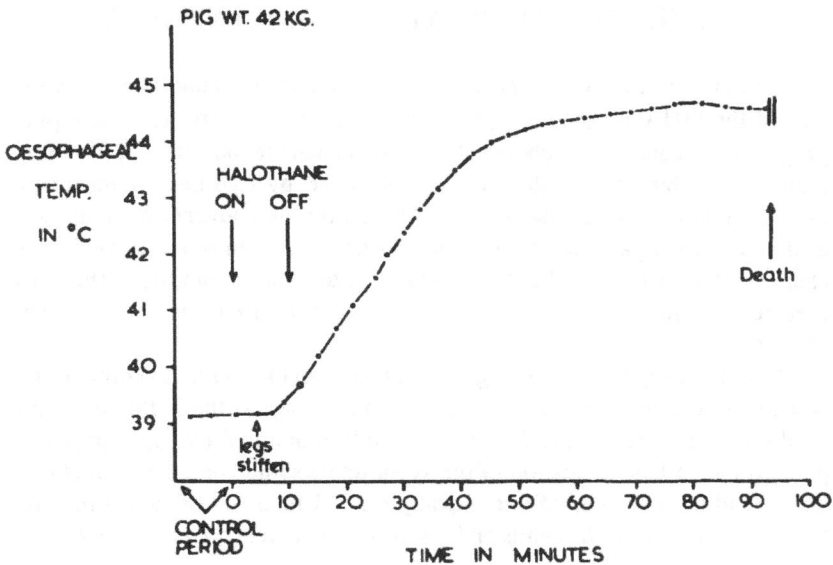

FIGURE 1. Esophageal temperature recorded in a Landrace pig during halothane-induced MH following a 30-min control period of thiopentone anesthesia. N_2O (60%)/O_2 (40%) was administered throughout by IPPV. Maximum rate of temperature rise 0.15°C/min or 1°C/6 min, 42 s. (From Harrison, G. G., Saunders, S. J., Biebuyck, J. F., Hickman, R., Dent, D. M., Weaver, V., and Terblanche, J., *Br. J. Anesth.*, 41, 844, 1969. With permission.)

A. MODIFICATIONS OF THE SYNDROME

When the unpremedicated MHS pig is anesthetized with halothane in this manner, the MH reaction commences within minutes, as soon as halothane concentration in the tissues rises. Subjecting the animal to manhandling stress or severe exercise sensitizes the triggering reaction and shortens the onset time markedly.[19] On the other hand, for reasons that are not yet clearly understood (see Section IX), pretreatment of the MHS pig with hypnotic[20] or anxiolytic drugs causes a variable delay in the onset of MH in response to the exhibition of halothane and may prevent that by stress.[21,22] However, once triggered, the speed of progression of the syndrome is unaltered. Usually of the order of 15 to 20 min, this delay or latent period may extend for 45 min or more, and in some circumstances the triggering of MH by halothane alone may even be prevented. Such pretreatment does not affect the triggering of the syndrome by the additional administration of succinylcholine.

The sensitivity of the MH-triggering mechanism is also affected by the genetic factors already discussed. Gradations in genotype-determined triggering sensitivity documented range from those that exhibit delay to those that fail to be triggered by halothane alone.[16] The latter, like Hall's historic pigs,[23] require the superimposition of succinylcholine depolarization to trigger the syndrome.

V. THE BIOCHEMICAL ACCOMPANIMENTS

Observed in the laboratory *in vivo* under controlled conditions, "switch on" of the MH syndrome is signaled by an array of interrelated and rapidly progressive changes in biochemical parameters that are indicative of the abrupt ignition of a hypermetabolic state accompanied by rigorous contracture in skeletal muscle. These changes are reflected by the conventional indices of acid/base, blood gas, electrolyte, and substrate status in blood as well as by changes observed in serial liquid nitrogen frozen muscle biopsies. They proceed to extreme values ahead of the physical rise in muscle and core temperature.[24,29]

Profound, rapidly worsening lactacidosis together with concomitant hypercapnea, the result of its physiological buffering, is the hallmark of this syndrome (see Chapter 5). The latter, readily monitored by capnography, is perhaps the earliest indication of the syndrome's switch on. A rise in plasma lactate and in oxygen uptake are equally early. Blood and tissue pH may fall from control levels to 6.8 units and lower in a time as short as 10 min (Figure 2).

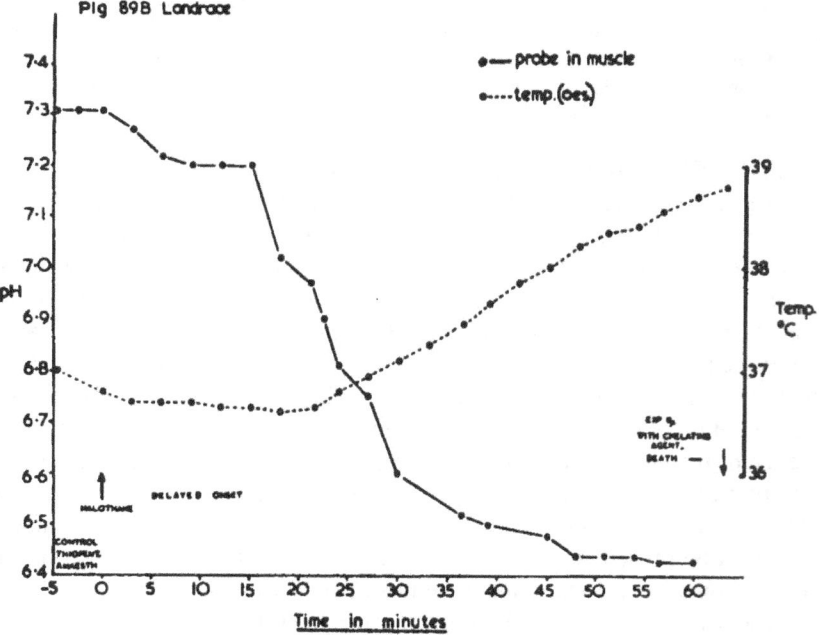

FIGURE 2. Simultaneous record of muscle pH (free-lying pH probe deep in thigh muscle) and esophageal temperature from Landrace pig during halothane-induced MH following 30-min control period of thiopentone anesthesia. N_2O (60%)/O_2 (40%) was administered throughout by IPPV. Note virtual "free fall" of pH that precedes commencement of temperature rise by 5 min. Death of this pig followed promptly on administration of Ca^{2+} chelating agent. (From Harrison, G. G., *Int. Symp. Malignant Hyperthermia*, R. A. Gordon, B. A. Britt, and W. Kalow, Eds., Charles C Thomas, Springfield, IL, 1973, 271. With permission.)

That the rise in plasma lactate precedes the rise in muscle and core temperature distinguishes MH from heatstroke and heat injury. In these conditions the rise in lactate is a late phenomenon occurring only after core temperature exceeds 41°C and correlates with the breakdown of compensatory mechanisms.

Though PaO_2 may not be reduced much, marked increase in tissue oxygen utilization results in an early and marked decrease in mixed venous PO_2 long before the terminal drop in cardiac output and the prominence of central cyanosis as a clinical sign.

Early elevation of plasma protein and Na^+ concentration tally with a shift of water into the cells. Elevation of plasma K^+ and Mg^{2+} also occurs early, the rise in the former being clinically important in the generation of the cardiac arrhythmias that characterize the terminal phases of the syndrome. Plasma Ca^{2+} and inorganic phosphate also rise, though the former has been reported variable.

Commencement of accelerated glycogenolysis and glycolysis is signaled by a rise in plasma glucose that correlates with depletion in muscle glycogen, itself stoichiometric with the increase in plasma lactate. Examination of serial muscle sections shows the whole glycolytic pathway to be accelerated with no single enzymatic step being specifically activated.[30] *Pari passu* with excessive glycolysis within skeletal muscle, the level of creatine phosphate falls within minutes, to be followed by that of ATP as both glycogen and creatine phosphate become exhausted. While ADP levels remain unaltered, AMP and inosine increase as the syndrome progresses, the end result being continuous unrequited nucleotide hydrolysis. This is a process that ends in producing the ante mortem biochemical conditions that characterize rigor mortis.[25]

Increasing permeability of the sarcolemma (SL) becomes evident in the rising plasma levels of the muscle enzymes, specifically CPK but also LDH, AST, and ALT.[26,28] In treatment-salvaged pigs, a severalfold rise in serum CPK 24 h after the experimentally induced syndrome serves as confirmation of the previous induction of MH.[31]

A surging increase in circulatory catecholamines accompanies onset of the syndrome and is doubtlessly responsible for the early tachycardia and later cardiac arrhythmias. It must be noted that chronologically this rise in circulating catecholamines follows that of lactate and PCO_2.[27]

VI. PATHOGENESIS

This progression of biochemical changes is the outcome of a single event — the induction of an abrupt and sustained rise in myoplasmic free Ca^{2+}. The validity of this hypothesis, founded until comparatively recently on experimental inference, has now been confirmed by direct observation. Utilizing ion-specific microelectrode impalement of MHS myocytes, Lopez and coworkers have demonstrated a rise in myoplasmic free Ca^{2+} to accompany the onset of MH rigor and a fall, induced by dantrolene, to accompany control of the syndrome and relaxation of muscle (Figure 3).[33,34]

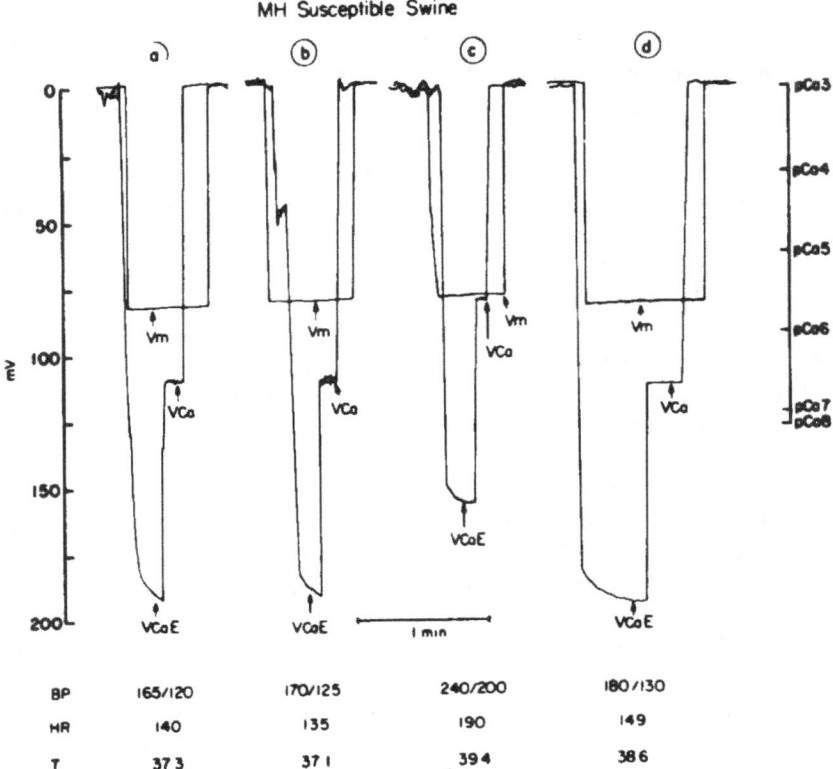

FIGURE 3. Changes in membrane potential, resting myoplasmic free calcium concentration, blood pressure (BP), heart rate (HR), and temperature (T) recorded during MH in MHS swine and its reversal with dantrolene. Responses were recorded (a) before halothane exposure during control anesthesia with thiopentone/fentanyl/N$_2$O, O$_2$/pancuronium; (b) after halothane exposure; (c) after reversal of pancuronium effect with muscle contracture well established; and (d) after dantrolene (2 mg/kg). Vm = resting membrane potential (KCl microelectrode); VCa = myoplasmic resting free calcium concentration (VCaE − Vm); and VCaE = potential measured by Ca^{2+}-specific microelectrode (Vm + VCa). (From Lopez et al., *Muscle Nerve*, 11, 82, 1988. With permission.)

The attainment of a threshold concentration in myoplasmic free Ca^{2+}, approximately 6 to 9 × 10^{-7}M, activates the ATPase-dependent troponin/actin/myosin interaction leading to muscle contraction, soon to persist as contracture when the free Ca^{2+} concentration is not only sustained but rises even higher to 10^{-5}M.[35] This reaction becomes progressively independent of Ca^{2+} when muscle temperature exceeds 40°C, an event among many that results in the syndrome's ultimate irreversibility.[36]

The early rise in plasma lactate (15- to 20-fold) and modest increase in oxygen uptake,[24,27] which accompany the vast increase in heat output (up to 17-fold),[37] signal the early onset of anaerobiasis. That this occurs in the absence of hypoxia long constituted an enigma.[38] Now, this too is seen as but one further sequela of the sustained rise in the level of myoplasmic free Ca^{2+}.

The sequestration of Ca^{2+}, for which mitochondria have a high affinity, is an energy consuming, respiration-dependent process that takes primacy over and replaces that of phosphorylation. Exposed to the high Ca^{2+} load, the mitochondria of MHS muscle display only 60% of the ATP-generative capacity of normal muscle.[39,40] *Ab initio*, the increased consumption of ATP by skeletal muscle adenine nucleotide hydrolysis exceeds the mitochondrial capacity for its regeneration. This situation may be worsened late in the syndrome when reduction in muscle blood supply for various reasons may actually reduce available oxygen.[41] The rapid depletion of muscle ATP content is a major factor in the establishment of the vicious cycle that finally becomes irreversible when ATP concentration falls to half the original resting level (Figure 4).[38]

Precise identification of the thermogenic reactions involved and their respective contributions has not been possible. The reason is that we are unable to observe steady-state conditions in metabolism and circulation during the acutely progressing MH syndrome as well as because of uncontrolled heat losses. Factors that have been identified as contributory to the heat generation (equivalent to maximal muscle exertion) are[25,38,42]

1. Hydrolysis of adenine nucleotides
2. Aerobic and anaerobic glycolysis
3. Buffering of the resultant H^+ ion production
4. Entropy of muscle contraction

It is relevant here to mention two attractive early hypotheses of the mechanisms of heat production in MH that are now discounted. Historically, the first serious hypothesis of a pathogenesis for MH[43] proposed the induction of uncoupling of oxidative phosphorylation, a proposal subsequently extensively investigated. The subsequent demonstration by many investigators of normal respiratory control in MHS muscle mitochondria has long since confirmed Wang and coworkers' original objections to this hypothesis on purely theoretical grounds.[44] The bulk of evidence now does not support a role for abnormalities in mitochondrial respiration in the pathogenesis of MH.[45]

The second hypothesis proposed a role for, and produced some evidence of, the futile recycling of fructose $6PO_4$ and fructose 1,6-diphosphate, the mechanism responsible for the preflight warming to operating temperature of bumble bee flight muscle.[46] Sadly, the amount of heat released by the rate of cycling observed in MHS pig muscle was insufficient to account for the heat output observed in MH. Further, the accelerated substrate cycling of glycolysis in MH is not futile but is in response to the additional ATP demands of the Ca^{2+} pumps.[42]

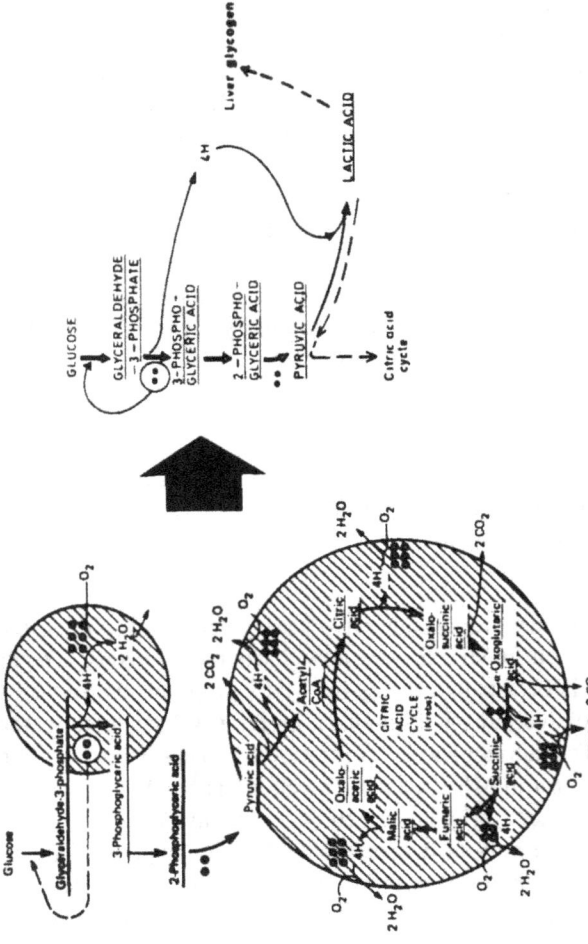

FIGURE 4(A). The key biochemical characteristics of MH, early and severe lactacidosis (despite adequate oxygenation) with concomitant energy substrate — glycogen and ATP — depletion are based on Ca^{2+} load depression of mitochondrial ATP generation, reducing the ATP yield of 1 mol of glucose from 38 with mitochondrial activity to 2 mol without. In this abbreviated diagram of cytosolic (Emden-Meyerhoff) and mitochondrial (Krebs) energy transduction pathways, the latter reactions are enclosed in the shaded circles. Underlining indicates that two molecules are formed from one of glucose. ATP generation is indicated by one black dot/mol. (From Nunn, J. F., *Applied Respiratory Physiology*, 2nd ed., Butterworths, London, Boston, 1977, pp. 378, 379. With permission). (B) The effect *in vitro* on ATP concentration of muscle from normal and MHS swine of incubation in Krebs-Ringer solution and exposure to halothane. (From Harrison, G. G., *Porcine Malignant Hyperthermia in Malignant Hyperthermia*, Little, Brown, Boston, 1979, 25. With permission.)

THE DISCOVERY OF MALIGNANT HYPERTHERMIA IN
PIGS - SOME PERSONAL RECOLLECTIONS.

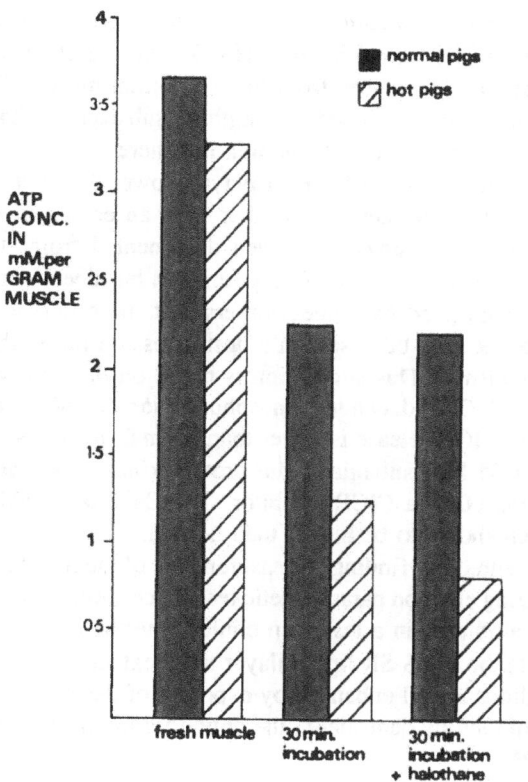

FIGURE 4(B).

A. MYOPLASMIC FREE Ca²⁺

The abrupt and runaway rise in myoplasmic free Ca^{2+} that drives the events of the MH crisis appears to be the response to triggering of the excitation/contraction/coupling (ECC) mechanisms of skeletal muscle afflicted by genetically induced dysfunctions of one or more of its complex sequential reactions. Indeed, dysfunction has been identified in MHS muscle at many ECC steps and in the organelles involved, some of primary import, others secondarily induced.

B. SARCOPLASMIC RETICULUM

Most relevant to the MH crisis is dysfunction of the sarcoplasmic reticulum (SR), the organelle which plays the principal role in the regulation of ECC myoplasmic Ca^{2+} fluxes. Though studies of the Ca^{2+} transport, uptake, and binding functions of MHS-SR have failed to yield a convincing explanation for the initiation of the MH process, recent characterization of SR Ca^{2+} release mechanisms and their modifications in MHS muscle now seems to provide the basis for an acceptable hypothesis of this event.[45,47]

The phenomenon of calcium-induced calcium release (CICR) exhibited by the triadic terminal cisternal SR of MHS skeletal muscle has been shown to exhibit substantial differences from that of normal muscle. These differences are described and discussed at length in subsequent chapters in this volume and accordingly are briefly summarized here.

This CICR function of MHS-SR displays a lower than normal threshold Ca^{2+} concentration for triggering, together with an enhanced rate of Ca^{2+} release.[35,48-52] Parallel findings have been documented from studies of the ryanodine receptor with which the CICR function has been identified.[53]

It has been suggested by some workers that the observed faster Ca^{2+} release by MHS-SR may be based on a desuppression rather than an actual activation mechanism.[54] This suggestion is based on the observation that in MHS pig SR, Ca^{2+}/CaM-dependent phosphorylation of a 60-kDa protein that normally inhibits CICR release is lower than normal. Responsible for this is a reduction in a 55-kDa subunit of the protein kinase that catalyzes phosphorylation of the 60-kDa CICR inhibitor. The Ca^{2+} permeability of MHS SR has also been shown to be higher than normal.

Associated with these findings, measurements of the SR membrane order parameter, utilizing electron paramagnetic resonance spectroscopy, have demonstrated that halothane, in a less than clinical anesthetic concentration, induces disorder in the MHS SR lipid bilayer to an extent greater than normal. These abnormalities are all enhanced by exposure of the SR to halothane and are uniquely inhibited by dantrolene, the only drug known to control the MH phenomenon.[49-52]

C. THE VICIOUS CYCLE

The rapid establishment of the vicious cycle which characterizes the PMH and SS syndromes can be more readily explained today in the light of recent elucidation of the structure, properties, and function of the ryanodine receptor. This receptor, a tetrameric protein which spans the sarcotubular gap, serves as the principal Ca^{2+} release channel of the SR.[50a] It is encoded by a 15.3 kb gene located in swine on chromosome 6. In all five breeds of swine which manifest it, the MHS phenotype is associated with a single point mutation (bp 1843) of a T/A for C/G.[4] The resultant codon encodes cysteine instead of arginine — a change which renders the ryanodine receptor channel leaky, in degree varying with the homo- or heterozygous expression of the gene. The channel also displays a greater sensitivity (of an order of magnitude) to the action of channel opening agents such as Ca^{2+}, ATP, and caffeine. It is postulated that the anesthetic triggers of MH and/or the endocrine responses to stress could act either directly on this abnormal channel or indirectly by raising the myoplasmsic concentration of physiological channel gating agents. Once opened, this MHS channel is unresponsive to Ca^{2+} and Mg^{2+} induced closure, so engendering the sustained rise in myoplasmic [Ca^{2+}] which drives the vicious cycle (Figure 5).

The abrupt termination of the syndrome by dantrolene, which itself lacks any effect on SR Ca^{2+} reuptake, implies that continued Ca^{2+} release, as against impairment of SR Ca^{2+} uptake, is fundamental to the genesis of MH. Once this is terminated by dantrolene, the functions of other Ca^{2+}-modulating mechanisms of the SR and mitochondria, are sufficient to return free Ca^{2+} concentration to resting levels — at least early in the syndrome — permitting relaxation of muscle and termination of the syndrome.

D. THE MILIEU OF IRREVERSIBILITY

Though dysfunction of SR itself provides a sufficient basis for the establishment of the MH vicious cycle; other functions (normal) and dysfunctions (peculiar to MHS genotype) of ECC mechanisms and the organelles involved also contribute to the milieu of irreversibility.

A primary role in the initiation of MH is no longer assigned to reduction in SR Ca^{2+} reuptake function, but, secondarily induced, it may well contribute significantly to perpetuation of the syndrome once established.

Inhibition, with ultimate inactivation, of SR Ca^{2+} reuptake occurs in response to the biochemical sequelae of the MH syndrome through three mechanisms.

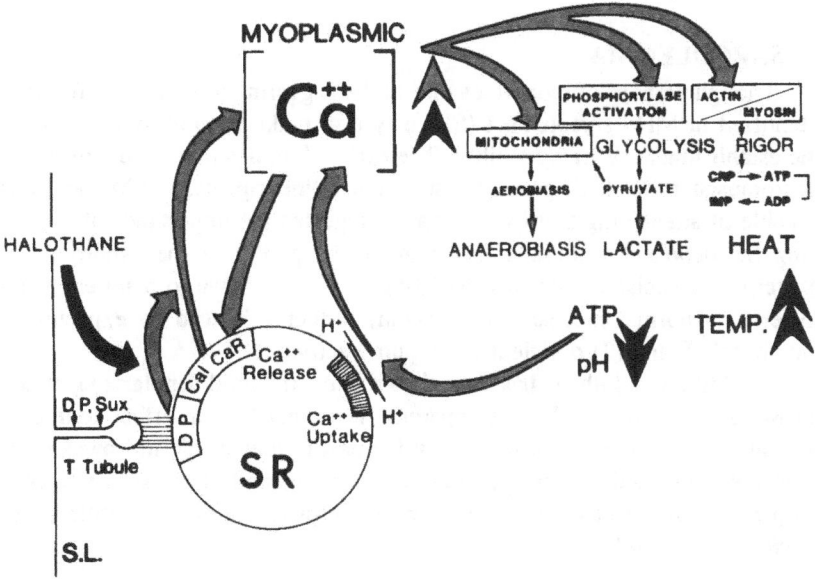

FIGURE 5. The vicious cycle of MH (see text for description): SL = sarcolemma; SR = sarcoplasmic reticulum; DP = depolarization; Sux = Succinylcholine; H$^+$ = protonation of SR; CICR = calcium-induced calcium release; CRP = creatine phosphate; ATP = adenosine triphosphate; ADP = adenosine diphosphate; IMP = inosine monophosphate; and Temp. = Temperature.

1. Proton or acid inactivation of SR Ca^{2+} transport induced by the early, rapid fall in intracellular pH, the threshold for which is itself raised in the presence of halothane;[55,56] while this phenomenon is a function of normal muscle, in MHS swine it may well be enhanced by reduced lactate clearance consequent on the defective hepatic gluconeogenesis they have been shown to manifest[57]
2. Substrate depletion consequent on the exhaustion of ATP[38]
3. Increase in membrane permeability secondary to the free fatty acid (FFA) release engendered by excessive Ca^{2+}-activated membrane associated phospholipase A_2 activity[58]

E. MITOCHONDRIA

Though a primary role in the pathogenesis of MH for enhanced endogenous levels of calmodulin-dependent phospholipase A_2, as postulated by Cheah[58] is not considered likely,[42] an increase in membrane Ca^{2+} permeability secondary to the FFA engendered by its Ca^{2+} activation (as in 3 above) may well promote the irreversibility of the established syndrome. The consequent failure of the mitochondria as a major intracellular Ca^{2+} sump is then manifested by (1) the reduction (8- to 10-fold) in mitochondrial Ca^{2+} accumulating ability observed in the MHS genotype[59] and (2) the increased rate (normal × 2) of mitochondrial Ca^{2+} efflux induced by anaerobiasis in MHS swine, an important event in the production of PSEP in MHS slaughter animals.[60]

F. SARCOLEMMA

Though perhaps of more relevance to the triggering of MH, a dysfunction identified in MHS sarcolemma (SL) may also make its contribution toward the establishment of irreversibility. The earlier findings that nondepolarizing neuromuscular blockade prevented succinylcholine triggering of MH and was capable of attenuating that by halothane suggested the importance of continuing SL depolarization as a factor in the triggering of the syndrome by exercise.[1] Associated with this, MHS-SL has been shown to manifest: (1) a lower than normal mechanical threshold, further enhanced by exposure to halothane[61,62] and (2) deficient Ca^{2+} pump activity.[63]

In addition, halothane has been shown to exert a mild depolarizing action on MHS-SL (5 to 15 mV) not apparent on normal SL, an effect countered by dantrolene.[64] Though postulated in the past to play a role in "awake" or anaesthetic-induced triggering,[42] this action has recently been shown to play no part, per se, in halothane induction of contracture in MHS muscle either *in vitro* or *in vivo*.[65]

G. CONTRACTILE PROTEINS

While the above mechanisms may all contribute *ab initio* to the establishment of the vicious cycle, another phenomenon demonstrable in normal muscle plays a part later, once muscle temperature has risen to 40°C and above. This is thermal inactivation of the Ca^{2+} dependence of the actin/myosin contractile interaction; a reaction which, under the circumstances of MH, is potentiated by the sharp decline in ATP content.[36]

H. OTHER MEMBRANES

Demonstrable dysfunction in the membranous elements of all the organelles involved in muscle ECC suggests the possibility that the MHS/PSS state may be associated with a generalized genetic membrane defect. To date, blood is the only tissue of which studies by many investigators has produced consistent evidence for such a hypothesis.[42]

The finding that MHS swine erythrocytes display an increased osmotic fragility[66-68] has been proposed as support for such a hypothesis. However, the importance of this finding, in a primary sense, to any general concept of the pathogenesis of MH is immediately called in question by the fact that it is not mirrored in the human patient susceptible to MH.[69]

Recently more subtle abnormalities have been identified in the plasmalemma of MHS swine lymphocytes[70,71] and erythrocytes[72,73] that are present also in those of human MHS subjects. These concern a halothane-induced increase in membrane Ca^{2+} permeability associated with evidence derived from electron paramagnetic resonance spectroscopy that halothane induces a greater degree of fluidity in MHS membranes than in those of normal animals. These changes induced by halothane in MHS plasmalemma are of a similar nature to those induced in MHS-SR[49,51,52] with the difference that, whereas in the latter they occur in response to less than clinical anesthetic concentrations of halothane, the former require a concentration of halothane severalfold in excess. While this evidence may strengthen the case for the existence in the MHS state of a more generalized genetic membrane defect involving tissues other than muscle, it is most unlikely — from this evidence — that this plays any part in the pathogenesis of the MH crisis.

VII. THE ROLE OF THE
SYMPATHETIC NERVOUS SYSTEM

The readiness with which MH can be evoked in MHS swine by excitement, stress, and exercise, considered together with the prominence of tachycardia and other sympathetic phenomena as the first clinical signs of its onset and the correlated increase observed in circulating catecholamines,[27,74] all suggest that activity of the sympathetic nervous system and endogenous catecholamine secretion must play a major role in the genesis of PMH. However, the question of whether sympathetic activity plays a primary role or is a secondary event has long been the subject of controversy.[42]

In spite of the extensive theory developed by Williams and colleagues and Lucke and coworkers incriminating norepinephrine as the primary factor in MH both as a basic abnormality and as a trigger,[75,76] the bulk of evidence favors a secondary role.

This evidence includes the complementary demonstrations that rigor and the biochemical markers of MH were induced by halothane in an isolated perfused MH muscle preparation,[77] that the syndrome was provoked by halothane in totally sympathectomized MHS swine with no rise in circulating catecholamine,[78] and the corollary that the syndrome was not initiated by the infusion into MHS swine of adrenergic agonists.[32,79] Further, as already mentioned (see Section V), the rise observed in circulating catecholamines is documented to chronologically follow the first metabolic changes observed.[27]

Though assigned a secondary role, when viewed in the context of the physiological effects catecholamines have on skeletal muscle — amplification of glycogenolysis energy transduction and 3,5 cyclic AMP-mediated change in the rate of SR Ca^{2+} uptake[80] — activity of the sympathetic nervous system must be accepted as playing an important amplifying role in the development of MH.

VIII. CAPTURE MYOPATHY

As it bears a superficial resemblance to PSS/PMH, a brief consideration of the life-threatening, stress-related syndrome manifested by wild game, particularly ungulates and birds, known as "capture myopathy"[81] is relevant here. Lacking the genetic constraints of PSS, this syndrome is precipitated in normal animals by the alarm, stress, and extreme muscular exertion of the flight from pursuit that precedes capture, or the darting and sedation-induced immobilization necessary for capture, of wild game. It presents as shock, prostration, muscle stiffness, or "spastic paresis", with moderate hyperthermia preceding coma and death. The principal biochemical derangement is a profound lactacidosis which, together with raised serum levels of muscle enzymes, points to the initiation of anaerobic glycolysis in muscle and membrane damage. Postmortem skeletal muscle may have an appearance very similar to PSEP.[82]

However, it has been noted that while capture myopathy does manifest an MH-like, end-stage vicious cycle, this can be aborted by the simple expedient of combating the acidosis alone by the administration of $NaHCO_3$.[83] Further, it can be reliably prevented by adequate precapture sedation with a variety of anxiolytic drugs, if such is achieved with minimal alarm and pursuit stress. It is suggested that, in the circumstances of capture myopathy, entry into the MH-like vicious cycle is by way of proton inactivation of SR Ca^{2+} reuptake (see Section IV.D). The ultimately uncompensated lactacidosis being the result of excessive muscular activity, is also amplified by the effects of the persistently stress-raised levels of circulating catecholamines.

IX. THE TRIGGERING OF PMH

In the description earlier in this chapter of the clinical characteristics of PMH/PSS, attention was drawn to the variations in triggering sensitivity that are produced by certain circumstances. These were, on the one hand, the enhancement of triggering sensitivity produced by stress, excitement, and exercise and, on the other, its attenuation in response to sedation, anxiolysis, and anesthesia. It is likely that these responses are but a reflection of the induction or inhibition of the capture myopathy scenario in the milieu of MHS muscle with its dysfunctional CICR and other ECC mechanisms. Circumstances most relevant to the enhancement of the sensitivity of triggering would follow from prolonged increases in myoplasmic free Ca^{2+} secondary to continuing multiple depolarizations, accentuated by catecholamine facilitation of prejunctional release and amplification of glycogenolysis.[80]

X. DRUG SCREENING IN MHS SWINE

The identification of drugs with MH-triggering potential depended — at least initially — on anecdote, "personal communication", and unpublished data, often uncorroborated. As ethical considerations prohibited any thought of prospective controlled clinical trials in humans, it is probable in the context of the polypharmacy inherent in modern anesthesia, that many such identifications were not valid. Once incorrectly identified as exhibiting MH-triggering potential, a drug could remain permanently so labeled, its identification as such being copied uncritically from text to text. Objective, retestable data from the pharmacological screening of drugs in MHS swine have ameliorated this situation.

MHS swine can be inbred to display a uniformity of response and sensitivity of the MH-triggering mechanism that is not found in humans.[1,10] Further, in such a model, drugs can be tested singly in contrast to the environment of polypharmacy that pertains in human clinical anesthesia. For the clinical anesthetist, it is of importance to note that human MHS patients react positively to all drugs that test positive as triggers of MH in the MHS pig model, though the converse does not hold.[84] This circumstance is most likely explainable by the above circumstances rather than by inherent species differences in drug response.

In the MHS pig model, the most potent triggers of MH are the newer volatile halogenated alkanes and ethers: halothane, ethrane, isoflurane, and sevoflurane. Of historical interest, so too is chloroform. Fluroxene (now withdrawn) and cyclopropane feature as weak and inconsistent triggering agents.[1] Strangely, methoxyflurane, trichlorethylene, diethyl ether, and nitrous oxide — all documented as MH triggers in the human — do not act this way in swine. Indeed, in swine nitrous oxide fails to display any MH-triggering activity even when administered under hyperbaric conditions.[85] (Harrison and Watson, unpublished data)

In the pig model, MH triggering has not been ascribed to any of the conventional i.v. anesthetic agents, including ketamine which has been questionably associated with initiation of human MH.[86] Indeed two such agents, althesin (now withdrawn) to a greater extent[20] and thiopentone to a lesser extent,[87] block or attenuate MH initiation by volatile anesthetics. Propofol, the most recent introduction into clinical anesthetic practice, has tested neutral to MH, neither stimulating nor attenuating its initiation.[88]

Of muscle relaxant drugs, depolarizing succinylcholine alone manifests the potential to trigger the syndrome. In the most highly reactive strains (those that react to halothane alone) succinylcholine alone also initiates the syndrome, though this may require two pulse doses. In those less reactive strains in which the syndrome is not precipitated by exposure to volatile anesthetics alone, succinylcholine acts as the specific added stressor to trigger the syndrome. None of the nondepolarizing relaxants trigger the syndrome, and, as already mentioned, pretreatment with them effectively blocks succinylcholine triggering.[1,84]

The attribution of MH-triggering potential to several drugs by anecdotal clinical association backed, perhaps, by some theoretical consideration of their effects on membrane Ca^{2+} fluxes, has been mentioned. Recent MHS pig screening of some of these drugs has revealed such inference to be invalid in the case of several clinically very useful drugs.

Perhaps first among these is lignocaine and the amide-linked group of local anesthetics (LA). Arguably, the most widely used LA agents in clinical practice and in many hospitals the only local anesthetic agents available, amide-linked LAs have long been documented as putative MH-triggering agents. That this important group of drugs is, in conventional doses, safe to use in the MHS patient has now been validated by a failure to trigger MH in the pig model with amide-linked LAs infused i.v. to monitored toxic levels.[89,90]

Digitalis is another such drug. In a sophisticated MH pig model utilizing cardiopulmonary bypass to obviate the drug's cardiotoxic effects, Gronert and coworkers[91] have demonstrated that digitalis infused i.v. to supratoxic, cardiac arresting levels (61 ng/ml) lacks any effect on whole body metabolism, and by inference that of skeletal muscle.

Similarly, in the same preparation $CaCl_2$ infused to cardiac arresting levels (15 mEq/l) was also shown to lack the MH-triggering potential it was long assumed to have.

Last, and perhaps most importantly, the MHS pig model has served as the pharmacological test bed in which the strange specificity of dantrolene in the control and prevention of MH was established.[92] The demonstration in rats by Ellis and coworkers[93] that the skeletal muscle relaxing properties of dantrolene stemmed from a selective depressive action on the ill-understood intrinsic mechanisms of ECC motivated his suggesting its therapeutic trial on the MH syndrome established in susceptible swine. In these animals, dantrolene proved to be the only drug capable of reliably terminating the MH syndrome and of completely blocking its inception by volatile anesthetics and/or succinylcholine. As triggering agents switched MH on in the susceptible animal, so dantrolene switched it off. These findings were subsequently successfully applied to the treatment of human MH.[92] Dantrolene, we now know, binds to and acts on the SR and T-tubular membranes, reducing the rate and amount of calcium release from the former, altering the T-tubular/ SR coupling "charge movements" of the latter and reducing at least the halothane component of CICR.[53,54]

These actions of dantrolene, superficially those of a Ca^{2+} channel blocker, are exceedingly complex and are still poorly understood. They are clearly distinguishable from those of the conventional Ca^{2+} channel blocking drugs, e.g., verapamil, nifedipine, diltiazem, etc., which act at an SL site and have no effect on MH,[94] and also the classic SR Ca^{2+} channel blockers, e.g., procaine and amethocaine, which do have a blocking but poor therapeutic effect on MH.[92] This virtual specificity of the actions of dantrolene in preventing and controlling the MH syndrome carries with it the implication that on their elucidation depends our final concept of the pathogenesis of the syndrome.

XI. FUTURE DIRECTIONS

Since its original identification in 1960, MH has provided a continuing stimulus for research by investigators in many disciplines, from the clinical scientist to the membrane chemist. Now that these endeavors have brought a worldwide awareness of the condition, a basic broad understanding of its pathogenesis, and a proven specific pharmacological cure, one may well question the direction of future research relevant to MH. For the clinician, priority must surely be given to the development of a diagnostic test for susceptibility to MH that is noninvasive and widely available, yet specific and sensitive. For the biological scientist, there remains the more intricate task of further unraveling the molecular mechanisms of SR calcium release. The solution to these problems in the future will doubtlessly come from the continued study of MH in swine.

ACKNOWLEDGMENTS

I wish to express my thanks to Mary Harrison for help with this manuscript and Phillipa Johnson for the art work in Figure 5.

REFERENCES

1. **Harrison, G. G.,** Porcine malignant hyperthermia — the saga of the "hot" pig, in *Malignant Hyperthermia,* B. A. Britt, Ed., Martinus Nijhoff, Boston, 1987, 103.
2. **Rutberg, H., Henriksson, K.-G., Jorfeldt, L., Larsson, J., Martensson, J., and Schildt, B.,** Metabolic changes in a case of malignant hyperthermia, *Br. J. Anaesth.* 55, 461, 1983.

3. **Lucke, J. N., Hall, G. M., and Lister, D.,** Body temperature and malignant hyperthermia, *Lancet,* i, 1405, 1976.
4. **Fujii, J., Otsu, K., Zorzato, F., DeLeon, S., Khanna, V. K., Weiler, J. E., et al.,** Identification of a mutation in porcine ryanodine receptor associated with Malignant Hyperthermia, *Science,* 253, 448, 1991.
4a. **MacLennan, D. H., Duff, C., Zorzato, F., Fujii, J., Phillips, M., Korneluk, G., et al.,** Ryanodine receptor gene is a candidate for predisposition to Malignant Hyperthermia, *Nature,* 343, 2244, 1990.
5. **Lawrie, R. A., Catherum, D. P., and Hale, H. P.,** Abnormally low pH in pig muscle, *Nature,* 182, 807, 1958.
6. **Wismer-Pedersen, J. and Briskey, E. J.,** Rate of anaerobic glycolysis versus structure in pork muscle, *Nature,* 189, 318, 1961.
7. **Williams, C. H.,** The development of an animal model for fulminant hyperthermia porcine stress syndrome, in *Malignant Hyperthermia — Current Concepts,* E. O. Henschel, Ed., Appleton-Century-Crofts, New York, 1977, 117.
8. **Kalow, W.,** Inheritance of malignant hyperthermia — a review of published data, in *Malignant Hyperthermia,* B. A. Britt, Ed., Martinus Nijhoff, Boston, 1987, 155.
9. **Topel, D. G., Bicknell, E. J., Preston, K. S., Christian, L. L., and Matsushima, C. Y.,** Porcine stress syndrome, *Mod. Vet Pract.,* 49, 40, 1968.
10. **Nelson, T. E., Flewellen, E. H., and Gloyna, D. F.,** Spectrum of susceptibility to malignant hyperthermia — diagnostic dilemma, *Anesth. Analg.,* 62, 545, 1983.
11. **Williams, C. H., Shanklin, M. D., Hedrick, H. B., Muhrer, M. B., Stubbs, D. H., Krause, G. F. et al.,** The fulminant hyperthermia syndrome: genetic aspects, in *Second Int. Symp. Malignant Hyperthermia,* A. Aldrete and B. A. Britt, Eds., Grune & Stratton, New York, 1978, 113.
12. **Woolf, N., Hall, L., Thorne, C., Down, M., and Walker, R.,** Serum creatine phosphokinase levels in pigs reacting abnormally to halogenated anaesthetics, *Br. Med. J.,* 3, 386, 1970.
13. **Heffron, J. J. A. and Mitchell, G.,** Diagnostic value of serum creatine phosphokinase activity for the porcine malignant hyperthermia syndrome, *Anesth. Analg.,* 54, 536, 1975.
14. **Sybesma, W. and Eikelenboom, G.,** Methods of predicting pale, soft, exudative pork and their application in breeding programmes, *Meat Sci.,* 2, 79, 1978.
15. **Britt, B. A.,** Muscle assessment of malignant hyperthermia susceptible patients, in *Malignant Hyperthermia,* B. A. Britt, Ed., Martinus Nijhoff, Boston, 1987, 193.
16. **Britt, B. A., Kalow, W., and Endrenyi, I. L.,** Malignant hyperthermia: pattern of inheritance in swine, in *Second Int. Symp. Malignant Hyperthermia,* A. Aldrete and B. A. Britt, Eds., Grune & Stratton, New York, 1978, 195.
17. **Rasmussen, B. A. and Christian, L. L.,** H blood types in pigs as prediction of stress susceptibility, *Science,* 191, 947, 1976.
18. **Eikelenboom, G., Minkema, D., Van Eldik, P., and Sybesma, W.,** Inheritance of the malignant hyperthermic syndrome in Dutch Landrace swine, in *Second Int. Symp. Malignant Hyperthermia,* A. Aldrete and B. A. Britt, Eds., Grune & Stratton, New York, 1978, 141.
19. **Van Den Hende, C., Lister, D., Muylle, E., Ooms, L., and Oyaert, W.,** Malignant hyperthermia in Belgian Landrace pigs, rested or exercised before exposure to halothane, *Br. J. Anaesth.,* 48, 821, 1976.
20. **Harrison, G. G.,** Althesin and malignant hyperpyrexia, *Br. J. Anaesth.,* 45, 1019, 1973.
21. **McLoughlin, J. Y., Somers, C. J., Ahern, C. P., and Wilson, P.,** Porcine MH syndrome: effectiveness of spiperone and dantrolene in prevention and treatment, *Acta Agric. Scand.,* Suppl. 21, 343, 1979.
22. **McGrath, C. J., Rempel, W. E., Addis, P. B. et al.,** Acepromazine and droperidol inhibition of halothane-induced malignant hyperthermia (porcine stress syndrome) in swine, *Am. J. Vet. Res.,* 42, 195, 1981.

23. **Hall, L. W., Woolf, N., Bradley, J. W., and Jolly, D. W.,** Unusual reaction to suxamethonium chloride, *Br. Med. J.*, 2, 1305, 1966.

24. **Berman, M. C., Harrison, G. G., Bull, A. B., and Kench, J. E.,** Changes underlying halothane induced malignant hyperpyrexia in Landrace pigs, *Nature*, 225, 653, 1970.

25. **Berman, M. C. and Kench, J. E.,** Biochemical features of malignant hyperthermia in Landrace pigs, in *Int. Symp. Malignant Hyperthermia*, R. A. Gordon, B. A. Britt, and W. Kalow, Eds., Charles C Thomas, Springfield, IL, 1973, 287.

26. **Jones, E. W., Nelson, T. E., Anderson, I. L., Kerr, D. D., and Burnap, T. K.,** Malignant hyperthermia in swine, *Anesthesiology*, 36, 42, 1972.

27. **Gronert, G. A. and Theye, R. A.,** Halothane induced porcine malignant hyperthermia: metabolic and haemodynamic changes, *Anesthesiology*, 44, 36, 1976.

28. **Verburgh, M. P., Oerlemans, F. T., Van Bennekom, C. A., Gielen, M. J., De Bruyn, C. H., and Crul, J. F.,** *In vivo* induced malignant hyperthermia in pigs. I. Physiological and biochemical changes and the influence of dantrolene sodium, *Acta Anaesth. Scand.*, 28, 1, 1984.

29. **Harrison, G. G.,** The effect of procaine and curare on the initiation of anaesthetic induced malignant hyperpyrexia, in *Int. Symp. Malignant Hyperthermia*, R. A. Gordon, B. A. Britt, and W. Kalow, Eds., Charles C Thomas, Springfield, IL, 1973, 271.

30. **Berman, M. L., Conradie, P., and Kench, J. E.,** The mechanism of accelerated muscle glycolysis during malignant hyperthermia in swine, *S. Afr. Med. J.*, 46, 1785, 1972.

31. **Harrison, G. G.,** Prophylaxis of malignant hyperthermia by oral dantrolene sodium in swine, *Br. J. Anaesth.*, 49, 315, 1977.

32. **Harrison, G. G., Saunders, S. J., Biebuyck, J. F., Hickman, R., Dent, D. M., Weaver, V., and Terblanche, J.,** Anaesthetic induced malignant hyperpyrexia and a method for its prediction, *Br. J. Anaesth.*, 41, 844, 1969.

33. **Lopez, J. R., Allen, P., Alamo, L., Jones, D., and Sreter, F.,** Myoplasmic free Ca^{2+} concentration during a malignant hyperthermia episode in swine, *Muscle Nerve*, 11, 82, 1988.

34. **Lopez, J. R., Allen, P., Alamo, L., Ryan, J. R., Jones, D., and Sreter, F.,** Dantrolene prevents the malignant hyperthermic syndrome by reducing free intracellular calcium concentration in skeletal muscle of susceptible swine, *Cell Calcium*, 8, 385, 1987.

35. **Endo, M.,** Calcium release from sarcoplasmic reticulum, *Phys. Rev.*, 57, 71, 1977.

36. **Fuchs, F.,** Thermal inactivation of calcium regulating mechanism of human muscle, *Anesthesiology*, 42, 584, 1975.

37. **Williams, C. H., Houchins, C., and Shanklin, M. D.,** Pigs susceptible to energy metabolism in the fulminant hyperthermia stress syndrome, *Br. Med. J.*, 3, 411, 1975.

38. **Heffron, J. J.,** Malignant hyperthermia: biochemical aspects of the acute episode, *Br. J. Anaesth.*, 60, 274, 1988.

39. **Stadhouers, A. M., Veiring, W. A. L., Verburgh, M. P., Ruitenbeek, W., and Sengers, R. C. A.,** *In vivo* induced malignant hyperthermia in pigs. III. Localisation of calcium in skeletal muscle mitochondria by means of electron microscopy and microprobe analysis, *Acta Anaesth. Scand.*, 28, 14, 1984.

40. **Ruitenbeek, W., Verburgh, M. P., Janssen, A. J. M., Stadhouers, A. M., and Sengers, R. C. A.,** "*In vivo*" induced malignant hyperthermia in pigs. II. Metabolism of skeletal muscle mitochondria, *Acta Anaesth. Scand.*, 28, 9, 1984.

41. **Hall, G. M., Lucke, J. N., Orchard, C., Lovell, R., and Lister, D.,** Porcine malignant hyperthermia. VIII. Leg metabolism, *Br. J. Anaesth.*, 54, 941, 1982.

42. **Gronert, G. A., Mott, J., and Lee, J.,** Aetiology of malignant hyperthermia, *Br. J. Anaesth.*, 60, 253, 1988.

43. **Wilson, R. D., Nichols, R. J., Dent, T. E., and Allen, C. R.,** Disturbances of oxidative phosphorylation mechanism as a possible etiologic factor in sudden unexplained hyperpyrexia occurring during anesthesia, *Anesthesiology*, 27, 231, 1966.

44. **Wang, J. R., Moffit, E. A., and Rosewear, J. W.**, Oxidative phosphorylation in acute hyperthermia, *Anesthesiology*, 30, 439, 1969.

45. **Ellis, F. R. and Heffron, J. J.**, Clinical and biochemical aspects of malignant hyperpyrexia, in *Recent Advances in Anaesthesia and Analgesia*, R. C. Atkinson and A. P. Adams, Eds., Churchill Livingstone, Edinburgh, 1985, 173.

46. **Clarke, M. G., Williams, C. H., Pfeifer, W. F., Bloxham, D. P., Holland, P. C., Taylor, C. A. et al.**, Accelerated substrate cycling of fructose 6 phosphate in muscle of MH pigs, *Nature*, 245, 99, 1973.

47. **Nelson, T. E.**, Skeletal muscle sarcoplasmic reticulum in malignant hyperthermia, in *Malignant Hyperthermia*, B. A. Britt, Ed., Martinus Nijhoff, Boston, 1984, 43.

48. **Endo, M., Yagi, S., Ishizuka, T., Horiuti, K., Koga, Y., and Amaha, K.**, Changes in Ca^{2+} induced Ca^{2+} release mechanism in SR of muscle from patients with MH, *Biomed. Res.*, 4, 83, 1983.

49. **Ohnishi, S. T., Taylor, S., and Gronert, G. A.**, Calcium induced Ca^{2+} release from sarcoplasmic reticulum of pigs susceptible to malignant hyperthermia: the effects of halothane and dantrolene, *FEBS Lett.*, 161, 103, 1983.

50. **Kim, D. H., Sreter, F. A., Ohnishi, S. T., Ryan, J. F., Roberts, J., Allen, P. D. et al.**, Kinetic studies of Ca^{2+} release from sarcoplasmic reticulum of normal and MHS pig muscles, *Biochim. Biophys. Acta*, 775, 320, 1984.

50a. **Zorzato, F., Fujii, J., Otsu, K., Phillips, M., Green, N., Lai, F., et al.**, Molecular cloning of cDNA encoding human and rabbit forms of Ca^{2+} release channel (ryanodine receptor) of skeletal muscle SR, *J. Biol. Chem.*, 265, 2244, 1990.

51. **Ohnishi, S. T., Waring, A. J., Fang, S. G., Horiuchi, K., Flick, J. L., Sadanaga, K. K. et al.**, Abnormal membrane properties of the sarcoplasmic reticulum of pigs susceptible to malignant hyperthermia: modes of action of halothane, caffeine, dantrolene and two other drugs, *Arch. Biochem. Biophys.*, 247, 294, 1986.

52. **Ohnishi, S. T.**, The effect of halothane, caffeine, dantrolene and tetracaine on the calcium permeability of skeletal sarcoplasmic reticulum of malignant hyperthermic pigs, *Biochim. Biophys. Acta*, 897, 261, 1987.

53. **Mickelson, J. R., Gallant, E. M., Litterer, L. A., Johnson, K. M., Rempel, W. E., and Louis, C. F.**, Abnormal sarcoplasmic reticulum ryanodine receptor in malignant hyperthermia, *J. Biol. Chem.*, 263, 9310, 1988.

54. **Kim, D. H., Sreter, F. A., and Ikemoto, N.**, Involvement of the 60 kDa phosphoprotein in the regulation of Ca^{2+} release from sarcoplasmic reticulum of normal and malignant hyperthermic susceptible pig muscles, *Biochim. Biophys.*, 945, 246, 1988.

55. **Berman, M. C., McIntosh, D. B., and Kench, J. E.**, Proton inactivation of calcium transport by sarcoplasmic reticulum, *J. Biol. Chem.*, 252, 994, 1977.

56. **Diamond, E. M. and Berman, M. C.**, The effect of halothane on the stability of Ca^{2+} transport activity of isolated fragmented SR, *Biochem. Pharmacol.*, 29, 375, 1980.

57. **Dimarco, N. M., Britz, D. C., Young, J. W., Topel, D. G., and Christian, L. L.**, Gluconeogenesis from lactate in liver of stress susceptible and stress resistant pigs, *J. Nutr.*, 106, 710, 1976.

58. **Cheah, K. S.**, Mitochondria and malignant hyperthermia, in *Malignant Hyperthermia*, B. A. Britt, Ed., Martinus Nijhoff, Boston, 1987, 79.

59. **Britt, B. A., Endrenyi, I. L., Cadman, D. L., Fan, H. M., and Fung, H. Y.-K.**, Porcine malignant hyperthermia: effects of halothane on mitochondrial respiration and calcium accumulation, *Anesthesiology*, 42, 292, 1975.

60. **Cheah, K. S. and Cheah, A. M.**, The trigger for PSE condition in stress susceptible pigs, *J. Sci. Food Agric.*, 27, 1137, 1976.

61. **Bryant, S. H. and Anderson, I. L.**, Mechanical activation and electrophysiological properties of intercostal muscle fibres from MH susceptible pigs, *Soc. Neurosci.*, 3, 213, 1977.

62. **Gallant, E. M., Gronert, G. A., and Taylor, S. R.,** Cellular membrane potentials and contractile threshold in mammalian skeletal muscle susceptible to malignant hyperthermia, *Neurosci. Lett.,* 28, 181, 1982.

63. **Mickelson, J. R., Ross, J. A., Hyslop, R. J., Gallant, E. M., and Louis, C. F.,** Skeletal muscle sarcolemma in malignant hyperthermia: evidence for a defect in calcium regulation, *Biochim. Biophys. Acta,* 897, 364, 1987.

64. **Gallant, E. M., Godt, R. E., and Gronert, G. A.,** Role of plasma membrane defect of skeletal muscle in malignant hyperthermia, *Muscle Nerve,* 2, 491, 1979.

65. **Gallant, E. M.,** Porcine malignant hyperthermia. No role for plasmalemmal depolarisation, *Muscle Nerve,* 11, 785, 1988.

66. **Harrison, G. G. and Verburg, C.,** Erythrocyte osmotic fragility in hyperthermia susceptible swine, *Br. J. Anaesth.,* 45, 131, 1973.

67. **Heffron, J. J. A. and Mitchell, G.,** Influence of pH, temperature, halothane and its metabolites on osmotic fragility of erythrocytes of MHS and resistant pigs, *Br. J. Anaesth.,* 53, 499, 1981.

68. **O'Brien, P. J., Rooney, M. T., Reik, T. R., Thatte, H. S., Remple, W. E., Addis, P. P., and Louis, C. F.,** Porcine hyperthermia: erythrocyte osmotic fragility, *Am. J. Vet. Res.,* 46, 1451, 1985.

69. **Zsigmond, E. K., Penner, J., and Kothary, S. P.,** Normal erythrocyte fragility and abnormal platelet aggregation in MH families, in *Second Int. Symp. Malignant Hyperthermia,* J. A. Aldrete and B. A. Britt, Eds., Grune & Stratton, New York, 1977, 213.

70. **Klip, A., Britt, B. A., Elliott, M. E., Pegg, W., Frodis, W., and Scott, E.,** Anaesthetic induced increase in ionised calcium in blood mononuclear cells from malignant hyperthermia patients, *Lancet,* II, 1463, 1987.

71. **Klip, A., Ramlal, T., Walker, D., Britt, B. A., and Elliott, M. E.,** Selective increase in cytoplasmic calcium by anaesthetic in lymphocytes from malignant hyperthermia susceptible pigs, *Anesth. Analg.,* 66, 381, 1987.

72. **Ohnishi, S. T. and Ohnishi, T.,** Halothane induced disorder of red cell membranes of subjects susceptible to malignant hyperthermia, *Cell Biochem. Funct.,* 6, 257, 1988.

73. **Ohnishi, S. T., Katagi, H., Ohnishi, T., and Brownell, A. K. W.,** Detection of malignant hyperthermia susceptibility using spin label techniques on red blood cells, *Br. J. Anaesth.,* 61, 565, 1988.

74. **Lister, D., Hall, G. M., and Lucke, J. N.,** Catecholamines in suxamethonium induced malignant hyperthermia in Petrain pigs, *Br. J. Anaesth.,* 46, 803, 1974.

75. **Lucke, J. N., Denny, H., Hall, G. M., Lovell, R., and Lister, D.,** Porcine malignant hyperthermia. VI. The effect of bilateral adrenalectomy and pretreatment with bretylium on the halothane induced response, *Br. J. Anaesth.,* 50, 241, 1978.

76. **Williams, C. H., Dozier, S. E., Buzello, W., Gehrke, C. W., Wong, J. K., and Gerhardt, K. O.,** Plasma levels of norepinephrine and epinephrine during malignant hyperthermia in susceptible pigs, *J. Chromatogr.,* 344, 71, 1985.

77. **Harrison, G. G., Berman, M. C., Hickman, R., Bull, A. B., Terblanche, J., and Kench, J. E.,** Anaesthetic induced malignant hyperpyrexia: some observations of the syndrome in Landrace pigs, in *Proc. III Asian Australasian Congr. Anaesthesiol.,* L. Shea and B. Dwyer, Eds., Butterworths, Australia, 1970, 158.

78. **Gronert, G. A., Milde, J. H., and Theye, R. A.,** The role of sympathetic activity in porcine malignant hyperthermia, *Anesthesiology,* 47, 411, 1977.

79. **Gronert, G. A., Milde, J. H., and Taylor, S. R.,** Porcine responses to carbachol, alpha and beta adrenoreceptor agonists, halothane and hyperthermia, *J. Physiol. (London),* 307, 319, 1980.

80. **Bowman, W. C. and Nott, M. W.,** Reaction of sympatheticomemetic amines and their antagonists on skeletal muscle, *Pharm. Rev.,* 21, 27, 1969.

81. **Harthoorn, A. M.**, *The Chemical Capture of Animals*, Bailliere Tindall, London, 1976, 77.
82. **Harthoorn, A. M., Louw, G. M., and Du Preez, J. J.**, Incipient capture myopathy as revealed by blood chemistry of chased zebras, *Madoqua Ser.*, 1, 45, 1973.
83. **Harthoorn, A. M., Van Der Walt, K., and Young, E.**, Possible therapy for capture myopathy in captured wild animals, *Nature*, 247, 577, 1974.
84. **Gronert, G. A.**, Malignant hyperthermia, in *Anesthesia*, R. D. Miller, Ed., Churchill Livingstone, Edinburgh, 1986, 1971.
85. **Gronert, G. A. and Milde, J. H.**, Hyperbaric nitrous oxide and malignant hyperthermia, *Br. J. Anaesth.*, 53, 1238, 1981.
86. **Gronert, G. A.**, Malignant hyperthermia, *Anesthesiology*, 53, 395, 1980.
87. **Hall, L. W., Trimm, M. N., and Woolf, N.**, Further studies in porcine malignant hyperthermia, *Br. Med. J.*, 2, 145, 1972.
88. **Raff, M. and Harrison, G. G.**, The screening of propofol in MHS swine, *Anesth. Analg.*, 68, 750, 1989.
89. **Harrison, G. G. and Morrell, D. F.**, Response of MHS swine to intravenous infusion of lignocaine and bupivacaine, *Br. J. Anaesth.*, 52, 385, 1980.
90. **Wingard, D. W. and Bobco, S.**, Failure of lidocaine to trigger porcine malignant hyperthermia, *Anesth. Analg.*, 58, 99, 1979.
91. **Gronert, G. A., Ahern, L. P., Milde, J. H., and White, R. D.**, Effect of CO_2, calcium, digoxin and potassium on cardiac and skeletal muscle metabolism in malignant hyperthermia susceptible swine, *Anesthesiology*, 64, 24, 1986.
92. **Harrison, G. G.**, Dantrolene — dynamics and kinetics, *Br. J. Anaesth.*, 60, 279, 1988.
93. **Ellis, K. O. and Carpenter, J. F.**, Mechanism of control of skeletal muscle contraction by dantrolene sodium, *Arch. Med. Rehabil.*, 55, 362, 1974.
94. **Harrison, G. G., Wright, I. G., and Morrell, D. F.**, The effects of calcium channel blocking drugs on halothane initiation of malignant hyperthermia in MHS swine and on the established syndrome, *Anaesth. Intens. Care*, 16, 197, 1988.

Chapter 9

CANINE MALIGNANT HYPERTHERMIA/ CANINE STRESS SYNDROME

Peter J. O'Brien

TABLE OF CONTENTS

I.   Anesthetic-Induced Malignant Hyperthermia in Dogs............106

II.   Canine Stress Syndrome 108

III.   Evidence for Muscle and Blood Cell Membrane Defects 108

IV.   Summary and Conclusions.....................................112

References..114

I. ANESTHETIC-INDUCED MALIGNANT HYPERTHERMIA IN DOGS

Although malignant hyperthermia (MH) was first diagnosed in man in 1960, it was not recognized in dogs until 1973.[1] Since then, at least 27 cases of canine MH susceptibility have been described,[2-14] of which 10 were fulminating MH reactions resulting in death.[2-4,7-9,12] The incidence is unknown, although the anesthetic deaths or complications have been estimated to occur at a rate of 1 in 2000 to 4000 veterinary anesthesias.[15]

As described below, the triggers, symptoms, laboratory findings, treatment, and inheritance of MH in dogs are similar to those observed for MH in people and swine. In dogs definitively diagnosed as being MH susceptible (MHS) by the caffeine contracture test or by their reaction to halothane, several preanesthetic features have been noted: family history of anesthetic death, working or sporting breed, muscular build, nervous and hyperactive temperament, and mild elevations of resting temperature, serum creatine kinase, serum aspartate transaminase (AST), and erythrocyte osmotic fragility.[8,13,14,16-19]

There appears to be a sex predilection for susceptibility to MH in dogs. Of 23 dogs that definitively have been diagnosed as MHS, 16 (70%) were male. The working and sporting breeds that appear to be most commonly afflicted with MH susceptibility are greyhound, border collie, springer spaniel, pointer, Irish wolfhound, and Labrador retriever. It has also been reported in crossbred doberman pinschers and spaniels.

Susceptibility to MH in dogs has been demonstrated to be inherited in an autosomal dominant pattern.[8] Gradations in susceptibility to halothane anesthesia, caffeine-induced contracture, and erythrocyte fragility have been observed.[8,12,13,16]

Episodes of MH in dogs have been characterized by sudden and unexplainable tachycardia, tachypnea, hyperthermia, and trismus (Table 1). Generalized rigidity is often present. In a full blown episode the tail is elevated,

TABLE 1
Major Clinical Signs of Canine
Malignant Hyperthermia

Rapid and sustained temperature elevation
Rigidity of jaw, body wall, and extensor muscles
Tachycardia and tachypnea
Cyanotic oral mucous membranes
Metabolic and respiratory acidosis
Hyperkalemia and hyperphosphatemia
Hemoconcentration with hypernatremia and polycythemia
Hypoxia and hypercarbia
Often fatal with rapid onset of rigor mortis

the ears pricked, the legs rigid and extended, and the mouth clamped shut.[8,12] The excessive rates of muscle metabolism result in increased oxygen consumption, thermogenesis, release of phosphate from adenosine triphosphate (ATP), and production of carbon dioxide, protons, and potassium. Body temperatures reach maximal values of 42 to 45°C. The anesthetic machine soda-lime canister also becomes hot as the lime is rapidly exhausted by the increased production of carbon dioxide.

The increase in heart and respiratory rates have been misinterpreted as a lightening of anesthesia and the halothane concentration has been increased, thereby accelerating the development of the syndrome. Death usually results from heart failure in association with the hyperthermia, acidosis, hyperkalemia, and hypercatecholemia. Rigor mortis develops rapidly after death due to exhaustion of muscle glycogen, creatine phosphate, and ATP.

Because MH often is not recognized during its early stages and because veterinarians are usually not prepared for its treatment, the fatality rate is nearly 100%. Therapy is successful only if initiated immediately after the onset of MH. Symptomatic treatment in conjunction with i.v. administration of dantrolene (1 to 3 mg/kg) and cessation of gaseous anesthesia are necessary for survival. Cooling with ice baths to reduce core temperature and i.v. infusion of sodium bicarbonate to lower serum hydrogen and potassium concentrations are usually necessary. If the syndrome is treated early, further symptomatic therapy may not be required. Three cases of successful treatment of canine MH with dantrolene, bicarbonate, and discontinuation of halothane administration have been reported.[5,12] More advanced cases may require treatment for cardiac dysrhythmias, pulmonary and central nervous system edema, rhabdomyolytic nephrosis, and disseminated intravascular coagulation.

Postmortem findings have included foci of fragmentation with loss of cross-striation and edema in cardiac and skeletal muscle, pulmonary and central nervous system edema, and splenic and hepatic congestion.[8,12]

Veterinary usage of commercially available i.v. dantrolene may be cost prohibitive; however, this may be relatively easily prepared from an inexpensive oral preparation and made available for emergency use during surgery.[20] The active ingredient can be isolated by manipulation of pH and using filtration.

Signs of MH have not been observed during the first 15 min of routine halothane anesthesia. The MH-protective effects of acetylpromazine and thiamylal used in anesthesia premedication and induction may be responsible for this delay in onset of signs. In fact, fulminating MH does not always occur during the first halothane anesthesia.[8] In unpremedicated dogs, MH may be triggered in less than 10 min.[12]

As in other species, succinylcholine[3,5] and enflurane[2] have also been implicated as triggers of MH in the dog, although methoxyflurane has not. In one MHS dog, it was used repeatedly with no symptoms developing despite the fact that the dog died from MH during a subsequent halothane anesthesia.[8] In man and in swine methoxyflurane is a weak trigger.

TABLE 2
Major Clinical Signs of Canine Stress Syndrome

Exercise intolerance
Exercise-induced hyperthermia
Apparent cramping of hind limb muscle
Dyspnea with rapid, labored, and stertorous respirations
Mixed metabolic acidosis with compensatory respiratory alkalosis
Marked hyperlactemia and hypocarbia with mild hyperoxia
Mild to moderate hemoconcentration
Usually reversible

Dogs with susceptibility to MH may be anesthetized safely with certain nontriggering agents. A satisfactory drug combination that has been used without complications is oxymorphone, acetylpromazine, thiamylal, and N_2O.[12] Use of i.v. diazepam and fentanyl droperidol has been associated with adverse reactions in four MHS dogs, two of which developed MH-like reactions.[8,11,12] The reason for this association is unclear as these have generally been regarded as nontriggering agents.

II. CANINE STRESS SYNDROME

Sudden and unexplained deaths were reported in a colony of MHS dogs.[8] Two dogs died during a period of stress associated with a change in their housing and a third died from undetermined causes.[12] Based on these deaths, an MH-related canine stress syndrome (CSS) analogous to porcine stress syndrome was postulated.[8]

Two awake dogs have developed severe hyperthermic reactions the day following anesthesia with nontriggering agents. Both were greyhounds, one of which was a littermate of a confirmed MHS dog. It is likely that stress played an important role in triggering MH in these dogs. The CSS was reversed by treatment with i.v. administration of dantrolene[11] and/or by surface cooling with ice.[10]

Three cases of exercise-induced hyperthermia have been reported in dogs.[13,14,18] The stress of moderate exercise consistently caused a reversible MH-like syndrome characterized by apparent muscle cramping, dyspnea, and hyperthermia. The marked degree of hyperlactemia and depression of serum bicarbonate indicated pronounced metabolic acidosis. However, this was compensated for by the development of respiratory alkalosis due to panting (Table 2).

III. EVIDENCE FOR MUSCLE AND BLOOD CELL MEMBRANE DEFECTS

The occurrence of hypersensitivity of fresh muscle biopsy specimens to the contracture-producing effect of caffeine, with or without halothane, can be used in diagnosis of MH-susceptibility in dogs. Though the caffeine/

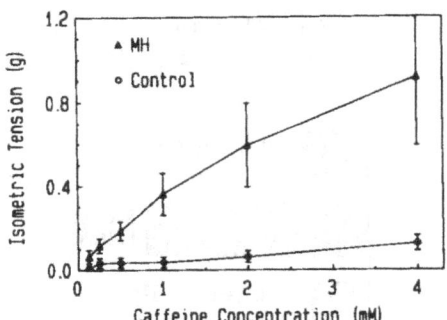

FIGURE 1. Dose-response curve for caffeine-induced increase in isometric tension of muscle biopsy specimens from MH-susceptible and control dogs. Muscle biopsy specimens were acquired from six MH-susceptible and five control dogs and incubated at 37°C in oxygenated physiologic saline. The isometric tensions developing in response to additions of 0.125, 0.25, 0.50, 1.0, 2.0, and 4.0 mM of caffeine were recorded using a force-displacement strain gauge connected to a Grass polygraph. Mean tensions (±SEM) in g are reported.

halothane contracture test has not been used frequently in dogs, it should be considered the best *in vitro* preanesthetic diagnostic test available at this time. The caffeine concentration required to produce a 0.1 or 0.2 g rise in tension (Figure 1) has distinguished MHS from normal dogs better than the caffeine-specific concentration (CSC; caffeine concentration causing 1 g increase in tension). Addition of halothane apparently increases the sensitivity of the caffeine contracture test but also decreases the precision of the assay. In one case where interpretation of the CSC was equivocal in a dog with a family history of MH, the caffeine and halothane contracture test was unequivocally positive (CSC of 1.5).[8]

In the 10 control dogs that we have subjected to the contracture tests, the CSC was 9.41 ± 5.0 (mean ± standard deviation).[8,38] That this value is higher than the CSC reported for people without MH susceptibility[21] may be due to the greater proportion of fast twitch fibers in canine compared to human muscle.[8] In three dogs with unequivocal MH susceptibility, the CSC was 3.0 ± 2.1.

In one case of CSS,[38] the biopsy specimen was resistant to the contracture-producing effects of caffeine (CSC of 21.3 mM caffeine). This was associated with an increased yield of light and heavy sarcoplasmic reticulum (SR) and with increased specific activity of calcium-transport ATPase in heavy SR (Figure 2). Furthermore, calcium was released at an increased rate and in an increased amount. A similar but smaller increase in Ca-ATPase has been seen in the muscle of MHS swine, apparently compensating for a hypersensitive calcium-release mechanism.[22] Perhaps such compensation in this canine case has occurred to an extent that it results in resistance to the calcium-increasing effect of caffeine. Caffeine-resistance and a nonrigid form of MH occurs in the Wausau variant of MH susceptibility found in people.[23]

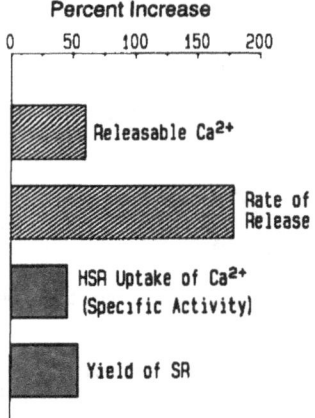

FIGURE 2. Calcium sequestration and release by SR isolated from a dog with susceptibility to MH. The specific activity of Ca-ATPase (U/mg SR protein) was used as a marker of calcium uptake and was measured as described in Figure 5. Calcium release from heavy SR (HSR) was measured at room temperature using a rapid filtration system. Vesicles were passively calcium-loaded by incubation in a medium containing 120 mM KCl, 10 mM histidine, and 10 mM CaCl$_2$ (with 50 μCi ^{45}Ca). They were applied to Millipore filters and release was stimulated by rapidly passing 90 mM caffeine at pH 7.0 in 120 mM KCl and 10 mM histidine through the filter. The ^{45}Ca remaining on the filters was measured. The bar graphs indicate the percent increase in SR activity of the MH-susceptible dog compared to the mean value for five control dogs. The amount of calcium released by SR from the MH-susceptible dog due to caffeine and the rate at which it is released is indicated in the upper bar graphs. The lowest bar indicates the total yield of SR from MH-susceptible muscle.

A mild, unexplained, and persistent increase in serum creatine kinase (CK) activity has been found in 9 out of 10 MHS dogs tested (416 ± 71 compared to reference range of <187; Figure 3). AST was increased in 8 of these 10 MHS dogs (51 ± 13 compared to reference range of <39). These

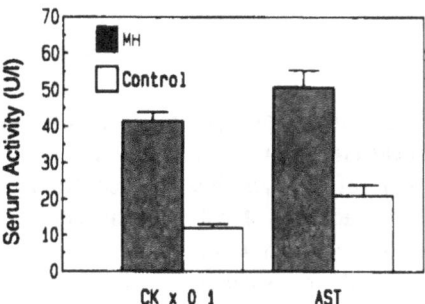

FIGURE 3. Activities of muscle enzymes in serum from MH-susceptible and control dogs. Values are shown for ten MH-susceptible and ten control dogs. Mean activities (±SEM) of creatine kinase and AST are shown.

increases occurred in the absence of other factors that are known to increase serum muscle enzymes, such as trauma, overt myopathy, rapid growth phase, or unaccustomed exercise. This may indicate either the presence of leaky sarcolemmal membranes or a propensity to mild, subclinical muscle injury in these dogs. As in people or swine, chronic elevation of muscle enzymes in serum is not a specific indicator of MH susceptibility; however, in dogs this indicator appears to be more sensitive than for MHS people or swine.[24,25]

Percutaneous muscle biopsy may reveal nonspecific histological changes such as increased internal nuclei counts, fiber caliber variation, and mitochondrial loss.[8] An increased percentage of fibers with internal nuclei (>2%) may be the most reliable histologic indicator of MH susceptibility. In contrast, cardiac muscle histomorphometric parameters have been reported as normal in MHS dogs.[26]

As has been described in MHS swine,[25] an erythrocyte membrane defect is associated with MH susceptibility in dogs. In three MHS dogs, erythrocyte osmotic fragility has been determined and found to be abnormally increased (Figure 4).[13,16] This membrane abnormality was associated with a decreased activation energy and increased thermostability of the membrane Ca-ATPase and an abnormal membrane transition temperature (Figure 5).[13] Furthermore, the membrane Ca-ATPase activity was found to be 100% increased in the MHS dogs, possibly to counter an increased calcium influx from the extracellular fluid due to the membrane defect. Similar findings have been made for MHS swine erythrocytes; namely increased calcium pumping activity[27] and lower activation energy of membrane probe motion[28] at temperatures greater than 23°C. In marked contrast, the Mg-ATPase activity was not different between the control and MHS dogs. These alterations in erythrocyte membranes apparently resulted in their decreased survival, as indicated by mild increases in reticulocyte counts.[16]

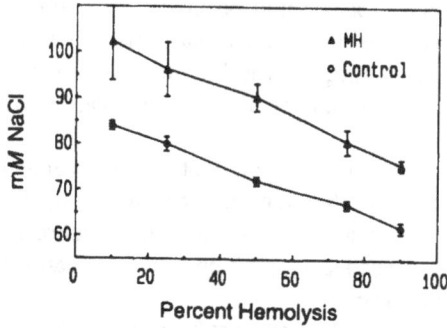

FIGURE 4. Erythrocyte osmotic fragility of MH-susceptible and control dogs. The concentrations of NaCl causing 10, 25, 50, 75, and 90% hemolysis after 30 min incubation in 5 mM Na phosphate at 22°C and pH 7.4 are plotted. Values are reported as mean ± SEM for three MH-susceptible and ten control dogs.

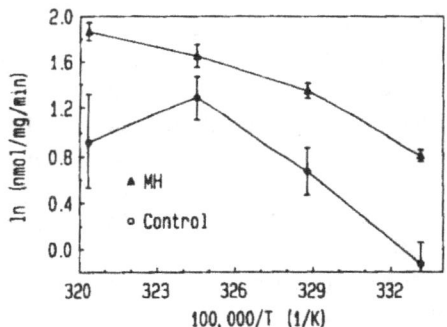

FIGURE 5. Temperature dependence of Ca-ATPase activity of erythrocytes from MH-susceptible and control dogs. The Ca-ATPase activity was defined as the increase in phosphate liberation caused by replacing 1 mM EGTA with 50 μM CaCl$_2$, in the incubation medium of 120 mM KCl, 4 mM mg ATP, and 20 mM imidazole at pH 7.0. The natural logarithm of activity is plotted against the reciprocal Kelvin temperature $\times$ 10^5. Activity was measured at 27, 31, 35, and 39°C for two MH-susceptible and four control dogs. Mean ($\pm$ SEM) values are plotted. The slope of the curves indicates the enthalpy of activation; the inflection point of the curves indicates the transition temperature.

A lymphocyte test has been recently reported for diagnosis of MH susceptibility in people and pigs.[29,30] In this assay lymphocytes are isolated from peripheral blood and exposed to halothane to assess whether they are hypersensitive to the calcium-increasing effects of halothane. Cytoplasmic free calcium concentrations are measured before and after exposure to the anesthetic, using fluorescent calcium dyes. In the three dogs tested thus far, the cells were hypersensitive to the halothane effect (Figure 6).[38]

IV. SUMMARY AND CONCLUSIONS

Dogs may be susceptible to anesthetic-induced MH. Although the actual incidence is unknown, documented occurrence of canine MH is rare. The disease has been reported in twice as many male dogs as females and has been reported in only sporting or working breeds or crossbreeds thereof. The disease is inherited in an autosomal dominant pattern with a spectrum of susceptibility.

The clinical syndrome is similar to that seen in man and swine. The most effective treatment, as in other species, consists of rapid cessation of anesthesia, cooling, and administration of sodium bicarbonate and dantrolene. Specific treatments of secondary problems such as cardiac dysrhythmias or nephrosis may be necessary.

Definitive diagnosis of MH susceptibility depends on documentation of the MH anesthetic reaction or positive caffeine/halothane contracture tests. Use of these tests may be cost or risk prohibitive. Alternatively, MH susceptibility may be tentatively diagnosed on the basis of a family history of MH susceptibility and evidence for subclinical membrane defects in skeletal muscle and blood cells (Table 3).

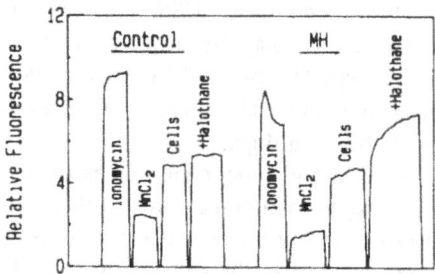

FIGURE 6. Halothane-induced increase in cytoplasmic calcium of lymphocytes isolated from MH-susceptible dogs. Lymphocytes were loaded with the fluorescent calcium indicator Indo-1 by incubation for 30 min at 37°C in 2 μM Indo-1/AM and RPMI medium. Cells were washed in RPMI medium and resuspended in 10 mM HEPES, 10 mM glucose, 140 mM NaCl, 3 mM KCl, and 1 mM MgCl$_2$ and 1 mM CaCl$_2$, pH 7.3. Typical spectrofluorograph tracings showing calcium-dependent fluorescence at 37°C with additions of (1) the calcium ionophore ionomycin to show maximum fluorescence, (2) MnCl$_2$ to displace calcium from the fluorescent dye and show minimum fluorescence, (3) no additions, and (4) halothane. (Figure provided courtesy of Dr. A. Klip, Hospital for Sick Children, University of Toronto.)

TABLE 3
Preanesthetic Diagnosis of Susceptibility to Malignant Hyperthermia in Dogs

Associated Characteristics
Sporting or working breed (greyhound, border collie, spaniel, pointer, retriever, doberman)
Generalized increased muscle bulk, strength, and tone
Mildly increased body temperature
Nervous and hyperactive temperament
Male (16/23 confirmed cases)

Family History of Anesthetic Death or Exercise-Induced Hyperthermia

Evidence for Subclinical Membrane Defect in Skeletal Muscle
Positive caffeine contracture test: caffeine causing a 0.2 g rise in tension at <0.5 mM (1 g tension usually at <6 mM)
Mild unexplained and persistent increase (9/10 cases) in serum creatine kinase (>187 U/l) and AST (>39 U/l)
Increased fibers with internal nuclei (>2% fibers)
Marked hyperthermia (>42°C), hyperlactemia (>10 mM) and dyspnea following moderate exercise
Abnormally increased calcium-release by isolated SR

Evidence for Subclinical Membrane Defect in Blood Cells
Unexplained increase in reticulocyte count (>1.5%)
Increased erythrocyte osmotic fragility (50% hemolysis occurring at >78 mM NaCl)
Increased erythrocyte Ca-ATPase activity with decreased activation energy and increased thermostability
Decreased intracellular calcium concentration of lymphocytes with increased sensitivity to calcium-increasing effects of halothane

MHS dogs are also susceptible to CSS, a disease analogous to porcine stress syndrome. Affected dogs may die unexpectedly or may exhibit exercise intolerance marked by hyperthermia and hyperlactemia following moderate exercise. An exercise tolerance test appears to be an effective method to screen for MH susceptibility in dogs.

Results of biochemical and functional studies of MHS dog muscle and erythrocyte and lymphocyte membranes are similar to those seen in MHS swine (Table 3). Results of studies of MHS canine muscle are compatible, with the primary defect being in the calcium release channel, as has been proposed for MHS swine and humans.[31-37]

REFERENCES

1. **Short, C. E. and Paddleford, R. R.,** Malignant hyperthermia in the dog, *Anaesthesiology*, 39, 462, 1973.
2. **Short, C. E.,** The significance of malignant hyperthermia in animal anaesthesia in *Second Int. Symp. Malignant Hyperthermia*, J. A. Aldrete and B. A. Britt, Eds., Grune & Stratton, New York, 1978, 1975.
3. **Bagshaw, R. J., Cox, R. H., Knight, D. H., and Detweiler, D. K.,** Malignant hyperthermia in a greyhound, *J. Am. Vet. Med. Assoc.*, 172, 61, 1978.
4. **Olfert, E. D., White, R. J., and Cribb, P. H.,** A malignant hyperthermia-like syndrome in the dog in 1978, *Proc. Can. Assoc. Lab. Anim. Sci.*, 360, 1978.
5. **Bagshaw, R. J., Cox, R. H., and Rosenberg, H.,** Dantrolene treatment of malignant hyperthermia, *J. Am. Vet. Med. Assoc.*, 178, 1029, 1981.
6. **Sawyer, D. C.,** Malignant hyperthermia, *J. Am. Vet. Med. Assoc.*, 179, 341, 1981.
7. **McGrath, C. J., Crimi, A. J., and Ruff, J.,** Malignant hyperthermia in dogs, *Vet. Med. Small Anim. Clin.*, 77, 218, 1982.
8. **O'Brien, P. J., Cribb, P. H., White, R. J., Olfert, E. D., and Steiss, J. E.,** Canine malignant hyperthermia: diagnosis of susceptibility in a breeding colony, *Can. Vet. J.*, 24, 172, 1983.
9. **Steidl, V. T., Apelt, H. J., and Kube, B.,** Ein Beitrag zur malignen Hyperthermie Kleintierpraxis, 28, 177, 1983.
10. **Leary S. L., Anderson L. C., Manning, P. J., Bache, R. J., and Zweber, B. A.,** Recurrent malignant hyperthermia in a greyhound, *J. Am. Vet. Med. Assoc.*, 182, 521, 1983.
11. **Kirmayer, A. H., Klide, A. M., and Purvance, J. E.,** Malignant hyperthermia in a dog: case report and review of the syndrome, *J. Am. Vet. Med. Assoc.*, 185, 978, 1984.
12. **Cribb, P. H., Olfert, E. A., and Reynolds, F. B.,** Erythrocyte osmotic fragility testing and the prediction of canine malignant hyperthermia susceptibility, *Can. Vet. J.*, 27, 517, 1986.
13. **Rand, J. S. and O'Brien, P. J.,** Exercise-induced malignant hyperthermia in an English springer spaniel, *J. Am. Vet. Med. Assoc.*, 190, 1013, 1987.
14. **Kalow, B. I. and O'Brien, P. J.,** Canine stress syndrome, *Can. Vet. J.*, 30, 595, 1989.
15. **Cohen, C. A.,** Malignant hyperthermia in a greyhound, *J. Am. Vet. Med. Assoc.*, 172, 1254, 1978.

16. O'Brien, P. J., Forsyth, G. W., Olexson, D. W., Thatte, H. S., and Addis, P. B., Canine malignant hyperthermia susceptibility: erythrocytic defects — osmotic fragility, glucose-6-phosphate dehydrogenase deficiency and abnormal Ca^{2+} homeostasis, *Can. J. Comp. Med.*, 48, 381, 1984.

17. O'Brien, P. J., Preanaesthetic diagnosis of canine malignant hyperthermia susceptibility, *Minn. Vet.*, 25, 43, 1985.

18. O'Brien, P. J. and Rand, J. S., Canine stress syndrome, *J. Am. Vet. Med. Assoc.*, 186, 432, 1985.

19. O'Brien, P. J., Malignant hyperthermia in dogs, *Can. Vet. J.*, 28, 302, 1987.

20. O'Brien, P. J. and Forsyth, G. W., Preparation of injectable dantrolene for emergency treatment of malignant hyperthermia-like syndromes, *Can. Vet. J.*, 24, 8, 1983.

21. Nelson, T. E., Flewellen, E. H., and Gloyna, D. F., Spectrum of susceptibility to malignant hyperthermia — diagnostic dilemma, *Anesth. Analg.*, 62, 545, 1983.

22. O'Brien, P. J., Porcine malignant hyperthermia susceptibility: increased calcium sequestering activity of skeletal muscle sarcoplasmic reticulum, *Can. J. Vet. Res.*, 50, 329, 1985.

23. Kalow, W., Britt, B. A., and Richter, A., The caffeine test of isolated human muscle in relation to malignant hyperthermia, *Can. Anaesth. Soc. J.*, 24, 678, 1977.

24. Britt, B. A., Malignant hyperthermia, *Can. Anaesth. Soc. J.*, 32, 665, 1985.

25. O'Brien, P. J., Rooney, M. T., Reik, T. R., Thatte, H. S., Rempel, W. E., Addis, P. B., and Louis, C. F., Porcine malignant hyperthermia susceptibility: erythrocyte osmotic fragility, *Am. J. Vet. Res.*, 46, 1451, 1985.

26. O'Brien, P. J., Fletcher, T. F., Metz, A. L., Kurtz, H. J., Reed, B. K., Rempel, W. E., Clark, E. G., and Louis, C. F., Malignant hyperthermia susceptibility: cardiac histomorphometry of dogs and young and market-weight swine, *Can. J. Vet. Res.*, 51, 50, 1987.

27. Thatte, H. S., Mickelson, J. R., Addis, P. B., and Louis, C. F., Erythrocyte membrane ATPase and calcium pumping activities in porcine malignant hyperthermia, *Biochem. Med. Metab. Biol.*, 38, 355, 1987.

28. Thatte, H. S., Addis, P. B., Thomas, D. D., Bigelow, D. J., Mickelson, J. R., and Louis, C. F., Temperature-dependent abnormalities of the erythrocyte membrane in porcine malignant hyperthermia, *Biochem. Med. Metab. Biol.* 38, 366, 1990.

29. Klip, A., Elliot, M. E., Frodis, W., Britt, B. A., Pegg, W., and Scott, E., Anaesthetic-induced increase in ionised calcium in blood from malignant hyperthermia patients, *Lancet*, 1, 463, 1987.

30. O'Brien, P. J., Kalow, B. I., Brown, B. D., Lumsden, J. H., and Jacobs, R. M., Porcine malignant hyperthermia susceptibility: halothane-induced increase in cytoplasmic free calcium of peripheral blood lymphocytes, *Am. J. Vet. Res.*, 50, 131, 1989.

31. Ohnishi, S. T., Taylor, S., and Gronert, G. A., Calcium-induced calcium release from sarcoplasmic reticulum of pigs susceptible to malignant hyperthermia: the effects of halothane and dantrolene, *FEBS Lett.*, 161, 103, 1983.

32. Endo, M., Yagi, S., Ishizuka, T., Horiuti, K., Koga, Y., and Amaha, K., Changes in the calcium-induced calcium release mechanism in the sarcoplasmic reticulum of the muscle from a patient with malignant hyperthermia, *Biomed. Res.*, 4, 83, 1983.

33. Nelson, T. E., Abnormality in calcium release from skeletal sarcoplasmic reticulum of pigs susceptible to malignant hyperthermia, *J. Clin. Invest.*, 72, 862, 1983.

34. Kim, D. H., Sreter, F., Ohnishi, S. T., Ryan, J., Robert, J., Allen, P. D., Meszaros, L. G., Antoniu, B., and Ikemoto, N., Kinetic studies of Ca release from sarcoplasmic reticulum of normal and malignant hyperthermia susceptible pig muscles, *Biochim. Biophys. Acta*, 775, 320, 1984.

35. O'Brien, P. J., Porcine malignant hyperthermia susceptibility: hypersensitive calcium-release mechanism of skeletal muscle sarcoplasmic reticulum, *Can. J. Vet. Res.*, 50, 318, 1986.

36. **Ohnishi, S. T., Waring, A. J., Fang, S. G., Horiuchi, K., Flick, J. L., Sadanaga, K. K., and Ohnishi, T.,** Abnormal membrane properties of the sarcoplasmic reticulum of pigs susceptible to malignant hyperthermia: modes of action of halothane, caffeine, dantrolene and two other drugs, *Arch. Biochem. Biophys.,* 247, 294, 1986.

37. **Ohnishi, S. T.,** Effects of halothane, caffeine, dantrolene and tetracaine on the calcium permeability of skeletal sarcoplasmic reticulum of malignant hyperthermic pigs, *Biochim. Biophys. Acta,* 897, 261, 1987.

38. **O'Brien, P. J., Pook, H. A., Klip, A., Britt, B. A., Kalow, B. I., McLaughlin, R. N., Scott, E., and Elliot, M. E.,** Canine stress syndrome/malignant hyperthermia susceptibility: calcium homeostasis defect in muscles and lymphocytes, *Res. Vet. Sci.,* 48, 124, 1990.

Chapter 10

DRUG-INDUCED HYPERMETABOLIC SYNDROMES

Stanley N. Caroff, Stephan C. Mann,
Kenneth Sullivan, and Wayne Macfadden

TABLE OF CONTENTS

I.   Introduction 118

II.   Clinical Comparison of NMS and MH 118
        A.   Epidemiology 118
        B.   Clinical Manifestations 120
        C.   Treatment 121
        D.   Diagnostic Testing 121

III.   Related Drug-Induced Disorders 123

IV.   Pathogenesis of NMS 123
        A.   Dopamine Hypothesis 123
        B.   Central Nervous System 124
        C.   Systemic Factors 125
        D.   Skeletal Muscle 126

V.   Conclusions 129

References 129

0-8493-8093-6/94/$0.00 + $.50

I. INTRODUCTION

The relationship between anesthetic-induced malignant hyperthermia (MH) and other drug- and stress-related conditions that resemble MH has intrigued and puzzled many investigators. While MH-like syndromes have been reported in association with a variety of drugs, the neuroleptic malignant syndrome (NMS) associated with the use of antipsychotic agents has received particular attention. Further investigation of the relationship between MH, NMS, and similar conditions is important from both a clinical and theoretical point of view; for example, MH-susceptible patients are sometimes advised to avoid psychotropic drugs based on the assumption that reports of hyperthermic reactions to these drugs imply MH-triggering properties. Conversely, some investigators have proposed that patients who recover from NMS may be at risk for MH during anesthesia. Examination of these questions may clarify the extent of crossreactivity in susceptibility to these syndromes and enhance the scientifically based management of these patients.

In addition, research investigations in which the common and dissimilar aspects of these conditions are compared may shed light on the physiologic and molecular mechanisms involved in triggering hyperthermic episodes. In this context, pharmacologic studies comparing the effects of the various triggering drugs on membrane-related processes involved in central and peripheral components of the thermoregulatory and neuromuscular systems may be a valuable strategy.

In this chapter, we review the clinical features of NMS, compare these with MH and other drug-induced syndromes, and examine hypotheses concerning common pathophysiologic mechanisms. Because only limited experimental data are available for disorders other than MH, etiologic hypotheses remain speculative. Nevertheless, we propose that these similar hyperthermic drug reactions may be triggered initially by distinct pharmacologic actions, but culminate in a final common pathway of thermoregulatory failure related primarily to skeletal muscle hypermetabolism.

II. CLINICAL COMPARISON OF NMS AND MH

A. EPIDEMIOLOGY

Early observers noted the similarities between NMS and MH and proposed a common pathophysiology.[1-4] With increasing data in recent years, important differences have emerged as well. NMS may be more common than MH, although both are rare. Data from several recent surveys suggest that the incidence of NMS in neuroleptic treated patients is approximately 0.2% (range of .001 to 3.23%), whereas the incidence of MH ranges from 0.0005 to 0.01% (Table 1).[5,6] In both instances, lack of consensus in diagnostic criteria, differences in base populations, drugs administered, and investigator biases have probably limited precision in estimating true incidences. Analysis of the

TABLE 1
Clinical Comparison of NMS and MH

	NMS	MH
Incidence	0.001–3.23%	0.0005–0.01%
Sex	M > F	M > F
Age (mean)	38	15
Familial occurrence	None	Often
Triggering drugs	Neuroleptics	Inhalational anesthetics, depolarizing muscle relaxants
Onset	Hours–days	Minutes–hour
Hyperthermia	Yes	Yes
Rigidity	Yes	Yes
Autonomic changes	Yes	Yes
Mental status	Yes	Yes
Rhabdomyolysis	Yes	Yes
Acidosis	Yes	Yes
Hypoxia/hypercapnia	Yes	Yes
Treatment	Dantrolene, dopamine agonists	Dantrolene
Mortality	10%	10%

literature reveals that both syndromes are reported more frequently in males by a ratio of 2 to 1. NMS is reported more commonly in adults (mean = 38 years), whereas the mean age of reported MH cases is in adolescence,[5,6] although either disorder may occur at any age. These age differences may reflect the patterns of use of these drugs, e.g., children are far more likely to receive anesthetics than neuroleptics. However, when neuroleptics are used to treat children, as in the case of the institutionalized mentally retarded, the incidence of NMS may also be increased.[7] In contrast to reports of variable and multifactorial genetic patterns in some families with MH,[6] including sporadic and apparently acquired cases, there have been no reports of familial susceptibility to NMS.

Pharmacologic differences are clear. NMS has been reported in association with the use of therapeutic doses of all classes of neuroleptics, which share the property of central dopamine receptor antagonism. While it is strongly suspected that the risk of NMS correlates with neuroleptic potency, dose or rate of dosage increase, this has been difficult to prove. MH occurs during anesthesia involving potent and volatile inhalational anesthetics and depolarizing skeletal muscle relaxants. These differences are underscored by the lack of evidence for crossreactivity between the syndromes. Sensitivity to neuroleptics has not been reported in MH-susceptible patients. On the contrary, potent neuroleptics such as droperidol have been recommended for anesthetic use in MH-susceptible patients despite reports of NMS due to droperidol being used as an antipsychotic.[7] Neuroleptic drugs have had no effect on MH-susceptible swine[8] and nonspecifically delayed and attenuated MH episodes in susceptible swine exposed to halothane.[9] Similarly, there are no reports of MH during anesthesia in patients with prior NMS episodes or among members of their families even when MH-triggering anesthetics were used.[10]

An important and characteristic feature of both syndromes is the variable and unpredictable clinical expression of the disorder in susceptible patients treated with triggering drugs. Among 52 reported NMS patients with a history of previous neuroleptic treatment, only 9 (17%) had developed NMS during prior neuroleptic exposures.[5] After recovery from NMS, the risk of recurrence during subsequent neuroleptic treatment may be no more than 30%.[5] Similarly, in some retrospective studies, up to 70% of MH-susceptible patients did not develop hyperthermia during general anesthesia administered on previous occasions.[11]

These data suggest that other poorly defined state-related factors are essential in facilitating the development of hyperthermia. Some investigators have proposed that organic brain disorders, mood disorders, agitation, dehydration, ambient temperature, or concurrent treatment with other psychotropic drugs may predispose to NMS.[12] Based partially on parallels with the porcine stress syndrome, investigators have suspected that state anxiety, hormonal secretion, exercise, or ambient temperature may facilitate the onset of MH.[6,7] In addition, patients with pre-existing neuromuscular pathology may be at increased risk for MH.[13] Understanding of these cofactors is critical in clarifying the pathogenesis of these syndromes and may be important in determining the risk of developing hyperthermia in general.

B. CLINICAL MANIFESTATIONS

Delayed in onset compared to MH, NMS develops within hours to days, with 96% of cases developing within 30 days of the initiation of treatment.[5,7] In contrast, once MH is triggered, a fulminant hypermetabolic response ensues in which body temperature may increase by 10°C every 5 min, with elevated temperatures invariably present within 1 to 2h of induction.[7] Occasionally, MH may arise or recur insidiously in the postoperative period and NMS may present in a more fulminant form. The contrast in onset of MH and NMS may reflect differences in the pharmacokinetics and routes of administration of the triggering drugs, or fundamental differences in lag time between underlying myogenic (MH) and neurogenic (NMS) mechanisms.

Once developed, MH and NMS both present as a hypermetabolic syndrome characterized by pronounced muscle rigidity, rhabdomyolysis, autonomic activation and instability, and hyperthermia. Early changes in mental status typical for NMS cannot be evaluated in the anesthetized MH patient, although both syndromes may lead to coma. Similar laboratory abnormalities resulting from hypermetabolic processes, including elevated serum catecholamines and muscle enzymes, hypoxia, hypercapnia, and metabolic acidosis, have been reported. In addition, patients with either disorder are at risk for developing acute cardiovascular, respiratory, and renal complications. While both conditions remain potentially life threatening, the mortality rate has apparently declined for MH and NMS due probably to heightened awareness and specific treatment.

C. TREATMENT

Based on reports of successful use in MH, dantrolene has been used in the treatment of an increasing number of NMS cases. In a recent review of the literature,[5] dantrolene was reported as definitely effective in 77% of cases of NMS. While these results underscore the role of skeletal muscle in NMS and the common mechanisms involved in MH and NMS, it is well known that the effect of dantrolene in dampening hypermetabolic activity in skeletal muscle is nonspecific and does not necessarily implicate a myogenic etiology of NMS. Regardless of causal mechanisms, dantrolene appears to be effective in reversing hypermetabolism.[7]

Relaxation of muscle rigidity has also been achieved in some NMS cases using muscle relaxants such as curare and pancuronium,[7] suggesting that rigidity in NMS is neurogenic in origin. Further evidence of the differences between MH and NMS is provided by numerous clinical reports of the efficacy of centrally active dopaminergic drugs in reversing the manifestations of NMS.

D. DIAGNOSTIC TESTING

Several investigators have tested the association between MH and NMS directly at the tissue level utilizing the *in vitro* skeletal muscle contracture test to screen for MH susceptibility in NMS patients (Table 2). In these

TABLE 2
Skeletal Muscle Contracture Test for
MH Susceptibility in NMS Patients

Dx criteria	MH (+)		Ref.
	NMS	Controls	
Caff < 4mM	0/1	—	17
Hal, Caff, Sux, KCl	0/1	—	18
Hal 1%, Caff < 2mM	1/1	2/2	14
Hal, Caff	0/1	—	19
Hal, Caff	0/1	—	20
Hal 1–3%	5/7	0/6	13
Hal 2%, Caff < 2mM	0/6	—	22
Caff < 5mM	6/8	0/8	15
—	0/1	—	21
Hal 2%, Caff < 2mM	0/8	0/10	23
Caff	3/3	0/4	16

Note: Caff = caffeine, Hal = halothane, Sux = succinylcholine, and KCl = potassium chloride.
Drugs and doses not specified in all reports.

investigations, muscle specimens obtained by biopsy from patients with documented NMS episodes were challenged *in vitro* with caffeine or halothane. The results have been inconsistent. While Caroff et al.,[13] Denborough et al.,[14] Araki et al.,[15] and Lopez et al.[16] reported results indicating MH susceptibility among NMS patients, contradictory results have been obtained by other investigators.[17-23]

In part, conflicting data between studies have been confounded by procedural and diagnostic differences. For example, investigators have used different test drugs, dosages, and durations of exposure as well as heterogeneous criteria defining MH susceptibility by muscle contracture responses. However, recent efforts to standardize MH screening techniques promise to enhance comparability of data between studies. Results from more recent contracture studies using standardized methods and criteria have been negative for MH susceptibility in NMS patients.[22,23]

Positive contracture test results in NMS patients in some studies also underscore the need to assess the specificity of the screening test for MH susceptibility. Results in NMS patients may represent false positives secondary to muscle damage sustained during a prior NMS episode. In fact, histopathologic examination of muscle obtained from patients after NMS has revealed nonspecific changes that are also found in patients with MH, Parkinson's disease, and other neurologic and neuromuscular disorders. While control data based on normal muscle have supported the specificity of the contracture test in identifying true MH susceptibility,[7,24] data from control groups, including patients with neurogenic and myogenic muscle pathology, are essential in validating this test. To date, positive test results in patients with neuromuscular disorders have been assumed to signify MH susceptibility and actually have correlated with clinical MH episodes in a few instances.[7]

In summary, data from *in vitro* diagnostic investigations of NMS patients are inconsistent and difficult to interpret, although more recent studies using standardized criteria have not demonstrated MH susceptibility in NMS. Clinical evidence, including the effect of dopaminergic drugs and muscle relaxants in reversing signs of NMS, and the safe use of anesthetics in NMS patients and their families, indicates that MH and NMS are triggered by distinct pharmacologic mechanisms and supports the primary role of neurogenic mechanisms in the development of NMS. Nevertheless, the virtually identical clinical signs of MH and NMS, their response to dantrolene and variability in onset and recurrence, suggest that these disorders at least share a final common pathway of skeletal muscle hypermetabolism and thermogenesis. We propose that while these and other clinically similar drug-induced disorders may be triggered by drug actions at different levels of the thermoregulatory and neuromuscular axes, they culminate in abnormal stimulation of calcium-dependent contractile and metabolic processes in skeletal muscle resulting in excessive endogenous heat production. Meyers and Meyers[25] suggested that these conditions comprised a human "thermic stress syndrome" similar to the stress syndrome reported in domestic animals and wildlife.[26] In the absence of any supporting evidence, it is unlikely that these disorders reflect a common pharmacogenetic defect; it may be worthwhile, however, to consider them collectively as a human hypermetabolic syndrome that can be induced in various ways by drugs or other stressors. Comparative studies may reveal more about the confluence of physiologic factors necessary for the development of hyperthermia after the initial triggering event, and thereby, result in innovative preventive and therapeutic strategies.

III. RELATED DRUG-INDUCED DISORDERS

Increased skeletal muscle activity resulting in heat overload and clinical hyperthermia is not unique to neuroleptics and anesthetics.[7] Although some drugs predispose to heatstroke by inhibiting heat loss, those of interest in relation to MH and NMS induce hyperthermia primarily by increasing endogenous heat production. Thermogenesis may be induced by drugs in several ways; for example, intoxication with drugs that uncouple oxidative phosphorylation, such as salicylates and phenolic compounds, can directly increase heat production despite intact heat loss mechanisms and normal muscle contractility. Hyperthermia has also been associated with centrally active psychotropic drugs apart from neuroleptics. Drugs that inhibit central dopamine activity such as metoclopramide and amoxapine and withdrawal of dopaminergic drugs such as levodopa and cocaine have been reported to cause an NMS-like syndrome. Lithium alone does not ordinarily affect thermoregulation, but has been associated with an NMS-like syndrome when used in combination with neuroleptics. Central stimulants and psychedelic drugs may result in cases of hyperthermia probably due to extreme agitation, convulsions, and muscle rigidity. Overdose with tricyclic antidepressants and intoxication with monoamine oxidase inhibitors used alone or in combination with tricyclics, stimulants, or opiates have resulted in hyperthermia, indistinguishable from NMS in some cases. While the pathogenesis of antidepressant-related hyperthermia is unclear and may partially reflect anticholinergic effects, agitation, or convulsions, studies in laboratory animals suggest that hyperthermia may be mediated by drug enhancement of serotonergic activity in the brain.[7,27] Considered together with MH and NMS, these reactions may represent variants of a human drug-induced hypermetabolic syndrome. Despite diverse pharmacologic properties of the triggering drugs, they eventuate in skeletal muscle hypermetabolism and a breakdown in compensatory mechanisms.

IV. PATHOGENESIS OF NMS

A. DOPAMINE HYPOTHESIS
The evidence implicating neuroleptic blockade of dopamine receptors in NMS is compelling. All neuroleptics are dopamine antagonists. Evidence

from clinical reports suggests that the risk of NMS may correlate with the potency of neuroleptics as dopamine-receptor antagonists. In addition, dopamine agonists have proven useful in reversing NMS in many cases. Reports of NMS-like reactions to the use of other drugs that inhibit dopaminergic activity provide further evidence supporting the involvement of dopamine in the pathogenesis of NMS.

While direct experimental confirmation of dopaminergic mechanisms in NMS is lacking, anatomic and physiologic studies of dopamine pathways support this hypothesis. Recent evidence increasingly suggests that dopamine in the medial anterior hypothalamic preoptic area is involved in mediating hypothermia. Mann et al.[28] have suggested that neuroleptic blockade of dopamine receptors in this area could facilitate the development of hyperthermia in NMS. Furthermore, neuroleptic-induced disruption of mid-brain dopaminergic projections and peripheral dopamine receptors could account for other cardinal features of NMS. In fact, lesions affecting dopamine tracts in the hypothalamus, areas adjacent to the third ventricle, the anterior cingulate cortex, and the brainstem have resulted in NMS-like conditions. In relation to this, it is interesting that Draper et al.[29] have proposed that there is a disturbance of the dopaminergic system of the basal ganglia in MH-susceptible pigs based on lower dopamine concentrations found in brains from susceptible as opposed to resistant pigs. While several investigators have examined cerebrospinal fluid metabolites in a few NMS patients to further examine the dopamine hypothesis, the results are inconsistent and without adequate controls on which to base conclusions.[7]

While dopamine blockade provides a logical explanation of NMS symptoms, the reasons for the rare idiosyncratic and unpredictable occurrence of the syndrome remain unclear. State-related factors appear critical in facilitating the development of the syndrome. It may be that concurrent synergistic changes in one or more components of the thermoregulatory and neuromuscular systems are necessary for the development of hyperthermia. This could occur in the central nervous system, systemically, or in skeletal muscle.

B. CENTRAL NERVOUS SYSTEM

In the brain, the baseline state of dopamine systems may be a determining factor in NMS. For example, presynaptic dopamine depletion, inhibition of dopamine synthesis, or downregulation of postsynaptic receptors resulting from excessive dopamine activity in psychotic states may eventuate in NMS when combined with the dopamine-blocking effect of neuroleptics. Alternatively, changes in postsynaptic calcium-dependent and membrane-related second messenger systems may potentiate dopamine antagonism by neuroleptics, facilitating the development of NMS. The cyclic AMP system may be involved because neuroleptics can inhibit cyclic AMP formation through direct effects on dopamine receptors and by blocking the calcium-mediated membrane binding of calmodulin, which activates adenylate cyclase and increases cyclic AMP production. In combination with decreases in intra-neuronal calcium concentrations that may accompany psychosis, agitation, and dehydration, which commonly precede NMS, neuroleptic-induced alterations in cyclic AMP formation could precipitate NMS. Similarly, changes in calcium concentrations and neuroleptic effects on the phosphoinositide system could act to augment dopamine-receptor blockade. This mechanism also provides an explanation for the putative role of lithium in predisposing to NMS, since lithium inhibits inositol-1-phosphatase, a key enzyme involved in the phosphoinositide system.[7,28]

Apart from dopamine, other neurotransmitters may be involved in NMS. Based on the involvement of tricyclic antidepressants in some cases of NMS, results of neuroendocrine challenge tests, and dramatic elevations of peripheral catecholamines, several investigators have suggested that norepinephrine may play a role in NMS.[7] Data on the role of serotonin in heat production pathways[27] and in modulating dopaminergic functions,[30] as well as laboratory and clinical investigations of hyperthermic reactions to serotonergic drugs, e.g., LSD, fenfluramine, and monoamine oxidase inhibitors, suggest that the balance between serotonin and dopamine may be critical in determining NMS risk.[7] Other neurotransmitters, such as GABA, acetylcholine endogenous opioids, and prostaglandins, which may affect dopamine function, have also been implicated.[7,28]

C. SYSTEMIC FACTORS

Apart from biochemical changes in the brain that may augment the widespread consequences of dopamine blockade caused by neuroleptics, the metabolic condition of the body as a whole may be important in the development of NMS. From a physiologic point of view, NMS is an involuntary form of exertional heatstroke, in which endogenous heat production overwhelms heat loss mechanisms. As a result, the changes associated with heat acclimatization and conditioning may be relevant to NMS. Adaptation to work in the heat includes the capacity to increase and sustain an adequate cardiac output, hormonal secretion to maintain salt and water balance, a drastic alteration in the composition and volume of sweat, and changes in fluid volume, renal function, and blood composition.[31] Obviously, any pre-existing disease or condition that interferes with heat adaptation may predispose to heatstroke. Aside from chronic medical illness, risk factors include salt and water depletion, malnutrition, chronic inactivity, fever, obesity, fatigue, and exposure to certain drugs. Several investigators have noted that fever, dehydration, and agitation leading to exhaustion are frequent precursors of NMS and MH.[6,7,12] Other drugs, including anticholinergics and alcohol, are often used together with neuroleptics by psychiatric patients who are also usually sedentary. In one review,[5] NMS cases clustered during winter months suggesting that lack of acclimatization to heat may be a significant factor. Thus, the readiness of the thermoregulatory system to respond to thermal challenge and dissipate a heat load may be critical in whether or not NMS or other hypermetabolic conditions prevail.

D. SKELETAL MUSCLE

In addition to central nervous system and systemic factors, the relationship between NMS and MH has stimulated interest in the role of skeletal muscle dysfunction in the pathogenesis of NMS. Although neuroleptic-induced blockade of central dopaminergic neurotransmission appears to be the principal precipitating factor in NMS, underlying or state-related abnormalities of muscle may contribute to the evolution of an episode. This is also consistent with the view of NMS as a form of drug-induced hypermetabolism in which excessive thermogenesis in skeletal muscle occurs.

In contrast to other areas, more direct experimental data are available with which to test the hypothesis of skeletal muscle dysfunction in NMS; this includes studies of skeletal muscle obtained from NMS patients and studies of neuroleptic effects on contractility and metabolism of muscle. As mentioned above, several groups have investigated the *in vitro* response of muscle from NMS patients to NMS- and MH-triggering drugs.[13-23] Differences between NMS muscle and controls in response to halothane and caffeine have been inconsistent and inconclusive. These studies have been confounded by methodologic differences and questions concerning the validity of this pharmacologic model in patients with muscle damaged during a previous NMS episode. Histopathologic studies of muscle obtained after an NMS episode have revealed a variable pattern of nonspecific abnormalities including neurogenic atrophy, type II atrophy, moth-eaten fibers, and increased IIc fibers. These findings are similar to findings in muscle from MH patients, but cannot be used to distinguish between neurogenic and myogenic processes or between cause and effect of NMS. (T. D. Heiman-Patterson et al., unpublished data).[1,15]

Caroff et al.[13] and Adnet et al.[23] also tested the *in vitro* response of NMS muscle to neuroleptics and found no difference between NMS, MH, and normal muscle, although one patient showed an exaggerated response to fluphenazine.[32] In contrast, Imaeda et al.[33] observed contractures in response to haloperidol (0.05 to 0.3 mM) in NMS muscle but not in controls. In a unique series of experiments designed to examine the porcine stress syndrome as an animal model for NMS, Keck et al.[8] administered haloperidol to MH-susceptible and -resistant swine. They found that the syndrome did not develop after haloperidol was administered but was induced in 2 of 3 susceptible and 1 of 3 resistant swine when lithium was preadministered. Concurrent treatment with lithium is a suspected risk factor for NMS. To date, these preliminary studies of human and swine muscle using pharmacologic challenge with triggering drugs have not resolved the question of primary or acquired MH-like muscle dysfunction in NMS nor the role of neuroleptic-muscle interactions in pathogenesis. However, refinements in diagnostic testing procedures and the data of Keck et al.[8] suggest that further investigations may be warranted.

Complementing work on intact muscle preparations, Lopez et al.[16] measured sarcoplasmic calcium ion concentration in muscle from three NMS patients as compared to nine controls using calcium-selective microelectrodes. In muscle specimens from NMS patients, all of whom showed abnormal contracture responses to caffeine, the resting calcium concentration was 4.6 times higher than in controls, suggesting an imbalance in the mechanisms regulating calcium homeostasis within the muscle cell. The significant elevation in calcium concentration was similar to that found in MH-susceptible patients and swine and was reduced by incubation with dantrolene. As in the contracture studies, however, it is difficult to exclude the possibility that the NMS episode itself resulted in muscle damage and altered calcium regulation.

Lopez et al.[16] also measured the effect of neuroleptics on calcium concentration and found a dose-dependent increase in ionic calcium when chlorpromazine was added to muscle baths containing control fibers. At higher drug concentrations, the increment in calcium was associated with a slow, irreversible contracture. Dantrolene blocked both the increase in calcium and the contracture response to chlorpromazine. In earlier studies of frog muscle, haloperidol as well as chlorpromazine were found to elicit an irreversible muscle contracture accompanied by a significant increase in sarcoplasmic calcium.[34]

These findings in human and frog muscle parallel results from other studies of mammalian and amphibian skeletal muscle. Balzer et al.[35,36] studied the effect of chlorpromazine on calcium exchange across cell membranes in frog and rabbit muscle and found that both the influx and efflux of calcium was inhibited by low concentrations of the drug. At high concentrations, contractures were induced in association with elevated myoplasmic calcium concentrations that appeared to reflect inhibition of the active calcium pump and the rate of calcium uptake in isolated vesicular fragments of SR. Andersson,[37] studying chlorpromazine-induced contractures in frog muscle, found a lowering of the mechanical threshold for contracture but concluded that contracture was produced by release of calcium from intracellular stores. In further pharmacologic studies of the chlorpromazine-induced contracture, Kelkar et al.[38] ruled out involvement of depolarization, cholinergic receptors, inhibition of oxidative phosphorylation, and sodium exchange and demonstrated that the response was calcium dependent. In agreement with Balzer et al.[35,36] they speculated that inhibition of the calcium pump of SR is the mechanism underlying these effects of chlorpromazine on muscle. In experiments on skinned muscle fibers from the guinea pig, Takagi[39] showed that chlorpromazine enhanced activation of the contractile system and influenced the function of the SR. Having observed that inhibition of calcium loading of the SR was antagonized by magnesium, procaine, and calcium-free media, Takagi concluded that chlorpromazine acts to release calcium intracellularly by activation of the calcium-induced calcium release mechanism.

Collins et al.[40] found that neuroleptics inhibit calcium-dependent ATPase activity and ATP-dependent calcium uptake and accelerate efflux of calcium from isolated SR from control and MH-susceptible swine muscle, confirming similar findings obtained earlier in rabbit skeletal muscle by other investigators.[41,42] Collins et al.,[40] however, also suggested that the relatively high concentrations of drugs required to achieve such effects on SR calcium transport functions may reflect nonspecific actions of these hydrophobic drugs on membrane integrity and permeability. While these effects of neuroleptics on calcium transport correlate with *in vitro* pharmacologic responses of skeletal muscle, their relevance to therapeutic drug concentrations *in vivo* is less clear. In contrast to the above studies showing activation of calcium-mediated processes, Somers and McLoughlin[9] showed that neuroleptics may delay and attenuate the response to halothane in MH-susceptible swine and correlated this effect with neuroleptic-induced increases in calcium uptake and sequestration by mitochondria.

With the exception of Somers and McLoughlin,[9] these experimental studies suggest that calcium concentrations may be elevated in skeletal muscle from NMS patients and that neuroleptics may enhance muscle contractility in association with increases in sarcoplasmic calcium, at least *in vitro*. Whether these neuroleptic effects result from inhibition of calcium uptake, stimulation of calcium release by SR, or both, is unclear and warrants further investigation. As in the case of neuronal membranes, further investigations of calcium regulation and second messenger systems in skeletal muscle may help synthesize these findings and clarify the pathogenesis of NMS and other hypermetabolic syndromes. For example, neuroleptics have dose-dependent effects on the phosphoinositide system[43] that may be relevant to calcium-mediated processes involved in excitation-contraction coupling in skeletal muscle.[44,45] Moreover, rather than considering neurogenic and myogenic mechanisms separately, an argument could be made to consider NMS and other hypermetabolic syndromes as representing a disorder of cell regulatory and metabolic functions due to abnormalities in membrane-related calcium messenger systems.

Neuroleptics may have broader effects on skeletal muscle apart from calcium transport and contractility. There are data suggesting that neuroleptics uncouple oxidative phosphorylation,[38,46] block postsynaptic cholinergic receptors[47] or promote desensitization[48] at the neuromuscular junction, and reverse the inhibitory effects of dopamine on muscle contractility.[49] In addition to neuroleptic effects or pre-existing muscle pathology, skeletal muscle dysfunction in NMS may be multifactorial in origin. Thus, consideration of the influence on skeletal muscle of elevated systemic catecholamines,[50] body temperature,[51] and other factors that may stimulate contractile and energetic processes by altering calcium regulation and transport is essential in understanding the role of skeletal muscle in contributing to the development of clinical hypermetabolic states.

V. CONCLUSIONS

NMS and MH present clinically as hypermetabolic syndromes. Although these disorders are diagnosed by nearly identical clinical signs and share common features in course and response to treatment, current evidence suggests that they are initiated by different pharmacologic mechanisms. This is consistent with the fact that there have been no reports of patients with crossreactivity to both disorders.

Nevertheless, there may be heuristic value in considering MH, NMS, and related conditions as examples of a human hypermetabolic syndrome that represents a pathophysiologic final common pathway of contraction and thermogenesis in skeletal muscle. Further investigations of membrane regulation of intracellular calcium concentrations and second messenger systems in excitable tissues may be particularly promising in clarifying convergent mechanisms underlying these disorders and perhaps other syndromes as well.

In NMS, drug-induced changes in central regulatory systems involving dopamine appear to be the principal factors in triggering episodes; however, the rare and idiosyncratic occurrence of NMS suggests that other facilitating factors are necessary. These may include synergistic changes in other central neurotransmitter systems involved in thermoregulation and neuromuscular activity or metabolic conditions in the patient that predispose to thermoregulatory failure. Skeletal muscle dysfunction may also contribute to the development of hypermetabolism. Studies of muscle from NMS patients have demonstrated nonspecific histopathologic findings and variable responses to triggering drugs *in vitro*. Apparently more promising are molecular studies that have demonstrated increased sarcoplasmic calcium ion concentrations in NMS muscle and the potential of neuroleptics to alter the regulation of calcium concentrations in the muscle cell.

REFERENCES

1. **Bourgeois, M., Tignol, J., and Henry, P.**, Syndrome malin et morts subite an cours des traitements par neuroleptiques simple et retard, *Ann. Med. Psychol.*, 2, 729, 1971.
2. **Meltzer, H. Y.**, Rigidity, hyperpyrexia and coma following fluphenazine enanthate, *Psychopharmacologia*, 29, 337, 1973.
3. **Itoh, H., Ohtsuka, N., and Ogita, K.**, Malignant neuroleptic syndrome, *Folia Psychiatr. Neurol. Jpn.*, 31, 565, 1977.
4. **Caroff, S. N.**, The neuroleptic malignant syndrome, *J. Clin. Psychiatry*, 41, 79, 1980.
5. **Caroff, S. N. and Mann, S. C.**, Neuroleptic malignant syndrome, *Psychopharmacol. Bull.*, 24, 25, 1988.

6. **Britt, B. A.**, Hereditary and epidemiological aspects of malignant hyperthermia, in *Malignant Hyperthermia: Current Concepts*, M. A. N. Felipe, S. Gottmann, and H. J. Khambatta, Eds., Normed Verlag, Bad Homburg, 1989, 19.
7. **Lazarus, A., Mann, S. C., and Caroff, S. N.**, *The Neuroleptic Malignant Syndrome and Related Conditions*, American Psychiatric Press, Washington, D.C., 1989.
8. **Keck, P. E., Seeler, D. C., Pope, H. G., and McElroy, S. L.**, Porcine stress syndrome: an animal model for the neuroleptic malignant syndrome?, *Biol. Psychiatry*, 28, 58, 1990.
9. **Somers, C. J. and McLoughlin, J. V.**, Malignant hyperthermia in pigs: calcium ion uptake by mitochondria from skeletal muscle in susceptible animals given neuroleptic drugs and halothane, *J. Comp. Pathol.*, 92, 191, 1982.
10. **Hermesh, H., Aizenberg, D., Lapidot, M., and Munitz, H.**, Risk of malignant hyperthermia among patients with neuroleptic malignant syndrome and their families, *Am. J. Psychiatry*, 145, 1431, 1988.
11. **Britt, B. A. and Kalow, W.**, Malignant hyperthermia: a statistical review, *Can. Anaesth. Soc. J.*, 17, 293, 1970.
12. **Keck, P. E., Pope, H. G., Cohen, B. M., McElroy, S. L., and Nierenberg, A. A.**, Risk factors for neuroleptic malignant syndrome: a case-control study, *Arch. Gen. Psychiatry*, 46, 914, 1989.
13. **Caroff, S. N., Rosenberg, H., Fletcher, J. E., Heiman-Patterson, T. D., and Mann, S. C.**, Malignant hyperthermia susceptibility in neuroleptic malignant syndrome, *Anesthesiology*, 67, 20, 1987.
14. **Denborough, M. A., Collins, S. P., and Hopkinson, K. C.**, Rhabdomyolysis and malignant hyperpyrexia, *Br. Med. J.*, 28, 1878, 1984.
15. **Araki, M., Takagi, A., Higuchi, I., and Sugita, H.**, Neuroleptic malignant syndrome: caffeine contracture of single muscle fibers and muscle pathology, *Neurology*, 38, 297, 1988.
16. **Lopez, J. R., Sanchez, V., and Lopez, M. T.**, Sarcoplasmic ionic calcium concentration in neuroleptic malignant syndrome, *Cell Calcium*, 10, 223, 1989.
17. **Tollefson, G.**, A case of neuroleptic malignant syndrome: *in vitro* muscle comparison with malignant hyperthermia, *J. Clin. Psychopharmacol.*, 1, 266, 1982.
18. **Scarlett, J. D., Zimmerman, R., and Berkovic, S. F.**, Neuroleptic malignant syndrome, *Aust. N.Z. J. Med.*, 13, 70, 1983.
19. **Ellis, F. R. and Heffron, J. J. A.**, Clinical and biochemical aspects of malignant hyperpyrexia, in *Recent Advances in Anaesthesia and Analgesia*, R. S. Atkinson and A. P. Adams, Eds., Churchill Livingstone, Edinburgh, 1985, 173.
20. **Merry, S. N., Werry, J. S., Merry, A. F., and Birchall, N.**, The neuroleptic malignant syndrome in an adolescent, *J. Am. Acad. Child Psychiatry*, 25, 284, 1986.
21. **Truong, D. D., Sczesni, B., Fahn, S., Gross, J., Donovan, K., van Bakel, A., and Wiley, K. M.**, Das neuroleptische maligne syndrom: dopaminabhangige maligne hyperthermie, *Nervenarzt*, 59, 103, 1988.
22. **Krivosic-Horber, R., Adnet, P., Guevart, E., Theunynck, D., and Lestavel, P.**, Neuroleptic malignant hyperthermia: *in vitro* comparison with halothane and caffeine contracture tests, *Br. J. Anaesth.*, 59, 1554, 1987.
23. **Adnet, P. J., Krivosic-Horber, M., Adamantidis, M. M., Handecoeur, G., Adnet-Bonte, C. A., Saulnier, F., and Dupuis, B. A.**, The association between the neuroleptic malignant syndrome and malignant hyperthermia, *Acta Anaesthesiol. Scand.*, 33, 676, 1989.
24. **Allen, G. C., Rosenberg, H., and Fletcher, J. E.**, Safety of general anesthesia in patients previously tested negative for malignant hyperthermia susceptibility, *Anesthesiology*, 72, 619, 1990.
25. **Meyers, E. F. and Meyers, R. W.**, Thermic stress syndrome, *JAMA*, 247, 2098, 1982.
26. **Harthoorn, A. M.**, *The Chemical Capture of Animals*, Balliere Tindall, London, 1976, 103.

27. **Myers, R. D. and Waller, M. B.**, Thermoregulation and serotonin, in *Serotonin in Health and Disease, Volume II: Physiological Regulation and Pharmacological Action*, W. B. Essman, Ed., Spectrum Publications, New York, 1978, 1.
28. **Mann, S. C., Caroff, S. N., and Lazarus, A.**, Pathogenesis of neuroleptic malignant syndrome, *Psychiatr. Ann.*, 21, 175, 1991.
29. **Draper, D. D., Rothschild, M. F., Beitz, D. C., and Christian, L. L.**, Age and genotype-dependent differences in catecholamine concentrations in the porcine caudate nucleus, *Exp. Gerontol.*, 19, 377, 1984.
30. **Roth, R. H., Wolf, M. E., and Deutch, A. Y.**, Neurochemistry of midbrain dopamine systems, in *Psychopharmacology: The Third Generation of Progress*, H. Meltzer, Ed., Raven Press, New York, 1987, 81.
31. **Knochel, J. P.**, Heat stroke and related heat stress disorders, *Disease-a-Month*, 35, 301, 1989.
32. **Caroff, S., Rosenberg, H., and Gerber, J. C.**, Neuroleptic malignant syndrome and malignant hyperthermia, *Lancet*, 1, 244, 1983.
33. **Imaeda, M., Sakai, M., Misugi, N., and Fujiwara, T.**, Syndrome malin due to neuroleptics: clinical and muscle studies of three cases, *Yokohama Med. Bull.*, 32, 57, 1981.
34. **Lopez, J. R. and Parra, L.**, Effects of haloperidol and chlorpromazine on calcium in skeletal muscle fibers, *Biophys. J.*, in press.
35. **Balzer, H., Makinose, M., and Hasselbach, W.**, The inhibition of the sarcoplasmic calcium pump by prenylamine, reserpine, chlorpromazine and imipramine, *Naunyn-Schmeidebergs Arch. Pharmakol. Exp. Pathol.*, 260, 444, 1968.
36. **Balzer, H. and Hellenbrecht, D.**, Influence of chlorpromazine, prenylamine, imipramine and reserpine on calcium exchange muscle function, *Naunyn-Schmeidebergs Arch. Pharmakol. Exp. Pathol.*, 264, 129, 1968.
37. **Andersson, K. E.**, Effects of chlorpromazine, imipramine and quinidine on the mechanical activity of single skeletal muscle fibers of the frog, *Acta Physiol. Scand.*, 85, 532, 1972.
38. **Kelkar, V. V., Doctor, R. B., and Jindal, M. N.**, Chlorpromazine-induced contracture of frog rectus abdominis muscle, *Pharmacology*, 12, 32, 1974.
39. **Takagi, A.**, Chlorpromazine and skeletal muscle: a study of skinned single fibers of the guinea pig, *Exp. Neurol.*, 73, 477, 1981.
40. **Collins, S. P., White, M. D., and Denborough, M. S.**, The effects of calmodulin antagonist drugs on isolated sarcoplasmic reticulum from malignant hyperpyrexia susceptible swine, *Int. J. Biochem.*, 19, 819, 1987.
41. **Campbell, K. P. and MacLennan, D. H.**, A calmodulin-dependent protein kinase system from skeletal muscle sarcoplasmic reticulum, *J. Biol. Chem.*, 257, 1238, 1982.
42. **Ho, M. M., Scales, D. J., and Inesi, G.**, The effects of trifluoperazine on the sarcoplasmic reticulum membrane, *Biochim. Biophys. Acta*, 730, 64, 1983.
43. **Walenga, R. W., Opas, E. E., and Feinstein, M. B.**, Differential effects of calmodulin antagonists on phospholipase A and C in thrombin-stimulated platelets, *J. Biol. Chem.*, 256, 12523, 1981.
44. **Vergara, J., Tsien, R. Y., and Delay, M.**, Inositol 1-4-5 triphosphate: a possible chemical link in excitation contraction coupling in muscle, *Proc. Natl. Acad. Sci. U.S.A.*, 82, 6352, 1985.
45. **Kojima, I., Kojima, K., and Krentler, D.**, The temporal integration of the aldosterone secretary response to angiotensin occurs via two intracellular pathways, *J. Biol. Chem.*, 259, 14448, 1984.
46. **Berger, M., Strecker, H. J., and Waelsch, H.**, Action of chlorpromazine on oxidative phosphorylation of liver and brain mitochondria, *Nature*, 177, 1234, 1956.
47. **Sokoll, M. D., Gergis, S. D., Post, E. L., Cronnelly, R., and Long, J. D.**, Effects of droperidol on neuromuscular transmission and muscle membrane, *Eur. J. Pharmacol.*, 28, 209, 1974.

48. **Carp, J. A., Aronstam, R. S., Witkop, B., and Albuquerque, E. X.**, Electrophysiological and biochemical studies on enhancement of desensitization by phenothiazine neuroleptics, *Proc. Natl. Acad. Sci. U.S.A.*, 80, 310, 1983.

49. **Ferko, A. P.**, The inhibitory action of dopamine on the anterior tibialis muscle preparation antagonized by pimozide and chlorpromazine, *Arch. Int. Pharmacodyn. Ther.*, 221, 66, 1976.

50. **Bowman, W. C. and Nott, M. W.**, Actions of sympathomimetic amines and their antagonists on skeletal muscle, *Pharmacol. Rev.*, 21, 27, 1969.

51. **Fuchs, F.**, Thermal inactivation of the calcium regulatory mechanism of human skeletal muscle actomyosin: a possible contributing factor in the rigidity of malignant hyperthermia, *Anesthesiology*, 42, 584, 1975.

Chapter 11

FREE CALCIUM CONCENTRATION IN SKELETAL MUSCLE OF MALIGNANT HYPERTHERMIA SUSCEPTIBLE SUBJECTS: EFFECTS OF RYANODINE

Jose Rafael Lopez-Padrino

TABLE OF CONTENTS

I.   Introduction 134

II. Methods 134
     A. Ca^{2+}-Selective Microelectrodes 135
     B.   Striation Spacing 136
     C.   Recording Procedure 137
     D.   Solutions 138
     E.   Criteria for Collecting Data 138

III. Results.. 138
     A. $[Ca^{2+}]_i$ in Control and MH-Susceptible Muscle 138
     B. $[Ca^{2+}]_i$ in Damaged Muscle Fibers 139
     C.   Effects of Ryanodine on $[Ca^{2+}]_i$ in
          Control Muscle 140
     D.   Effects of Ryanodine on $[Ca^{2+}]_i$ in
          MH-Susceptible Muscle 140
     E.   Inhibitory Effects of Dantrolene 142

IV. Discussion 142
     A. $[Ca^{2+}]_i$ Measurements by Means of
          Ca^{2+} Microelectrodes 142
     B.   Intracellular Calcium Regulation in
          Skeletal Muscle 145
     C.   Resting $[Ca^{2+}]_i$ Control and MH Muscle Fibers 145
     D.   Effect of Ryanodine on $[Ca^{2+}]_i$ 147

Acknowledgments... 147

References.. 148

I. INTRODUCTION

Malignant hyperthermia (MH) is an uncommon genetically transmitted syndrome induced by volatile anesthetics and/or depolarizing muscle relaxants.[1] The clinical picture of an MH episode is characterized by tachycardia, muscle contracture, respiratory and metabolic acidosis, hyperpyrexia, changes in blood pressure, and elevated plasma levels of creatine phosphokinase (CK).[1]

The mechanism responsible of the pathophysiology of this disease is not fully understood, but it is now well established that the underlying mechanism is related to a malfunction of the intracellular calcium homeostasis.[2-5] An elevated intracellular free calcium concentration has been measured *in vitro* and *in vivo* in MH muscle fibers from patients[4-6] and swine.[7] A marked increase in intracellular calcium concentration has been shown to occur during experimentally induced MH episodes.[8] Muscle relaxants, in which the mechanism of action involves reduction in the intracellular Ca^{2+} concentration, can prevent or reverse the MH episode.[9-11] The presence of abnormal Ca^{2+} release channels has been demonstrated in isolated sarcoplasmic reticulum (SR) vesicles obtained from MH muscle.[12] More recently, a defect in the intracellular calcium regulation in leukocytes isolated from MH patients or swine has also been reported.[13]

Ryanodine is a plant alkaloid known to interfere with the excitation-contraction coupling in muscle, which usually is bound with high affinity to a receptor localized in the functional SR membrane.[14,15] Because ryanodine has been found to be a selective ligand to modulate the calcium release channel in the SR,[14] this study has examined the action of ryanodine on intracellular free calcium concentration ($[Ca^{2+}]_i$) in control and MH muscle fibers. In addition, we have re-examined the $[Ca^{2+}]_i$ in intact muscle fibers isolated from control and MH-susceptible patients.

II. METHODS

Intact external intercostal muscle biopsies were obtained under local anesthesia (tetracaine) from four patients (ages 4 to 25) who survived an MH episode and from six susceptible patients (ages 6 to 32) whose susceptibility was determined by a positive caffeine contracture test. In addition, similar muscle samples were obtained from 10 subjects (ages 15 to 45) without any antecedents of neuromuscular diseases, who served as controls. The infiltration with tetracaine was done on the superficial tissue, avoiding as much as possible contamination of the muscle fibers with this local anesthetic. The muscle biopsies were dissected free of adipose and connective tissues in a dissecting dish, bubbled with a gas mixture of 95% O_2 and 5% CO_2, with the aid of a stereo microscope, then divided into several small bundles of four to six intact muscle fibers for electrophysiological measurements. In all cases the muscle biopsies were performed after informed consent and approved by the institution's human studies committee.

A. Ca^{2+}-SELECTIVE MICROELECTRODES

Microelectrodes with an outside tip diameter of about 0.4 μm[16] were pulled from glass capillaries with filament (WPI TWI150F-4) previously washed with HCl and again with distilled water. Subsequently, the inner wall near the tip was siliconized by exposure to dimethyldichlorosilane vapors after drying for 2 h at 200°C to drive off water absorbed by the glass microelectrodes. The glass microelectrodes were then cooled and the tips backfilled with the liquid Ca^{2+} sensor ETH 1001[16] 24 h later. The remaining part of the Ca^{2+} microelectrode was similarly backfilled with pCa 7 solution.

The Ca^{2+}-selective microelectrodes were individually calibrated 24 h after they were made using a set of solutions of varying pCa (3 to 8) of a composition similar to those reported by Tsien and Rink[17] and Alvarez-Leefmans et al.,[18] with the addition of NaCl 8 mM. After 24 h the filled microelectrodes gave a supra-Nernstian response (more than 30.5 mV per decade change in [Ca^{2+}]$_i$ at 37°C). However, after storing these microelectrodes for 36 to 48 h in nitrogen or argon, the calibration curve in a few of them became Nernstian (30.5 mV per decade in [Ca^{2+}]). Only those microelectrodes that showed a Nernstian slope, between pCa 3 and 7, were used experimentally. Figure 1 shows a schematic drawing of calcium-selective microelectrode and the scanning electron micrograph of the terminal portion of a Ca^{2+} microelectrode. Figure 2 shows a typical calibration curve obtained with one of these microelectrodes, in which one can observe the Nernstian response between pCa 3 and 7. The slope became smaller when the pCa was decreased below 7 decade (10 to 12 mV). Due to the fact that the Ca^{2+} microelectrode properties remained fairly constant, recalibration was not necessary after each impalement, but was carried out after each five measurements. The values for the [Ca^{2+}]$_i$ were estimated from the calibration curve performed before and after the measurements.

The interferences of Mg^{2+}, Na$^+$, and H$^+$ were explored in some of the microelectrodes. In solutions of very low calcium concentration (pCa 8), a change of [Mg^{2+}] from 0 to 6 mM or [Na$^+$] from 0 to 20 mM produced a 0 to 1 mV or 4 mV increase in the microelectrode potential, respectively. Changes in pH between 7.8 and 6.4 gave 1 to 3 mV deflection in the Ca microelectrode potential. These ions showed no interference in the Ca^{2+} microelectrode output when similar experiments were carried out at pCa 7. The interference of these ions was considered to be negligible in the measurements of [Ca^{2+}]$_i$ done in the present study, because the majority of determinations were at pCa 7 or higher.

Although the Ca^{2+}-selective microelectrodes measure ion activities, we present the results as Ca^{2+} concentration, on the assumption that the extracellular medium has the same ionic strength as the intracellular one. Because care was taken to calibrate the Ca^{2+}-selective microelectrodes in solutions that had constant ionic strength, which is similar to that of the intracellular medium, the Debye-Huckel activity coefficient of Ca^{2+} should remain constant.

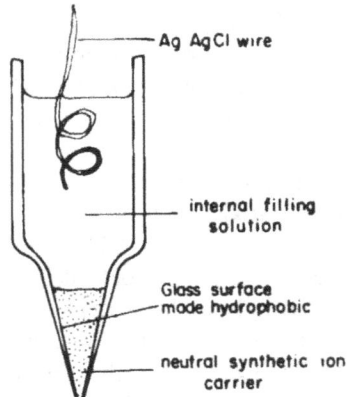

Ag AgCl wire

internal filling
solution

Glass surface
made hydrophobic

neutral synthetic ion
carrier

Microelectrode Terminal Segment

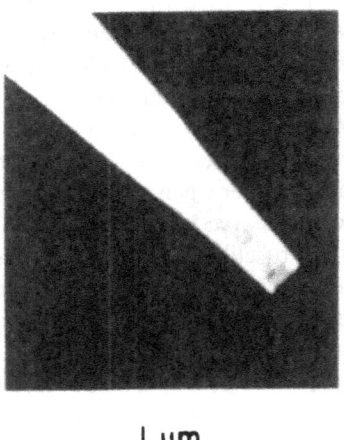

I μm

x 9.000
Measured
Via Philips 500 SEM.al 20 KV

FIGURE 1. Top: diagram of ion selective microelectrode; bottom: scanning electron micrograph of terminal segment of a selective microelectrode.

B. STRIATION SPACING

The striation spacing was determined by laser diffraction technique as described by Cleworth and Edman.[19] The diffraction patterns were taken in at least four different places along the muscle fibers.

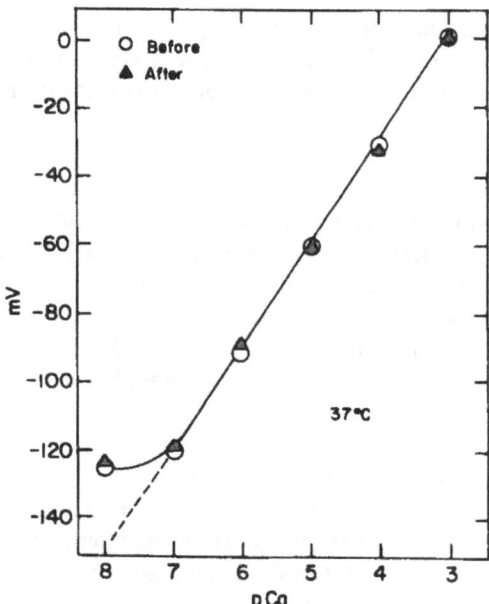

FIGURE 2. Calibration curves of a submicron tip Ca^{2+}-selective microelectrode before and after the $[Ca^{2+}]_i$ measurements were carried out. The ordinate shows the potential measured by the Ca^{2+} microelectrode and the abscissa shows the concentration of Ca^{2+} (pCa = negative log $[Ca^{2+}]$).

C. RECORDING PROCEDURE

Control and MHS muscle fibers were placed in a temperature-controlled bath (37°C) filled with Krebs solution constantly equilibrated with 95% CO_2 and then fixed between two stainless steel hooks mounted on two manipulators, which allowed us to adjust the striation spacing to 2.25 μm determined by the laser pattern. An equilibration period of at least 60 min was allowed prior to the measurements being performed. In addition, this period allowed the washing of any possible tetracaine contamination during the muscle biopsy performance.

Single muscle fibers were impaled first with a conventional 3M KCl microelectrode, and then the same fiber was impaled with the calcium microelectrode. The measurements of these two parameters were carried out in the same muscle fiber, which was verified by visual observation and by passing a hyperpolarizing pulse through the membrane potential microelectrode. The distance between both microelectrodes was about 200 to 300 μm. Muscle damage was assessed by impaling the fiber first with the 3M KCl microelectrode, which allowed us to observe whether subsequent impalement with a Ca^{2+}-selective microelectrode caused any change in membrane potential. The potential values of both the 3M KCl (Vm), and the calcium-selective microelectrode (VCaE) were recorded via a high impedance amplifier WPI

FD 223 and substracted electronically to give differential signal VCaE-Vm, which represented the $[Ca^{2+}]_i$ (VCa). Signals were displayed on digital voltmeters (Simpson M-465) and recorded on a two-channel recorder (Linear-M205).

D. SOLUTIONS

The composition of the Krebs solution was (in millimoles): NaCl, 118; KCl, 4; $CaCl_2$, 2.5; KH_2PO_4, 1.2; $MgSO_4$, 2.4.; $NaHCO_3$, 25; glucose, 10; pH 7.2. Ryanodine was added to the Krebs solution at the desired concentrations. Dantrolene was prepared just in one concentration ($5 \times 10^{-6} M$) because of its low solubility. The high calcium Krebs solution had a composition identical to the standard Krebs solution, but 12.5 mM of $CaCl_2$ was added instead of 2.5 mM.

E. CRITERIA FOR COLLECTING DATA

Data that fulfilled the following criteria were accepted: (1) the microelectrode calibration curve performed before and after measurements differed by no more than 4 mV between pCa 6 and 7 and (2) membrane potential of the muscle fibers was not less than -80 mV. Results are presented as the mean $\pm$ SEM. Student t test for paired and unpaired data was used between groups. Significance was assumed at the $p < 0.05$ level.

III. RESULTS

A. $[Ca^{2+}]_i$ IN CONTROL AND MH-SUSCEPTIBLE MUSCLE

Figure 3 shows a typical experiment in which Vm and $[Ca^{2+}]_i$ were recorded from a control (A) and MH-susceptible muscle (B). While there was no significant difference in the resting membrane potential, the resting $[Ca^{2+}]_i$ was 3.2 times greater in MH-susceptible muscles than in controls.

The mean resting $[Ca^{2+}]_i$ in the normal muscle fibers was 0.11 ± 0.01 μM (n = 20); (range 0.08 to 0.13 μM), while it was 0.35 ± 0.02 μM (n = 24); (range 0.26 to 0.42 μM) in the MH-susceptible fibers. No significant difference in the resting membrane potential between these two groups of muscle was detected (-84.4 ± 0.45 mV and -83.9 ± 0.44 mV, respectively).

In a second set of experiments, the possible leakage around the Ca^{2+} microelectrode by changing the $[Ca^{2+}]_o$ during the performance of $[Ca^{2+}]_i$ measurements in control and MH muscle fibers was explored. In 20 measurements in control muscle biopsy and 10 measurements from an MH biopsy the $[Ca^{2+}]_i$ was measured before and after the $[Ca^{2+}]_o$ was changed from 2.5 to 12.5 mM (high calcium Krebs solution). No difference was detected in$[Ca^{2+}]_i$ before and after in each group, which indicated that membrane sealing around the 3M KCl and Ca^{2+} microelectrode was adequate and no damage in the membrane was present. Therefore, the measurements of $[Ca^{2+}]_i$ were not

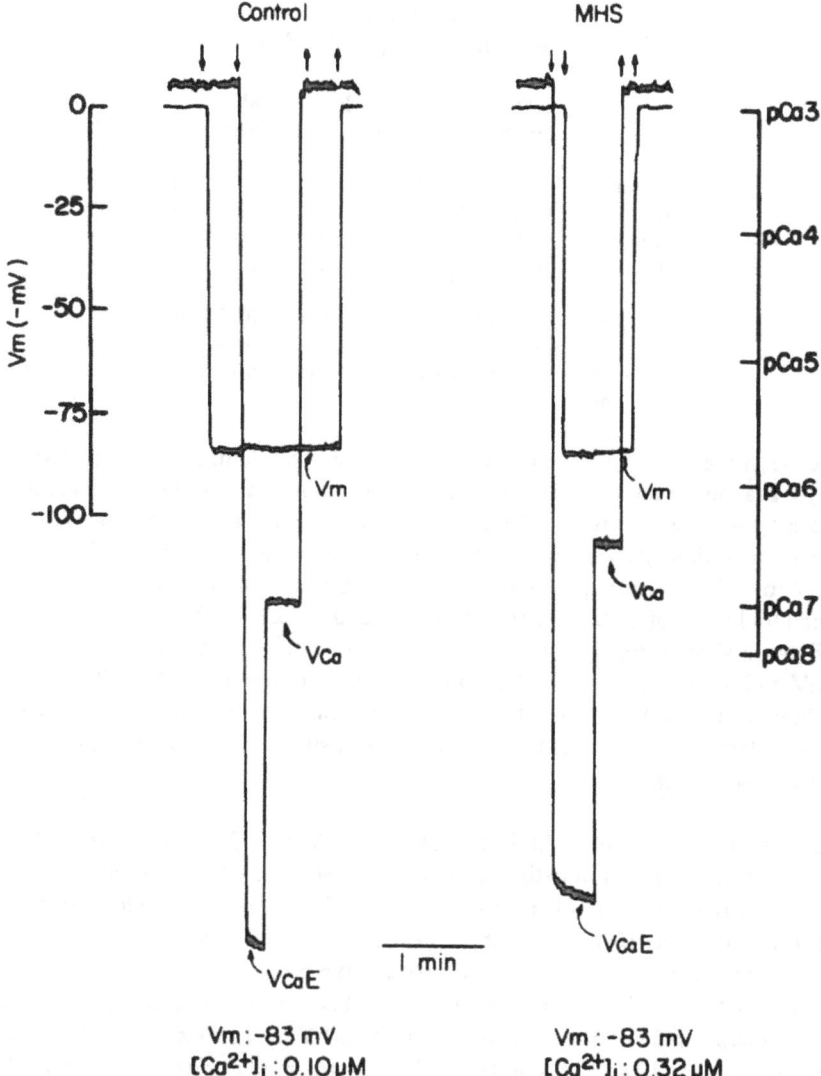

Control   MHS

FIGURE 3. Determinations of resting membrane potential (Vm) and intracellular calcium concentration ([Ca²⁺]ᵢ) in control and MH-susceptible muscle fibers.

contaminated by calcium leakage into muscle fibers due to a poor sealing around the microelectrodes. Table 1 shows the summary of $[Ca^{2+}]_i$ measurements in control and MH muscle under different experimental conditions.

B. $[Ca^{2+}]_i$ IN DAMAGED MUSCLE FIBERS

In 26 control and 20 MH determinations of $[Ca^{2+}]_i$, muscle damage was induced by making a gross impalement with a third microelectrode placed in

TABLE 1
Effects of $[Ca^{2+}]_o$ on $[Ca^{2+}]_i$

	Vm ($-$Vm)	$[Ca^{2+}]_i$ (μM)	$[Ca^{2+}]_o$ (mM)	n
Control	-82 ± 0.38	0.12 ± 0.01	2.5	20
MH	-84 ± 0.69	0.32 ± 0.02	2.5	13
Control	-83 ± 0.45	0.10 ± 0.01	12.5	20
MH	-82 ± 0.70	0.36 ± 0.02	12.5	18

Note: The values represent the mean $\pm$ SEM. $[Ca^{2+}]_i$ and $[Ca^{2+}]_o$ are the intra- and extracellular calcium concentrations, respectively; n = number of measurements.

between the Vm and the Ca^{2+} microelectrode. The damage was established by visual observation. The resting membrane potential was used as an indicator to establish the condition of the muscle membrane. In the control muscle, membrane damage was associated with a depolarization (from -85 ± 0.4 mV to -53 ± 6 mV), which was followed by an increment in $[Ca^{2+}]_i$ from an initial value of 0.10 ± 0.01 μM to 2.06 ± 0.92 μM. In the MH-susceptible fibers, a similar depolarization was observed from -83 ± 0.6 to -48 ± 9 mV and an increase in $[Ca^{2+}]_i$ from 0.32 ± 0.02 μM to 4.86 ± 0.73 μM. These results indicate that damage of the plasma membrane as a result of microelectrode impalement is associated with sustained depolarization and a large rise in $[Ca^{2+}]_i$.

C. EFFECTS OF RYANODINE ON $[Ca^{2+}]_i$ IN CONTROL MUSCLE

The addition of ryanodine (0.01 or 0.1 μM) to the bath solution did not induce any change in either Vm or $[Ca^{2+}]_i$. However, at ryanodine concentrations of 1 and 10 μM, we observed an increment in the $[Ca^{2+}]_i$ that was dose dependent. Figure 4 shows representative records of the ryanodine (10 μM) effects on $[Ca^{2+}]_i$. In this particular fiber, the increase in $[Ca^{2+}]_i$ was by a factor of 52.7 times, with no effects on Vm. The mean $[Ca^{2+}]_i$ after ryanodine 1 or 10 μM was added to the external medium were 0.39 ± 0.03 μM (n = 19; range 0.28 to 0.61 μM) and 4.31 ± 0.47 μM (n = 20); (range 2.09 to 6.83 μM), with no effect on Vm. The increment in $[Ca^{2+}]_i$ observed in the presence of ryanodine 10 μM was always associated with a slow and irreversible muscle contracture. Table 2 shows a summary of the effects of ryanodine at different concentrations of $[Ca^{2+}]_i$ in control muscle fibers.

D. EFFECTS OF RYANODINE ON $[Ca^{2+}]_i$ IN MH-SUSCEPTIBLE MUSCLE

Ryanodine at all of the concentrations tested (0.01, 0.1, 1, and 10 μM) produced increments in $[Ca^{2+}]_i$ in the MH-susceptible fibers that are dose dependent. Figure 5 shows a typical experiment in which Vm and $[Ca^{2+}]_i$

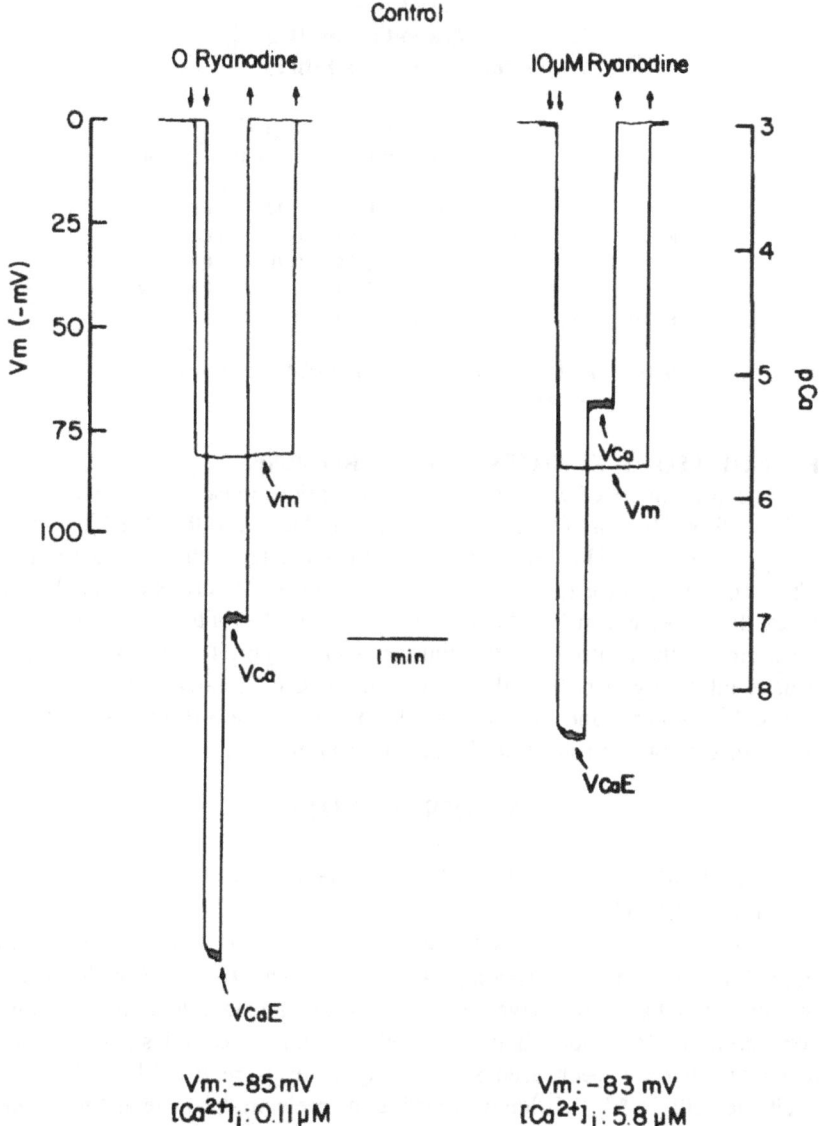

FIGURE 4. The effects of ryanodine on Vm and $[Ca^{2+}]_i$ in a control muscle fiber. On the left-hand side Vm and $[Ca^{2+}]_i$ were recorded in normal Krebs solution; on the right-hand side, in the presence of ryanodine (10 μM).

were recorded before and after ryanodine 10 μM was added to the external medium. At ryanodine higher than 0.1 μM, the increase in $[Ca^{2+}]_i$ was accompanied by a slow, but irreversible contracture. Table 3 shows the summary of the effect of ryanodine on $[Ca^{2+}]_i$ in MH muscle fibers.

TABLE 2
Effects of Ryanodine on $[Ca^{2+}]_i$
in Control Muscle Fibers

	Vm ($-Vm$)	$[Ca^{2+}]_i$ (μM)	n
Control	-84.4 ± 0.45	0.11 ± 0.01	20
R ($0.01 \times 10^{-6}\,M$)	-85.5 ± 0.64	0.12 ± 0.01	7
R ($0.1 \times 10^{-6}\,M$)	-84.5 ± 0.94	0.10 ± 0.01	8
R ($1 \times 10^{-6}\,M$)	-85.0 ± 0.54	0.39 ± 0.03	19
R ($10 \times 10^{-6}\,M$)	-84.3 ± 0.80	4.31 ± 0.47	20

Note: The values represent the mean $\pm$ SEM; R = ryanodine; n = number of measurements.

E. INHIBITORY EFFECTS OF DANTROLENE

The incubation of control and MH-susceptible muscle fibers with dantrolene ($5 \times 10^{-6}\,M$) induced a significant reduction in the $[Ca^{2+}]_i$ in both groups of muscles. This reduction was slightly greater in the MH-susceptible fibers than in control (40% vs. 53%). In addition, dantrolene was able to block the increment in $[Ca^{2+}]_i$ as well as the muscle contracture induced by ryanodine in the control and MH muscle fibers. Figure 6 illustrates the dantrolene inhibitory effects on the increment on $[Ca^{2+}]_i$ induced by ryanodine ($10\ \mu M$) in control and MH-susceptible muscle. Table 4 shows a summary of the effects of dantrolene on the action of ryanodine.

IV. DISCUSSION

A. $[Ca^{2+}]_i$ MEASUREMENTS BY MEANS OF Ca^{2+} MICROELECTRODES

There now seems to be a fairly general agreement that Ca^{2+} plays an important role in muscle physiology as well as in other tissues. A wide variety of techniques have been developed for measuring intracellular free calcium concentration.[20-22] Among them, Ca^{2+}-selective microelectrodes represent one technique that has been used successfully to measure $[Ca^{2+}]_i$ in different excitable cells.[16-18,23,24] Calcium-selective microelectrodes have as their main advantage the fact that they can measure $[Ca^{2+}]_i$ accurately at the concentration usually found in muscle cells at rest.[16,17,25] However, they face a number of fundamental difficulties, such as the seal around the microelectrodes (3M KCl or Ca^{2+}) at the site of impalement. Because of great inward electrochemical gradients on calcium, even a slight leak can raise the $[Ca^{2+}]_i$ near the microelectrode tip, generating a source of error in the $[Ca^{2+}]_i$ measurement. We changed the $[Ca^{2+}]_o$ by a factor of 3 or 4 times and watched the effect in $[Ca^{2+}]_i$ as one experimental criterion for detecting leaks around the microelectrodes tips. In fibers in which a leak did not exist around one of the microelectrode tips, changes in $[Ca^{2+}]_o$ was not followed by a sustained

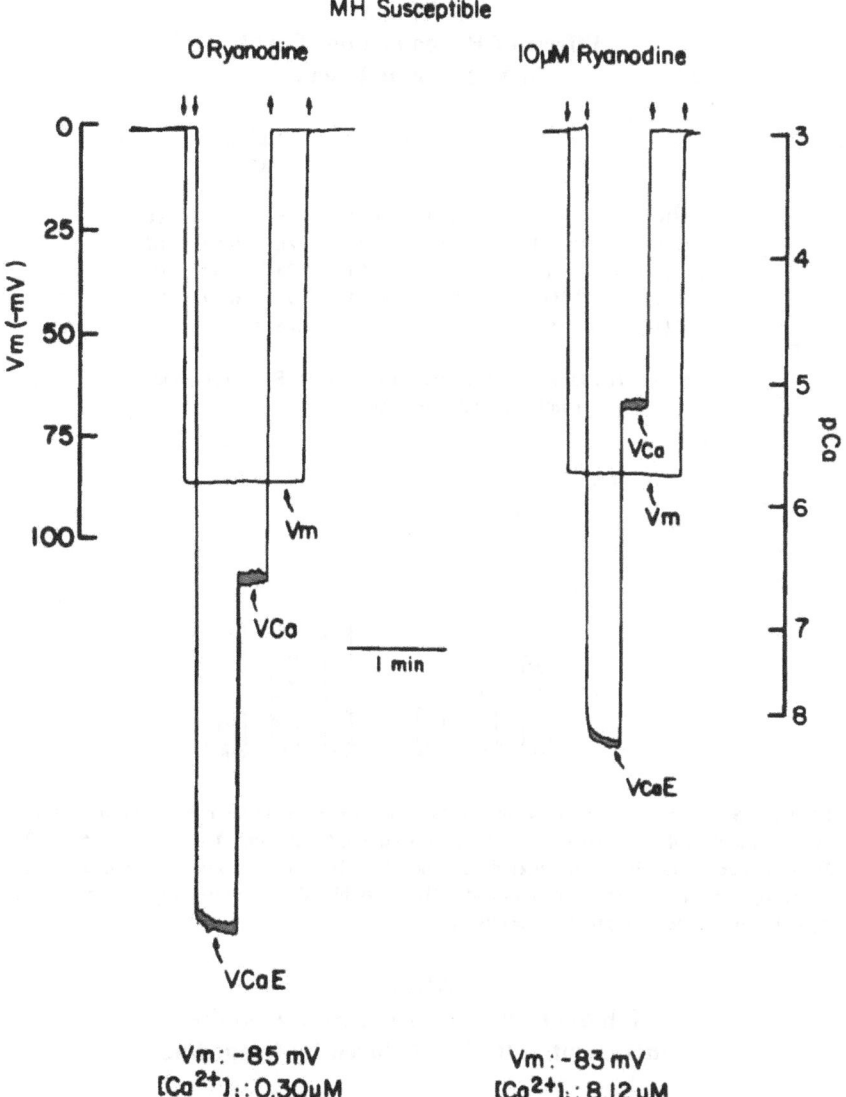

FIGURE 5. The effects of ryanodine on Vm and $[Ca^{2+}]_i$ in an MH muscle fiber. Vm and $[Ca^{2+}]_i$ were measured before (left) and after (right) ryanodine 10 μM was added to Krebs solution.

raise in $[Ca^{2+}]_i$. A second limitation is the microelectrode response time to changes in $[Ca^{2+}]_i$. Because of problems with diffusion and ion-binding kinetics at submicromolar calcium concentrations, the microelectrode response was on the order of 100 ms, which was too slow to follow transiently, but sufficient to measure resting calcium in a steady-state condition. A theoretical

TABLE 3
Effects of Ryanodine on $[Ca^{2+}]_i$ in MH Muscle Fibers

	Vm ($-Vm$)	$[Ca^{2+}]_i$ (μM)	n
MH	-83.9 ± 0.44	0.35 ± 0.01	24
R ($0.01 \times 10^{-6}\,M$)	-84.5 ± 0.72	0.80 ± 0.03	16
R ($0.1 \times 10^{-6}\,M$)	-83.5 ± 0.54	4.34 ± 0.43	16
R ($1 \times 10^{-6}\,M$)	-84.3 ± 0.74	3.99 ± 0.37	12
R ($10 \times 10^{-6}\,M$)	-85.5 ± 0.80	5.28 ± 0.32	12

Note: The values represent the mean $\pm$ SEM; R = ryanodine; n = number of measurements.

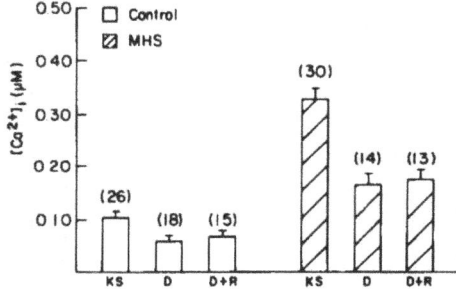

FIGURE 6. Effects of dantrolene on $[Ca^{2+}]_i$. The bars represent the mean $\pm$ SEM of $[Ca^{2+}]_i$ measured in the following conditions: (1) Krebs solution; (2) 10 min after dantrolene (5×10^{-6} M) was added; and (3) 10 min after dantrolene (5×10^{-6} M) and ryanodine (10 μM) were added together. The values for control and MH-susceptible fibers are represented in the left and right portion of the each graph, respectively.

TABLE 4
Inhibitory Effects of Dantrolene on the Increment in $[Ca^{2+}]_i$ Induced by Ryanodine

	Vm ($-Vm$)	$[Ca^{2+}]_i$ (μM)	n
Control	-85.0 ± 0.06	0.10 ± 0.01	26
Control + D	-83.2 ± 0.48	0.06 ± 0.01	18
Control D + R	-84.6 ± 0.65	0.09 ± 0.01	15
M. H.	-84.5 ± 0.88	0.32 ± 0.02	30
M.H. + D	-85.2 ± 0.97	0.15 ± 0.02	14
M.H. + D + R	-84.2 ± 0.42	0.14 ± 0.02	13

Note: The values represent the mean $\pm$ SEM; D = dantrolene (5×10^{-6}); R = ryanodine ($10 \times 10^{-6}\,M$); n = number on measurements.

problem is that the microelectrode reads a single point sample of the $[Ca^{2+}]_i$ at its tip, which may not represent the entire cell. However, there is no experimental evidence to suggest an intracellular Ca^{2+} gradient in resting skeletal muscle.

B. INTRACELLULAR CALCIUM REGULATION IN SKELETAL MUSCLE

In muscle, as well as in other excitable cells, the long-term maintenance of the Ca gradient between the intra- and extracellular medium is the result of the action of the plasma membrane transport systems.[26] Two Ca^{2+} transporting systems of the plasma membrane have been identified: Na^+/Ca^{2+} exchange[27] and the Ca^{2+}-dependent ATP pump.[28] The Na/Ca exchange is a large capacity, low affinity system.[27] Most of its characteristics have been obtained from work conducted in cardiac tissue[28,29] and the giant axon of the squid.[26] For example, it has been established that the system operates electrogenically, exchanging three Na^+ for one Ca^{2+},[26] and that the Km (Michaelis constant) for calcium is about 10 to 20 μM, although its Km can be decreased to 1 μM when the exchanger is activated by a kinase-linked phosphorylation.[26] The second mechanism at the plasma membrane level is the Ca^{2+} ATPase pump, which has a high affinity (Km about 0.5 μM), but has a low total calcium transport capacity.[30] In this regard, it has been reported that in sarcolemmal vesicles obtained from MH-susceptible swine, the total accumulating capacity of this mechanism is significantly more reduced than the control.[31] Experiments conducted in a similar preparation obtained from an MH-susceptible patient showed a similar deficiency in the total capacity than those observed in MH swine (unpublished observation).

Although the calcium transported by the plasma membrane is essential for the long-term maintenance of the calcium gradient, the largest portion of the calcium used for muscle contraction is derived from intracellular stores, the SR. Thus the SR represents the structure responsible for the fine regulation of Ca^{2+} in the myoplasm from moment to moment.[32] The SR membrane possesses an ATPase, with a Km below 0.5 μM. The possibility of alteration in the function of the SR in MH-susceptible subjects and swine is still controversial.[3,33-35] There appears to be agreement that the calcium release is faster and that the sensitivity to Ca^{2+}-induced release of calcium is higher in MH-SR membranes than controls.[36] However, conflicting reports have been published as to whether the calcium uptake by the SR is or is not reduced in MH muscle vesicles.[33-35]

C. RESTING $[Ca^{2+}]_i$ CONTROL AND MH MUSCLE FIBERS

The results presented in this paper show that the values for $[Ca^{2+}]_i$ in MH-susceptible skeletal muscle fibers are substantially higher than in controls (a factor of 3.6). This observation is in agreement with our previous reports[4-6,35] using a similar technique. We have suggested that this apparent imbalance in the resting intracellular calcium homeostasis might be a direct consequence of altering the intracellular mechanisms controlling the myoplasmic $[Ca^{2+}]_i$, either in the plasma membrane and/or the SR[4] and some considerations have been raised relating to this finding.[37,38] According to Gronert et al.[37] and Iaizzo et al.[38] the high resting calcium observed in the MH-susceptible muscle fibers from human and swine might be related to the invasive nature of the method. In a recent report by Iaizzo et al.[38] using Fura 2, no difference in resting $[Ca^{2+}]_i$ was detected between control and MH-susceptible swine muscle fibers and the values for $[Ca^{2+}]_i$ during muscle contracture induced by halothane were considerably lower than previously reported.[8] Iaizzo et al.[38] suggested that this discrepancy might be related to differences in experimental conditions, to damage of the cell membrane produced by the calcium microelectrode, and/or to the fact that Fura 2 is less sensitive than Ca^{2+} microelectrodes to measure $[Ca^{2+}]_i$. We believe that the most probable reason for the difference reported[38] is related to some limitation of Fura 2 as a calcium indicator. Fura 2 has a high affinity for Ca^{2+} and therefore the dye increases the Ca^{2+} buffering properties of the myoplasm, reducing the $[Ca^{2+}]$ at rest and during muscle activation given an artifactually reduced apparent $[Ca^{2+}]_i$.[39] The presence of a large fraction of Fura 2 (60 to 65%) bound to intracellular constituents, such as soluble myoplasmic proteins,[40] raises considerable uncertainty about the calibration of the dye signals in terms of absolute levels of $[Ca^{2+}]_i$.[39,41,42] The measurement of $[Ca^{2+}]_i$ reported in this paper as well as in the previous reports[4-6,35] has been conducted using Ca^{2+}-selective microelectrodes, which have allowed us to continuously direct measurements of $[Ca^{2+}]_i$ in muscle fibers during resting steady-state conditions. The linear response of the Ca^{2+} microelectrodes in the measured range of pCa 3 to 7 demonstrates no limitation of calcium measurements based on the microelectrode response. The plasma membrane damage responsible for the increase in resting $[Ca^{2+}]_i$ seen in MH-susceptible muscle can be ruled out by the fact that calcium determination included in those studied as well as in the present came from muscle with resting membrane potential greater than -80 mV. We have shown in this paper that the $[Ca^{2+}]_i$ in MH muscle fibers with damaged plasma membrane is several times higher than the values that we have previously reported for $[Ca^{2+}]_i$. In addition, the cell damage produces similar effects on Vm and $[Ca^{2+}]_i$ in both control and MH muscles. Therefore, plasma membrane damage cannot account for the differences in $[Ca^{2+}]_i$ between control and MH muscle fibers. Furthermore, experiments in which the $[Ca^{2+}]_o$ was changed up to five times its normal concentration did not show any alteration in the $[Ca^{2+}]_i$ (see results), which is a good indication that the seal around the microelectrode tip was adequate.

Gronert et al.[37] have raised some concern in relation to the fact that this high $[Ca^{2+}]_i$ is close to the threshold that could activate contractile activity. The $[Ca^{2+}]_i$ that we have reported in MH-susceptible subjects or swine have been in the range of 0.32 to 0.42μM. Such concentration is far from the actual value described for mechanical threshold in muscle preparation from animals as well as from humans.[43,44] Therefore, no increase in resting tension at this $[Ca^{2+}]_i$ would be expected. This increment in intracellular free $[Ca^{2+}]$ is not a unique feature of MH muscle fibers, because in other muscle pathology we have found similar alterations[43-46] and therefore possible use for diagnostic purposes of MH susceptibility[47] is not a consideration.

D. EFFECT OF RYANODINE ON $[Ca^{2+}]_i$

Ryanodine has been implicated as a specific ligand for the Ca^{2+} release channel of SR in skeletal muscle.[14] The ryanodine receptor has been localized to the terminal cisternae of SR in skeletal muscle.[14,15] This receptor has been purified from skeletal muscle[48] and shown to be identical to the feet structures localized between the terminal cisternae and the T tubule.[48]

The exposure of control and MH muscle fibers to ryanodine produced increments in $[Ca^{2+}]_i$ that were dose dependent. At concentrations higher than 10 μM in the control and 0.1 μM in the MH, the increments in the $[Ca^{2+}]_i$ were accompanied by a slow contracture. It is interesting to point out that the concentration of ryanodine required to induce either an increment in $[Ca^{2+}]_i$ or muscle contracture was much lower in the MH muscle group than in the control. It has been reported that ryanodine at micromolar concentrations in the presence of Ca^{2+} locks the channel in an open state.[49] At lower concentrations, the effect is similar but requires a longer time for its effect to be seen.[49] These results provide new evidence about the existence of an abnormal ryanodine receptor in the MH SR.[31]

It was found that dantrolene prevented the effects of ryanodine in control and MH muscle fibers. Dantrolene is a muscle relaxant that has no effect on neuromuscular transmission, on electrical activity, or on the inward spread of activation in skeletal muscle.[50,51] In addition, dantrolene does not affect the contractile response of the myofilaments to calcium.[52] The relaxant effect of dantrolene appears to be related to some action upon the T-tubule SR coupling mechanism or on the SR itself by inducing an inhibition of Ca^{2+} release.[53] Dantrolene reduces the amplitude of the transient Ca^{2+},[54] and it decreases the myoplasmic resting $[Ca^{2+}]$ in MH-susceptible patients,[5] neuroleptic malignant-susceptible patients,[55] MH-susceptible swine,[11] and frog skeletal muscle.[56] The fact that dantrolene was able to prevent the ryanodine effect might suggest that both drugs may exert opposing actions at morphologically related sites.

ACKNOWLEDGMENTS

The author thanks Dr. R. DiPolo for his helpful criticism. Special thanks to Mrs. Mariela Meneses and Mrs. Dhuwya Otero for their secretarial assistance and illustration. This work has been supported by grants from CONICIT of Venezuela S1-1277 and Angelini Pharmaceuticals (New York).

REFERENCES

1. **Gronert, C. A.**, Malignant hyperthermia, *Anesthesiology*, 53, 395, 1980.
2. **Britt, B. A.**, Malignant hyperthermia. A review, in *Handbook of Experimental Pharmacology, Pyretics and Antipyretics*, A. S. Milton, Ed., Springer-Verlag, Heidelberg, 1982, 547.
3. **Ellis, F. R. and Heffrom, F. F. A.**, Clinical and biochemical aspects of malignant hyperpyrexia, in *Recent Advances in Anesthesia and Analgesia*, R. S. Atkinson and A. P. Adams, Eds., Churchill Livingstone, Edinburgh, 1985, 173.
4. **López, J. R., Alamo, L., Caputo, C., Wikinski, J., and Ledezma, D.**, Intracellular ionized calcium concentration in muscles from humans with malignant hyperthermia, *Muscle Nerve*, 8, 355, 1985.
5. **López, J. R., Medina, P., and Alamo, L.**, Dantrolene sodium is able to reduce the resting ionic $[Ca^{2+}]_i$ in muscle from humans with malignant hyperthermia, *Muscle Nerve*, 10, 77, 1987.
6. **López, J. R., López, M., and Allen, P.**, Sarcoplasmic ionic $[Ca^{2+}]$ measured *in vivo* in malignant hyperthermia susceptible patients, *Biophys. J.*, 55, 486a, 1989.
7. **López, J. R., Jones, D., Alamo, L., Allen, P., and Sreter, F.**, $[Ca^{2+}]_i$ in muscles of malignant hyperthermia susceptible pigs. Determined *in vivo* with Ca^{2+} selective microelectrodes, *Muscle Nerve*, 9, 85, 1986.
8. **López, J. R., Allen, P. D., Alamo, L., Jones, D., and Sreter, F.**, Myoplasmic free $[Ca^{2+}]_i$ during a malignant hyperthermia episode in swine, *Muscle Nerve*, 11, 82, 1988.
9. **Flewellen, E. G. and Nelson, T. E.**, Dantrolene dose response in malignant hyperthermia susceptible (MHS) swine, *Anesthesiology*, 52, 303, 1980.
10. **Harrison, G. G.**, The prophylaxis of malignant hyperthermia by oral dantrolene sodium in swine, *Eur. J. Anesth.*, 49, 315, 1977.
11. **López, J. R., Allen, P., Alamo, L., Jone, D., and Sreter, F.**, Dantrolene prevents the malignant hyperthermic syndrome by reducing free intracellular calcium concentration in skeletal muscle of susceptible swine, *Cell Calcium*, 8, 385, 1987.
12. **Parra, L., Suarez Isla, B., and López, J. R.**, Large conductance calcium channel in malignant hyperthermia sarcoplasmic reticulum membranes is blocked by dantrolene, *Can. Anaesth. Soc. J.*, 36, S113, 1989.
13. **Klip, A., Britt, B. A., Elliot, M., Pegg, W., Frodis, W., and Scott, E.**, Anesthetic induced increase in ionised calcium in blood mononuclear cells from malignant hyperthermia patients, *Lancet*, 463, 466, 1987.
14. **Fleischer, S., Ogunbunmi, E. M., Dixon, M. C., and Fleer, E. A. M.**, Localization of Ca^{2+} release with ryanodine in junctional terminal cisternae of sarcoplasmic reticulum of fast skeletal muscle, *Proc. Natl. Acad. Sci. U.S.A.*, 82, 7456, 1985.
15. **Pessah, I. N., Waterhouse, A. L., and Casida, J. E.**, The calcium-ryanodine receptor complex of skeletal and cardiac muscle, *Biochem. Biophys. Res. Commun.*, 128, 449, 1986.
16. **López, J. R., Alamo, L., Caputo, C., DiPolo, R., and Vergara, J.**, Determination of ionic calcium in frog skeletal muscle fibers, *Biophys. J.*, 43, 1, 1983.
17. **Tsien, R. and Rink, T.**, Neutral carrier ion selective microelectrodes for measurements of intracellular free calcium, *Biochim. Biophys. Acta*, 599, 623, 1980.
18. **Alvarez-Leefmans, F. J., Rink, T. J., and Tsien, R.**, Free calcium ions in neurons of *Helix aspersa* measured with ion selective microelectrode, *J. Physiol.*, 315, 531, 1981.
19. **Cleworth, D. R. and Edman, K. A. P.**, Changes in sarcomere length during isometric tension development in frog skeletal muscle, *J. Physiol.*, 227, 1, 1972.
20. **Blinks, J. R., Wier, W., Hese, P., and Prendergast, F.**, Measurement of Ca^{2+} concentrations in living cells, *Prog. Biophys. Mol. Biol.*, 40, 1, 1982.

21. **Scarpa, A.**, Measurements of calcium ion concentrations with metallochromic indicators, in *Detection and Measurement of Free Ca²⁺ in Cells*, C. Ashley and A. Campbell, Eds., Elsevier/North-Holland, 1979, 85.

22. **Alvarez-Leefmans, F. J., Rink, T. J., and Tsien, R.**, Free calcium ions in neurones of *Helix aspersa* measured with ion selective microelectrode, *J. Physiol.*, 315, 531, 1981.

23. **Marban, E., Rink, R., and Tsien, R.** Free calcium in heart muscle at rest and during contraction measured with Ca²⁺-sensitive microelectrode, *Nature*, 286, 845, 1980.

24. **Alamo, L., López, J. R., Papp, L., and Sreter, F.**, Simultaneous measurements of free intracellular ionized calcium and magnesium concentration in rabbit muscle fibers, *Muscle Nerve*, 48, 472, 1986.

25. **Sreter, F., López, J. R., Alamo, L., Mabuchi, K., and Geryely, J.**, Changes in ionized calcium concentration in stimulated muscle, *Am. J. Physiol.*, 260, C296, 1987.

26. **DiPolo, R. and Beauge, L.**, Ca²⁺ transport in never fibers, *Biochim. Biophys. Acta*, 947, 549, 1988.

27. **Mullins, L. J.**, A mechanism of Na/Ca exchange, *J. Gen. Physiol.*, 70, 681, 1977.

28. **Carafoli, E. and Caroni, P.**, The calcium pumping ATPase of heart plasma membrane, in *Myocardial and Skeletal Muscle Bioenergetics*, N. Brautbar, Ed., Plenum Publishing, 1986, 563.

29. **Caroni, P. and Carafoli, E.**, The regulation of the Na⁺-Ca²⁺ exchanger of heart sarcolemma, *Eur. J. Biochem.*, 132, 451, 1983.

30. **Caroni, P., Zurini, M., Clark, A., and Carafoli, E.**, Further characterization and reconstitution of the purified Ca²⁺ pumping ATPase of heart sarcolemma, *J. Biol. Chem.*, 258, 708, 1983.

31. **Mickelson, J., Gallant, E., Litterer, L., Johnson, K., Rempel, W., and Louis, C.**, Abnormal sarcoplasmic reticulum ryanodine receptor in malignant hyperthermia, *J. Biol. Chem.*, 262, 1740, 1988.

32. **Martonosi, A.**, Mechanism of Ca²⁺ release from sarcoplasmic reticulum of skeletal muscle, *Physiol. Rev.*, 64, 1240, 1983.

33. **Isaacs, H. and Heffron, J.**, Morphological and biochemical defects in muscles of human carriers of the malignant hyperthermia syndrome, *Br. J. Anesth.*, 47, 475, 1975.

34. **Denborough, M. A.**, The pathopharmacology of malignant hyperpyrexia, *Pharmacol. Ther.*, 9, 357, 1980.

35. **Condrescu, M., López, J. R., Medina, P., and Alamo, L.**, Deficient function of the sarcoplasmic reticulum in malignant hyperthermia susceptible patients, *Muscle Nerve*, 10, 238, 1987.

36. **Ohnishi, T., Taylor, S., and Gronert, G.**, Calcium induced calcium release from sarcoplasmic reticulum of pigs susceptible to malignant hyperthermia, *FEBS Lett.*, 161, 103, 1983.

37. **Gronert, G. A., Mott, J., and Lee, J.**, Aetiology of malignant hyperthermia, *Br. J. Anaesth.*, 60, 253, 1988.

38. **Iaizzo, P., Klein, W., and Lehmann-Horn, F.**, Fura 2 detected myoplasmic calcium and its correlation with contracture force in skeletal muscle from normal and malignant hyperthermia susceptible pigs, *Pflugers Arch.*, 411, 648, 1988.

39. **Baylor, S. and Hollingworth, S.**, Fura-2 calcium transient in frog skeletal muscle fibers, *J. Physiol.*, 403, 151, 1988.

40. **Olson, A., Kunishi, M., Hollingworth, S., and Baylor S.**, Myoplasmic binding of Fura-2 investigated by steady state fluorescence emission anisotropy, *Biophys. J.*, 53, 600a, 1988.

41. **Highsmith, S., Bloebaum, P., and Snowdown K.**, Sarcoplasmic reticulum interacts with the Ca²⁺ indicator precursor Fura-2 AM, *Biochem. Biophys. Res. Commun.*, 138, 1153, 1986.

42. **Wier, W. G., Cannell, M. B., Berlin, J. R., Marban, E., and Lederer, W. J.**, Cellular and subcellular heterogenecity of $[Ca^{2+}]$ in single heart cells revealed by Fura-2, *Science*, 235, 325, 1987.

43. **Taylor, S. and Godt, R.**, Calcium release and contraction in vertebrate skeletal muscle calcium in biological systems, *Symp. Soc. Exper. Biol.*, 30, 361, 1976.

44. **Fabiato, A. and Fabiato, F.**, Myofilament generated tension oscillations during partial calcium activation and activation dependence of the sarcomere length-tension relation of skinned cardiac cells, *J. Gen. Physiol.*, 72, 667, 1978.

45. **López, J. R., Sanchez, V., Briceño, L., and Horvat, D.** Myoplasmic $[Ca^{2+}]_i$ in Duchenne muscular dystrophy patients, *Acta Cient. Venez.*, 38, 503, 1987.

46. **López, J. R., Briceño, L., Cordovez, G., Sanchez, V., and Linares, N.**, Intracellular free $[Ca^{2+}]_i$ in human skeletal muscle with myopathic carnitine deficiency, *Gen. Physiol. Biophys.*, 8, 91, 1989.

47. **Ording, H.**, Diagnosis of susceptibility to malignant hyperthermia in man, *Br. J. Anaesth.*, 60, 287, 1988.

48. **Invi, M., Saito, A., and Fleischer, S.**, Purification of the ryanodine receptor and identity with feet structures of functional terminal cistarnae of sarcoplasmic reticulum from fast skeletal muscle, *J. Biol. Chem.*, 262, 1740, 1987.

49. **Nagasaki, K. and Fleischer, S.**, Ryanodine sensitivity of the calcium release channel of sarcoplasmic reticulum, *Cell Calcium*, 9, 1, 1988.

50. **Putney, J. W. and Bianchi, C. P.**, Site of action of dantrolene in frog sartorius muscle, *J. Pharmacol. Exp. Ther.*, 189, 202, 1974.

51. **Helland, L. A., López, J. R., Taylor, S. R., Trube, G., and Wanek, L.** Effect of calcium "antagonist" on vertebrate skeletal muscle, *Proc. N.Y. Acad. Sci.*, 522, 259, 1988.

52. **Brocklehurst, L.**, Dantrolene sodium and skinned muscle fibers, *Nature*, 254, 364, 1974.

53. **Ohnishi, S., Taylor, S., and Gronert, G.**, Calcium induced Ca^{2+} release from sarcoplasmic reticulum in pigs susceptible to malignant hyperthermia, *FEBS Lett.*, 161, 103, 1983.

54. **Desmedt, J. and Halnaut, K.**, Inhibition of intracellular release of calcium by dantrolene in barnacle giant muscle fibers, *J. Physiol.*, 265, 565, 1977.

55. **López, J. R., Sanchez, V., and López, M. J.**, Sarcoplasmic ionic calcium concentration in neuroleptic malignant syndrome, *Cell Calcium*, 10, 223, 1989.

56. **Alamo, L., López, J. R., and Caputo, C.**, Dantrolene reduces the $[Ca^{2+}]_i$ increase in stretched skeletal muscle fibers, *Biophys. J.*, 51, 104A, 1987.

Chapter 12

MALIGNANT HYPERTHERMIA
AND FREE RADICALS

Garry G. Duthie and John R. Arthur

TABLE OF CONTENTS

I.   Introduction...152

II.   Free Radicals and Lipid Peroxidation............................152

III.   Formation of Oxygen Radicals...................................153

IV.   The Halothane Radical..155

V.   Antioxidant Defense Systems....................................156

VI.   Evidence for an Antioxidant Abnormality in MH.................158

VII.   Effects of Stress..159

VIII.   *In Vivo* and *In Vitro* Effects of Halothane 160

IX.   Can Membrane or Antioxidant Abnormalities Be Used
        for the Diagnosis of MH?......................................161

X.   Lipid Peroxidation and Calcium 162

XI.   The Nature of the Antioxidant Abnormality in MH..............165

XII.   Conclusion..165

Acknowledgments...165

References..166

Appendix: Erythrocyte Lipid Peroxidation as a Diagnostic
Test for MH...168

I. INTRODUCTION

Malignant hyperthermia (MH) is a pharmacogenetic disorder that is triggered in susceptible individuals by exposure to certain anesthetic agents, in particular halothane. It is characterized by a rapid rise in body temperature, cardiac arrhythmia, marked limb rigidity, the appearance of cyanotic areas on the skin, and destruction of muscle tissue. Etiologically similar syndromes are found in a number of species in which, in addition to halothane intubation, stresses such as transportation, exercise, mating, and parturition also trigger an MH response. The condition in swine is referred to as the porcine stress syndrome (PSS) and the pig is regarded as a useful animal model for the MH syndrome in humans. Recent reviews on clinical, biochemical, and physiological aspects of MH include: O'Brien,[1] Gronert et al.,[2] Harriman,[3] Heffron,[4] and Rosenberg.[5]

The primary biochemical defect responsible for the MH syndrome has not been identified. Due to the characteristic limb rigidity that occurs during an MH episode, many studies have looked for faults in Ca^{2+} homeostasis in the skeletal muscle of MH-susceptible humans and animals. Possible abnormalities in membrane depolarization, repolarization, Ca^{2+}-ATPase pumps, Na^+/Ca^{2+}-antiporters, and slow voltage Ca^{2+} channels have been proposed.[2,6] However, there is also considerable evidence that MH reflects a widespread membrane defect that is detectable not only in skeletal muscle but also in heart muscle, smooth muscle, platelets, lymphocytes, monocytes, and erythrocytes.[7] This suggests that the perturbations in Ca^{2+} in skeletal muscle may be a dramatic expression of ubiquitous membrane disorder. In this article we suggest that the defect in MH arises from an antioxidant abnormality that increases the susceptibility of cell membranes to damage by free radicals. The resulting rapid peroxidation of membrane lipids leads to an uncontrolled increase in myoplasmic Ca^{2+}, triggering contraction of the skeletal muscle and initiating the characteristic rise in body temperature.

II. FREE RADICALS AND LIPID PEROXIDATION

Free radicals are molecules or molecular fragments with an unpaired electron. The presence of an unpaired electron can convey considerable reactivity to the free radical, which by abstracting hydrogen can damage a wide range of biological molecules such as DNA, nucleotide coenzymes, and protein thiols. Polyunsaturated fatty acids (PUFA:H) are particularly susceptible to damage by free radicals and therefore cell membranes are very vulnerable to peroxidation. Abstraction of a hydrogen from a fatty acid initiates the potentially autocatalytic cascade of lipid peroxidation as follows:

PUFA:H   ⟶ PUFA· :Hydrogen abstraction
PUFA· + O_2 ⟶ PUFAOO· :Peroxyl radical
PUFAOO· + PUFA:H ⟶ PUFAOOH + PUFA· :Hydroperoxide + radical

Homolytic fission results in the formation of additional radicals:

$$PUFAOOH \longrightarrow PUFAO\cdot + OH\cdot$$

or

$$2 \times PUFAOOH \longrightarrow PUFAOO\cdot + PUFAO\cdot + H_2O$$

Consequently, in the absence of free radical scavenging antioxidants the formation of one peroxyl radical is sufficient to produce a rapid self-propagating cascade of lipid peroxidation.[8]

Over 60 byproducts of lipid peroxidation have been detected. Of these, conjugated dienes, lipid hydroperoxides, aldehydes, fluorescent conjugates, and hydrocarbons are commonly used to assess lipid peroxidation in plasma, samples of tissues, and whole animals. The formation of some of these products during the peroxidation of an ω-3 fatty acid is shown in Figure 1. The advantages and disadvantages of methods for the measurement of lipid peroxidation (Table 1) are discussed by Halliwell and Gutteridge[9] and Gutteridge.[10]

III. FORMATION OF OXYGEN RADICALS

Endogenous production of free radicals occurs as a consequence of normal aerobic metabolism. The superoxide anion O_2^- is produced during reductive processes associated with electron transport chains in the mitochondria and endoplasmic reticulum. In mitochondria, electron transport involves the sequential reduction of flavoproteins, ubiquinones, and cytochromes with resultant generation of ATP. The reoxidation of ubisemiquinone and reduced flavin dehydrogenase produces O_2^-.[11] The electron transport system of the endoplasmic reticulum involves transfer of an electron from a reduced flavin to the cytochrome P450 complex, with the transfer of a second electron to molecular oxygen thus forming O_2^-. Although many other cellular redox systems such as ischemia-derived xanthine oxidase, aldehyde oxidase, and membrane NADPH oxidases produce O_2^-, the endoplasmic reticulum and mitochondrial compartments probably make the greatest contributions to the intracellular O_2^- load. For example, approximately 1 to 4% of the total oxygen uptake by mitochondria may be used by O_2^- production, of which 20% may be ejected into the cell.[12]

O_2^- has a low rate constant for biomolecular reactions; however, it is capable of diffusing relatively large distances through the cell where transition metal ions (most probably Fe or Cu) can catalyze a Haber-Weiss reaction to produce the potentially very reactive hydroxyl (OH ·) radical.

$$Fe^{3+} + O_2^-\cdot \longrightarrow Fe^{2+} + O_2^-$$
$$Fe^{2+} + H_2O_2 \longrightarrow Fe^{3+} + OH^- + OH\cdot$$

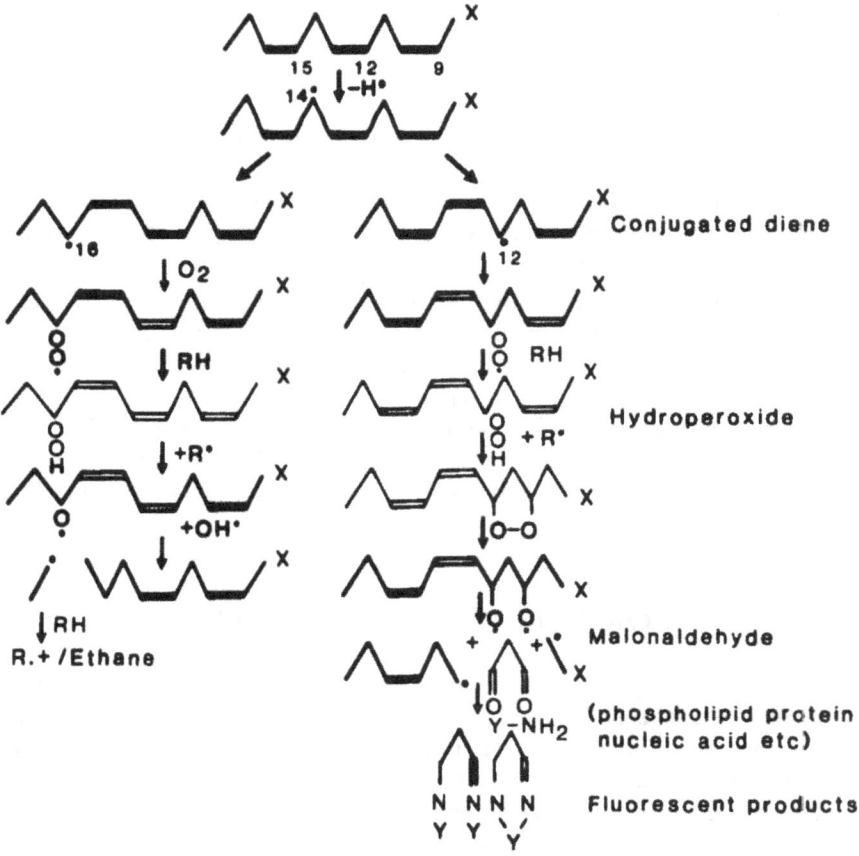

FIGURE 1. Proposed scheme of free radical-mediated peroxidation of an ω-3 polyunsaturated fatty acid.

TABLE 1
Some Methods for the Detection and Measurement of Lipid Peroxidation

Parameter	Method of Detection
Free radical	Electron spin resonance
Polyunsaturated fatty acid	GLC, HPLC
Conjugated diene	HPLC, UV absorbance
Lipid hydroperoxide	HPLC, thiobarbituric acid, iodometric titration
Aldehydes	HPLC, thiobarbituric acid, fluorescence
Hydrocarbon gases	GLC

The hydrogen peroxide (H_2O_2) required for the above reaction is formed in the cell from O_2^- either by spontaneous dismutation or by the enzyme superoxide dismutase (SOD).

$$O_2^- + O_2^- \longrightarrow H_2O_2 + O_2 \text{ (spontaneous or SOD)}$$

Hydroxyl or similar very reactive radicals have a small diffusion radius and rapidly react with adjacent molecules. Therefore OH · has the potential to be an initiator of lipid peroxidation if it is formed in the lipid membranes or their immediate vicinity.

IV. THE HALOTHANE RADICAL

The MH response is triggered in susceptible humans by exposure to halothane and other potent halogenated hydrocarbon anesthetics such as chloroform.[7] The prevalence of the MH response to general anesthetics is approximately 1:50,000,[13] but the mechanism by which these halogenated hydrocarbons induce the MH response is unclear. It may involve the blocking of synaptic transmissions by altering the conformation of synaptic membrane proteins. This may occur by direct interaction of the anesthetic and protein or by interference with the lipid matrix surrounding the protein.[14] However, another feature of some halogen-based anesthetics is their ability to form reactive free radicals capable of initiating lipid peroxidation. Pulse radiolysis can cause a one-electron reduction of halothane in aqueous solution to form a halothane radical and bromide ion as follows:

$$CF_3CHBrCl + 2e\text{-aqueous} \longrightarrow Br^- + CF_3C\cdot HCl$$

The resultant radical can react with oxygen to form a more reactive peroxy radical.

$$CF_3C\cdot HCl + O_2 \longrightarrow CF_3CHClOO\cdot$$

The peroxy radical has strong oxidizing properties and is capable of hydrogen abstraction from a wide range of biological molecules (X).

$$CF_3CHClOO\cdot + X \longrightarrow CF_3CHClOO^- + X^{+\cdot}$$

In vitro, the halothane peroxy radical reacts rapidly with fatty acids with the rate increasing with the degree of unsaturation of the fatty acid. The rate constants ($\times 10^6 \text{ m}^{-1} \text{ s}^{-1}$) for oleic acid (18:1), linoleic acid (18:2), linolenic acid (18:3), and arachidonic acid (20:4) are 0.3, 0.8, 1.3, and 1.5, respectively.[15]

In vivo, $CF_3C \cdot HCl$ is likely to arise from reactions of halothane with cytochrome P450. In addition to the aerobic formation of halothane peroxy radicals, CF_3C HCl may itself abstract hydrogen from molecules such as membrane lipids to give chlorotrifluoroethane, which has been detected in the expired breath of rabbits and human patients exposed to halothane.[9]

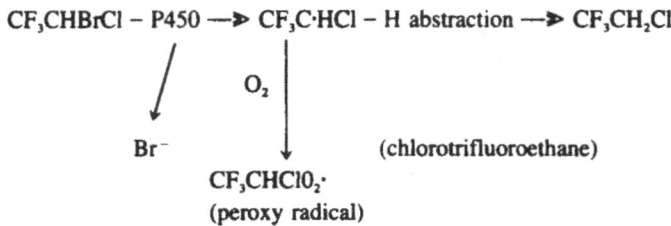

Moreover, electron spin resonance studies with spin-trapping compounds have demonstrated the formation of free radicals when halothane is metabolized by rat hepatic microsomes. Similar radicals have been detected when spin traps were administered to intact animals undergoing halothane anesthesia.[16,17] Therefore, there is little doubt that exposure to halothane produces potent free radicals. Compared with superoxide (O_2^-), the diffusion distance of the halothane radical through the cell is likely to be small and thus it would react with other molecules at or near its site of formation.[15] As halothane is lipid-soluble, formation of halothane radicals within the phospholipid component of the cell membranes may lead to lipid peroxidation with resultant alteration of membrane structure and function.

V. ANTIOXIDANT DEFENSE SYSTEMS

Living cells possess a variety of systems for the prevention of damage by free radicals. In the cell membrane, vitamin E is the major, if not the only, lipid-soluble antioxidant that breaks the chain reactions of lipid peroxidation. Vitamin E is the general name for a number of tocopherol and trienol isomers that can act as antioxidants, the most potent biologically being α-tocopherol (Figure 2). If vitamin E does not prevent formation of lipid hydroperoxides in the cell membrane, they can be released from phospholipids by phospholipase A_2 and then degraded by selenium-containing glutathione peroxidase in the cell cytoplasm. Additionally, another selenium-containing glutathione peroxidase has been isolated, this form of the enzyme being capable of metabolizing lipid hydroperoxides attached to phospholipids.[18] Hydrogen peroxide formed from O_2^- is prevented from forming OH $\cdot$ by glutathione peroxidase and by catalase. Other cell antioxidants include vitamin C, reduced glutathione, and carnosine, all of which have the ability to scavenge free radicals and may also participate in the regeneration of vitamin E, after it has reacted with a free radical. A simplified scheme of the cell antioxidant systems is shown in Figure 3.

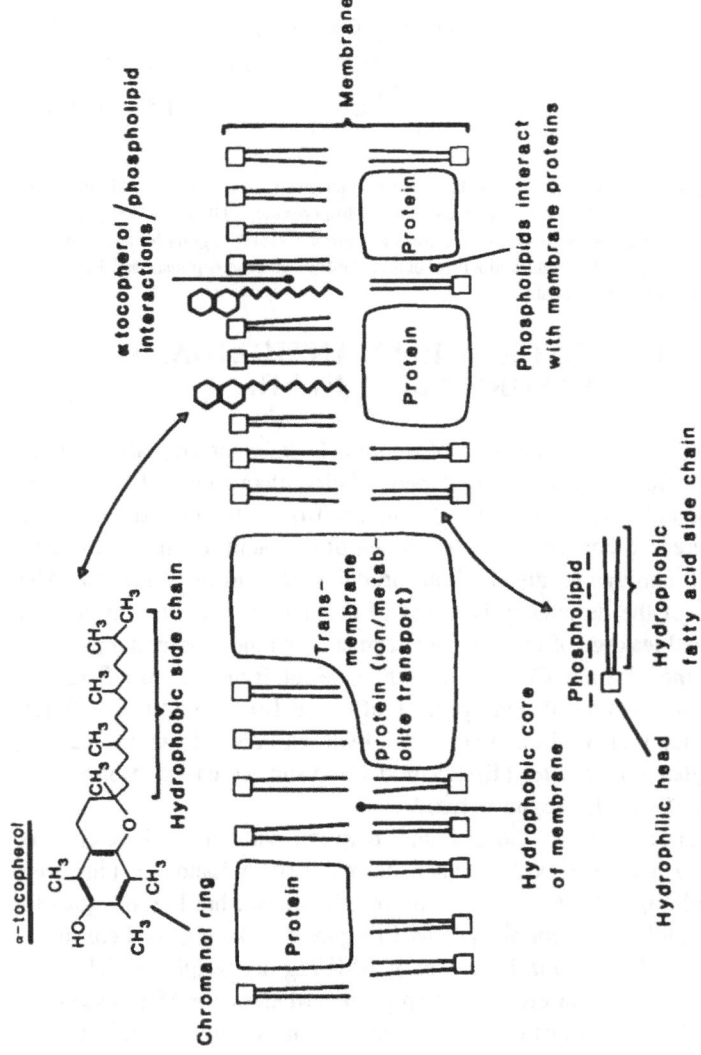

FIGURE 2. The structure of α-tocopherol and a scheme for its positioning in the cell membrane.

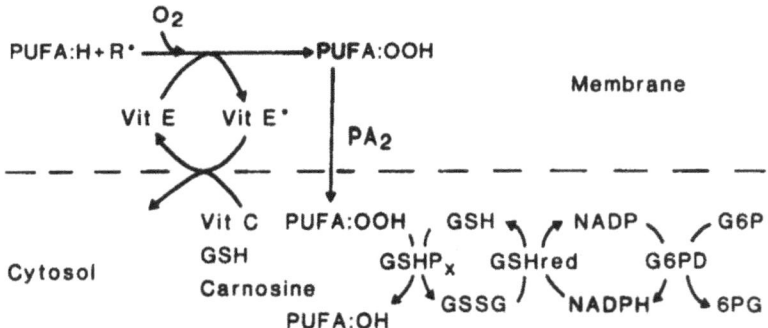

FIGURE 3. Some of the major antioxidant defense mechanisms within the cell. PUFA:H, polyunsaturated fatty acid; PUFA:OOH, fatty acid hydroperoxide; PUFA:OH, fatty acid hydroxide; GSH, reduced glutathione; GSSG, oxidized glutathione; GSHPx, glutathione peroxidase; PA₂, phospholipase A₂; GSH_red, glutathione reductase; G6PD, glucose-6-phosphate dehydrogenase; and 6PG, 6-phosphogluconate.

VI. EVIDENCE FOR AN ANTIOXIDANT ABNORMALITY IN MH

PUFAs in the cell membranes of vitamin E-deficient animals are more susceptible to free radical mediated peroxidation than those of vitamin E-supplemented individuals. As a result, plasma from vitamin E-deficient animals has increased concentrations of thiobarbituric acid reactive substances (TBARS) and conjugated dienes, both products of lipid peroxidation. Also characteristic of the deficiency is a loss of cell membrane integrity leading to the enhanced leakage of the muscle enzymes, creatine kinase and pyruvate kinase, into the plasma. Compared with material from vitamin E-supplemented animals, incubated homogenates of tissue from vitamin E-deficient animals produce increased amounts of the hydrocarbons ethane and pentane and erythrocytes show greater TBARS production and decreased deformability when incubated with hydrogen peroxide.[19]

Similar differences to those found between vitamin E-deficient and -sufficient animals were evident when normal British Landrace pigs were compared with pigs of the same age and breeding stock but homozygous for the gene that confers susceptibility to MH (Figure 4). The pigs had consumed identical diets with a vitamin E content of 10 IU/kg dry weight, which meets the normal vitamin E requirement of the pig. Nevertheless, the MH-susceptible pigs showed the same signs of a decreased capacity to prevent lipid peroxidation and cell damage as are found in vitamin E-deficient animals. Despite these differences the MH-susceptible pigs were not vitamin E-deficient insofar as plasma and tissue vitamin E concentrations were identical in the MH-susceptible and -resistant pigs.[21] However, supplementation with 20 times the assumed dietary requirement of vitamin E (as α-tocopherol acetate) produced decreases in plasma pyruvate kinase and creatine kinase activities. Moreover,

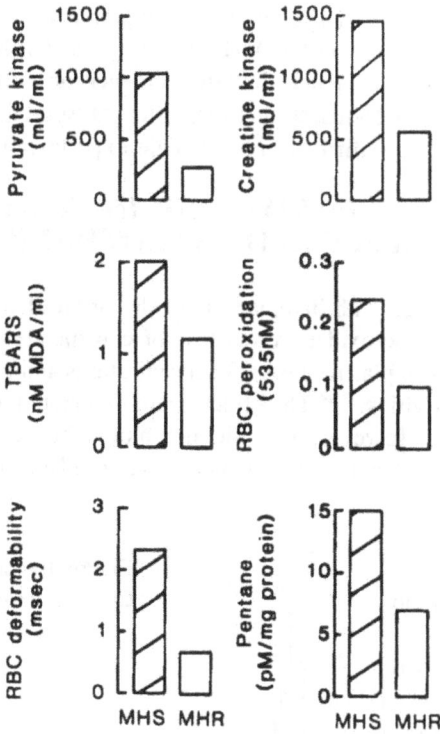

FIGURE 4. Indices of cell membrane damage and lipid peroxidation of MH-susceptible (MHS) and MH-resistant (MHR) pigs. Data from Duthie and Arthur.[20]

plasma TBARS concentrations, erythrocyte peroxidation, and pentane production by muscle homogenates of MH-susceptible pigs were markedly reduced by vitamin E supplementation.[22] These results are consistent with diminished free radical-mediated lipid peroxidation and improved membrane integrity of vitamin E-supplemented, MH-susceptible pigs.

VII. EFFECTS OF STRESS

Physical or pharmacological stress is likely to increase oxygen consumption and oxidative phosphorylation in the cell, thus increasing the production of potentially injurious free radicals. To assess whether stress, a trigger of MH in susceptible pigs, could further exceed the capacity of the apparently impaired antioxidant defense system, MH-susceptible and -resistant pigs were transported for 30 min prior to assessment of indices of cell membrane integrity and lipid peroxidation.[23] Additionally, some of the pigs were given large dietary supplements of vitamin E from weaning. Plasma creatine kinase activity and TBARS concentrations increased after transport of the MH-susceptible pigs; however, these changes were of smaller magnitude in susceptible pigs that had received the large vitamin E supplements (Figure 5). No effect of transport was observed in the MH-resistant pigs. Furthermore, Hoppe et al.[24] give preliminary evidence that supplementation with antioxidants decreases mortality of MH-susceptible pigs after transportation. These results, however, need to be confirmed in large scale experiments.

VIII. *IN VIVO* AND *IN VITRO* EFFECTS OF HALOTHANE

Intubation of pigs with halothane until the onset of limb rigidity causes an increase in lipid peroxidation and loss of cell membrane integrity manifested by increases in plasma TBARS concentrations and pyruvate kinase and creatine kinase activities.[23,24] The effects were moderated by supplementation with antioxidants. However, this did not block the development of limb rigidity, indicating that increasing dietary antioxidants may not avert the

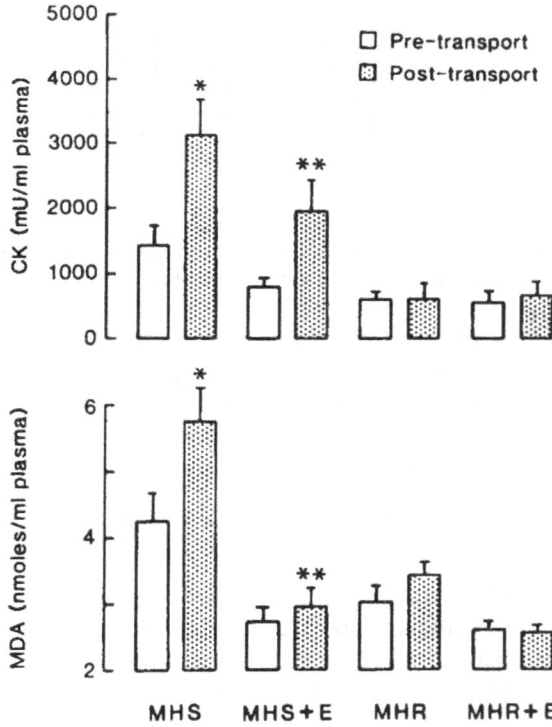

FIGURE 5. Effects of α-tocopherol supplementation and transport on plasma TBARS concentrations and creatine kinase activities. *, denotes significant difference pre- and post-transportation (p<0.05); **, denotes significant difference between α-tocopherol-supplemented and -unsupplemented MH-susceptible pigs pre- and post-transportation (p<0.05, creatine kinase; p<0.001, TBARS). Data from Duthie et al.[22]

progression to the fulminant MH attack following a major stress such as halothane inhalation.

Incubation of muscle biopsy samples from MH-susceptible animals with halothane produces contraction and changes in Ca^{2+} metabolism that have been used to diagnose the condition. Results from incubation of hepatic microsomal preparations from MH pigs have, however, given equivocal results. A marked enhancement of endogenous peroxidation was apparent in liver microsomes derived from some MH-susceptible pigs but not from others. In the preparations that peroxidized the activity is further stimulated in the presence of halothane (Figure 6). Why this effect was not observed in all MH-susceptible pigs is unclear. Halothane, however, does not stimulate peroxidation in hepatic microsomal preparations from stress-resistant pigs (Figure 6).

IX. CAN MEMBRANE OR ANTIOXIDANT ABNORMALITIES BE USED FOR THE DIAGNOSIS OF MH?

In the diagnosis of MH, a number of studies have attempted to exploit the impairment of cell membrane integrity found in susceptible individuals. Increased leakage of the muscle isozyme of creatine kinase into the plasma has been demonstrated in MH-susceptible pigs but the large natural variability in enzyme activities results in a large number of false classifications. Plasma pyruvate kinase activity is more effective than creatine kinase activity in discriminating between MH-susceptible and -resistant pigs,[25] but the

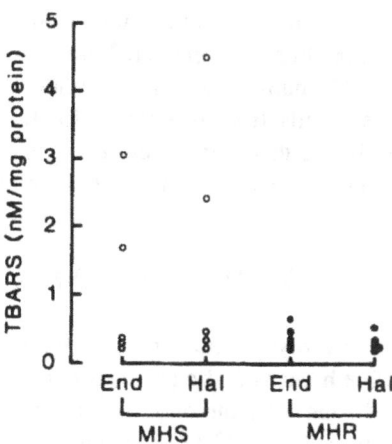

FIGURE 6. TBARS production by liver microsomes from MH-susceptible and -resistant pigs. Buffer contained 20 mM HEPES, 130 mM NaCl, and 2 mM $CaCl_2$, pH 7.4 (endogenous incubation), or was 50% saturated with halothane. Incubation time 1 h, temperature 37°C.

misclassification rate is still unacceptably high.[26] Methods that rely on variations in the susceptibility of erythrocytes to osmotic lysis have also been unsatisfactory. It is worth emphasizing that comparisons between MH-susceptible and -resistant animals should be made between groups of similar breed and genetic stock consuming the same basal diet; otherwise, any differences may be due to breed or diet and not to MH. It is less easy to obtain control values for observations made with MH-susceptible humans; this may explain the diversity of changes that have been associated with the syndrome.

Duthie et al.[27] assessed whether incubating red blood cells with hydrogen peroxide could be used as a diagnostic test for MH in pigs. This method was based on the hypothesis that the decreased membrane integrity in MH reflects an antioxidant abnormality that increases the susceptibility of cell membranes to damage by free radicals generated from hydrogen peroxide. Results were compared with measurements from the same pigs of plasma pyruvate kinase and creatine kinase activities and osmotically induced red cell lysis (Figure 7). Osmotically induced hemolysis was identical in MH-susceptible and -resistant pigs. Plasma pyruvate kinase and creatine kinase activities were significantly increased in the MH-susceptible pigs, but there was still a significant overlap of values between the two pig types. In contrast, there was no overlap between the pig types when red blood cells were subjected to peroxidation. Cells from MH-susceptible pigs produced significantly more TBARS than those from the MH-resistant animals on incubation with 0.9 or 1.5% hydrogen peroxide. Thus, this method offers a substantial improvement on the currently available means of identifying MH-susceptible pigs, avoiding the need to resort to testing by halothane anesthesia. It is not yet known whether age, vitamin E status, or intercurrent disease will confound the discrimination between pig types obtained by red cell peroxidation or whether this method will be useful in the identification of MH-susceptible humans. Using the fluorescent dye Quin 2, Klip et al.[28] have shown, that white blood cells from MH-susceptible humans or pigs accumulate Ca^{2+} on incubation with halothane, whereas cells from resistant individuals do not. This may provide another effective method for the detection of MH-susceptible individuals, but the influence of factors such as intercurrent disease have yet to be investigated.

X. LIPID PEROXIDATION AND CALCIUM

Klip et al.[6] report that myoplasmic concentrations of free Ca^{2+} are elevated in MH-susceptible humans and pigs, consequently, suggesting that the limb rigidity observed soon after the onset of the MH response arises from a sudden increase in myoplasmic Ca^{2+}. Skeletal muscle contraction is then triggered by Ca^{2+} binding to troponin C, a protein of the thin filament. The diverse mechanisms of intracellular Ca^{2+} regulation and the possible abnormalities of such mechanisms in MH-susceptible individuals are discussed

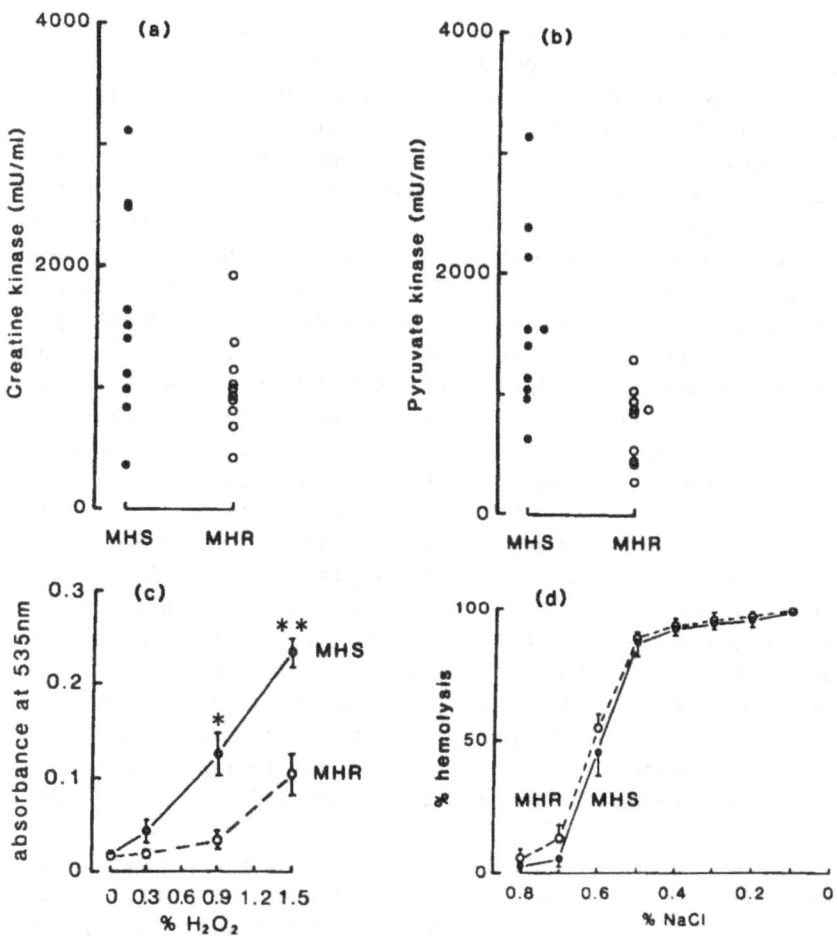

FIGURE 7. Tests used to discriminate MH-susceptible and -resistant pigs: (a) plasma creatine kinase activity; (b) plasma pyruvate kinase activity; (c) erythrocyte TBARS production in the presence of hydrogen peroxide; and (d) osmotically induced erythrocyte hemolysis. *, denotes significant differences MHS vs. MHR (p<0.005); **, MHS vs. MHR (p<0.001). Data from Duthie, G. G. et al., *Am. J. Vet. Res.*, 49, 508, 1988.

elsewhere in this volume. Briefly, low intracellular Ca^{2+} is maintained in relaxed muscle by the active transport of Ca^{2+} either into intracellular stores, such as the sacroplasmic reticulum (SR) and mitochondria, or through the plasma membrane. Mitochondria and SR have membrane-bound Ca-ATPase pumps to facilitate Ca^{2+} accumulation. As well as Ca-ATPase, efflux of Ca^{2+} through the plasma membrane involves a two way Na^+Ca^{2+} antiporter. Influx of Ca^{2+} into the myoplasm from external stores also involves the Na^+Ca^{2+} antiporter as well as slow voltage Ca^{2+} channels. The mechanisms by which Ca^{2+} is released from intracellular organelles are less well understood, although the process requires low priming concentrations of Ca^{2+} in the myoplasm and involves depolarization of the SR. In addition, inositol triphosphate, which is derived from receptor-activated hydrolysis of phosphatidylinositol 4,5-biphosphate, releases Ca^{2+} from the SR.[29]

Studies of abnormal Ca^{2+} release in MH have concentrated on the SR.[1] Aberrant responses to halothane that lead to depolarization of the terminal cisternae of the SR, enhanced sensitivity of Ca^{2+}-induced Ca^{2+} release channels, and stimulation of slow voltage Ca^{2+} channels are all possibly involved in triggering muscle contraction in MH.[30-35] Others have suggested that the abnormality resides in the mitochondrion and that increased phospholipase A_2 activity in mitochondrial membranes stimulates Ca^{2+} release.[36,37] Another possibility is that an antioxidant abnormality in MH leads to lipid peroxidation of plasma and/or organelle membranes causing a sudden increase in myoplasmic Ca^{2+} concentration. Braughler[38] demonstrated that Fe^{2+}-stimulated lipid peroxidation of synaptosomes was associated with rapid Ca^{2+} accumulation into the vesicles. Within 5 s of the onset of lipid peroxidation, the vesicle Ca^{2+} content increased fourfold, indicating that the change in Ca^{2+} permeability of the membrane was extremely rapid. Ca^{2+} blockers failed to inhibit Ca^{2+} accumulation suggesting that the influx was related to a general deterioration of membrane structure. In particular there was a loss of phosphatidylcholine, an important lipid component of cell membrane. *In vitro* Ca^{2+} concentrations as low as 0.1 μM accelerate the rate of lipid peroxidation of membrane vesicles. Consequently, if free radical-mediated damage caused even minor leakage of Ca^{2+} it may still be of sufficient magnitude to trigger Ca^{2+} release channels that may be primarily responsible for the rapid Ca^{2+} efflux observed in MH.[30-35]

Increased intracellular free Ca^{2+} arising from the initial leakage through damaged membranes may therefore exacerbate the peroxidative process. Ca^{2+} activates phospholipase A_2 that, as well as catalyzing the release of intact fatty acids such as arachidonic, preferentially removes lipid hydroperoxides from phospholipids. Consequently, increased cytoplasmic Ca^{2+} may further contribute to the peroxidative cascade by increasing the supply of substrate. Accelerated loss of membrane fatty acids would also contribute to the loss of membrane integrity. Increased phospholipase A_2 activity has been observed in muscle mitochondria from MH-susceptible pigs.[31]

Thus the apparent inadequacies of the antioxidant defense mechanisms in the MH-susceptible pig could be severely compromised by increased O_2^-/ $OH\cdot$ production during stress or by the formation of halothane radicals. As a result, lipid peroxidation of cell membranes may lead to the rapid destruction of phospholipid components, Ca^{2+} efflux, activation of the troponin complex, and triggering of muscle contraction. The subsequent uncoupling of mitochondrial electron transport from ATP production by the disruption of membrane structure would cause the rapid rise in body temperature typical of MH. However, some authors have indicated that uncoupling of mitochondria may not occur during an MH episode (see Reference 1).

XI. THE NATURE OF THE ANTIOXIDANT ABNORMALITY IN MH

The hypothesis that the MH syndrome reflects an antioxidant abnormality, although supported by evidence of subsequent membrane damage and lipid oxidation, has not been proved by the identification of any specific defect. Reported deficiencies in the antioxidant enzymes glutathione peroxidase and glucose-6-phosphate dehydrogenase in erythrocytes[34,42] have not been confirmed.[25] When MH-susceptible and -resistant pigs from the same genetic stock are compared glutathione peroxidase activities are in fact higher in some muscles from MH-susceptible pigs as are concentrations of the antioxidant glutathione.[22,27] These increases may represent a compensatory response to a sustained free radical load. Increases in free radicals cannot be attributed to changes in catalase, superoxide dismutase, or ceruloplasmin activities because these are similar in MH-susceptible and -resistant pigs.

Assuming that the antioxidant abnormality of MH is located within the cell membranes, it is possible that the increased indices of lipid peroxidation merely reflect increased amounts of polyunsaturated fatty acids, which are particularly susceptible to oxidative reactions. Although increased pentane production by homogenates of longissimus dorsi and semitendinosus muscles (Figure 4)[22] indicate increased peroxidation of ω-6 fatty acids, fatty acid profiles of muscle from MH-susceptible animals are no different from those of MH-resistant pigs.[20] Consequently, it is more likely that the efficiency of membrane antioxidants is impaired in MH-susceptible pigs. For example, structural defects within the cell membrane could impair access of vitamin E to free radicals or alternatively, a deficiency in a membrane-associated glutathione peroxidase of the type described by Ursini et al.[18] would increase the possibility of initiation of free radical damage to the cell membrane.

XIII. CONCLUSION

Although MH-related mortality in patients has been considerably decreased in recent years, due to an improvement in case management and use of premedicants such as dantrolene, the problem remains substantial within the swine industry. For example, in Europe up to 90% of some breeds of pigs, selected for lean carcass characteristics, are MH-susceptible and stress-related mortalities remain a considerable economic problem. Identification of the lesion responsible for MH is thus of considerable practical importance as well as being of great scientific interest. It is probable, whatever the precise nature of the lesion, that it will be closely related to antioxidant systems and membrane function.

ACKNOWLEDGMENTS

Our research described in this Chapter was supported by BASF, Germany.

REFERENCES

1. **O'Brien, P. J.**, Etiopathogenic defect of malignant hyperthermia: hypersensitive calcium release channel of skeletal muscle sarcoplasmic reticulum, *Vet. Res. Comm.*, 11, 527, 1987.
2. **Gronert, G. A., Mott, J., and Lee, J.**, Aetiology of malignant hyperthermia, *Br. J. Anaesth.*, 60, 253, 1988.
3. **Harriman, D. G. F.**, Malignant hyperthermia myopathy — a critical review, *Br. J. Anaesth.*, 60, 309, 1988.
4. **Heffron, J. J. A.**, Malignant hyperthermia: biochemical aspects of the acute episode, *Br. J. Anaesth.*, 60, 274, 1988.
5. **Rosenberg, H.**, Clinical presentation of malignant hyperthermia, *Br. J. Anaesth.*, 60, 268, 1988.
6. **Klip, A., Britt, B. A., Elliot, M. E., Walker, D., Ramal, T., and Pegg, W.**, Changes in cytoplasmic calcium caused by halothane. Role of plasma membrane and intracellular Ca^{2+} stores, *Biochem. Cell. Biol.*, 64, 1181, 1986.
7. **Britt, B. A.**, Malignant hyperthermia, *Can. Anaesth. Soc. J.*, 32, 666, 1985.
8. **Chow, C. K.**, Nutritional influence on cellular antioxidant systems, *Am. J. Clin. Nutr.*, 32, 1066, 1979.
9. **Halliwell, B. and Gutteridge, J. M. C.**, *Free Radicals in Biology and Medicine*, Clarendon Press, Oxford, 1985, 346.
10. **Gutteridge, J. M. C.**, Lipid peroxidation: some problems and concepts, in *Oxygen Radicals and Tissue Injury*, B. Halliwell, Ed., FASEB, Maryland, 1988, 9.
11. **Fridovich, I.**, Superoxide radical: an endogenous toxicant, *Annu. Rev. Pharmacol. Tox.*, 23, 239, 1983.
12. **Foreman, H. J. and Boveris, A.**, Superoxide and hydrogen peroxide in mitochondria, in *Free Radicals in Biology and Medicine*, Vol. 5, W. A. Pryor, Ed., Academic Press, New York, 1982, 65.
13. **McGrath, C. J.**, Malignant hyperthermia, *Semin. Vet. Med. Surg. (Small Anim.)*, 1, 238, 1986.
14. **Lechleiter, J., Wells, M., and Gruener, R.**, Halothane induced changes in acetylcholine receptor channel kinetics are attenuated by cholesterol, *Biochim. Biophys. Acta*, 856, 640, 1986.
15. **Forni, L. G., Packer, J. E., Slater, T. F., and Willson, R. L.**, Reaction of the trichlormethyl and halothane-derived peroxy radicals with unsaturated fatty acids: a pulse radiolysis study, *Chem. Biol. Interact.*, 45, 171, 1983.
16. **Poyer, J., McCay, P. B., Waddle, C. C., and Downs, P. E.**, *In vivo* spin-trapping of radicals formed during halothane metabolism, *Biochem. Pharmacol.*, 30, 1517, 1981.
17. **Plummer, J. L., Beckwith, A. L. J., Bastin, F. N., Adams, J. F., Cousins, M. J., and Hall, P.**, Free radical formation and hepatotoxicity due to anaesthesia with halothane, *Anesthesiology*, 57, 160, 1982.
18. **Ursini, F., Maiorini, M., and Gregolin, C.**, The selenoenzyme phospholipid hydroperoxide glutathione peroxidase, *Biochim. Biophys. Acta*, 839, 62, 1985.
19. **Duthie, G. G., Arthur, J. R., and Mills, C. F.**, Tissue damage in vitamin E-deficient rats is not detected by expired ethane and pentane, *Free Rad. Res. Comm.*, 4, 21, 1987.
20. **Duthie, G. G. and Arthur, J. R.**, The antioxidant abnormality in the stress susceptible pig: the effects of vitamin E supplementation, *Ann. N.Y. Acad. Sci.*, 570, 322, 1989.
21. **Duthie, G. G., Arthur, J. R., Mills, C. F., Morrice, P. C., and Nicol, F.**, Anomalous tissue vitamin E distribution in stress susceptible pigs after dietary vitamin E supplementation and effects on plasma pyruvate kinase and creatine kinase activities, *Livest. Prod. Sci.*, 17, 169, 1987.

22. **Duthie, G. G., Arthur, J. R., Nicol, F., and Walker, M. J.,** Increased indices of lipid peroxidation in stress susceptible pigs and effects of vitamin E, *Res. Vet. Sci.,* 46, 226, 1989.

22. **Duthie, G. G., Arthur, J. R., Nicol, F., and Walker, M. J.,** Increased indices of lipid peroxidation in stress susceptible pigs and effects of vitamin E, *Res. Vet. Sci.,* 46, 226, 1989.

23. **Duthie, G. G., Arthur, J. R., and Hoppe, P. P.,** Porcine stress syndrome, free radicals and vitamin E, in *Oxygen radicals in Biology and Medicine,* M. Simic, Ed., Plenum Press, New York, 1988, 605.

25. **Duthie, G. G. and Arthur, J. R.,** Blood antioxidant status and plasma pyruvate kinase activity of halothane-reacting pigs, *Am. J. Vet. Res.,* 48, 309, 1987.

26. **Duthie, G. G., Arthur, J. R., Simpson, P., and Nicol, F.,** Plasma pyruvate kinase activity vs. pyruvate kinase activity as an indicator of the porcine stress syndrome, *Am. J. Vet. Res.,* 49, 508, 1988.

27. **Duthie, G. G., Arthur, J. R., Bremner, P., Kikuchi, Y., and Nicol, F.,** Increased lipid peroxidation of erythrocytes of stress-susceptible pigs: an improved diagnostic test for porcine stress syndrome, *Am. J. Vet. Res.,* 50, 84, 1989.

28. **Klip, A., Britt, B. A., Elliott, M. E., Pegg, W., Frodis, W., and Scott, E.,** Anaesthetic-induced increase in ionised calcium in blood mononuclear cells from malignant hyperthermia patients, *Lancet,* i, 463, 1987.

29. **Berridge, M. J.,** Inositol triphosphate and calcium mobilisation, in *CIBA Foundation Symp. 122,* D. Evered and J. Whelan, Eds., (Wiley, Chichester, U.K.), 1986, 39.

30. **Ohnishi, S. T., Taylor, S., and Gronert, G. A.,** Calcium-induced calcium release from sarcoplasmic reticulum of pigs susceptible to malignant hyperthermia: the effects of halothane and dantrolene, *FEBS Lett.,* 161, 103, 1983.

31. **Endo, M., Yagi, S., Ishizuka, T., Horiuti, K., Koga, Y., and Amaha, K.,** Changes in the calcium-induced calcium release mechanism in the sarcoplasmic reticulum of the muscle from a patient with malignant hyperthermia, *Biomed. Res.,* 4, 83, 1983.

32. **Nelson, T. E.,** Abnormality in calcium release from skeletal sarcoplasmic reticulum of pigs susceptible to malignant hyperthermia, *J. Clin. Invest.,* 72, 862, 1983.

33. **Kim, D. H., Sreter, F., Ohnishi, S. T., Ryan, J., Robert, J., Allen, P. D., Meszaros, L. G., Antoniu, B., and Ikemoto, N.,** Kinetic studies of Ca release from sarcoplasmic reticulum of normal and malignant hyperthermia susceptible pig muscles, *Biochim. Biophys. Acta,* 775, 320, 1984.

34. **Ohnishi, S. T., Waring, A. J., Fang, S. G., Horiuchi, K., Flick, J. L., Sadanaga, K. K., and Ohnishi, T.,** Abnormal membrane properties of the sarcoplasmic reticulum of pigs susceptible to malignant hyperthermia: modes of action of halothane, caffeine, dantrolene and two other drugs, *Arch. Biochem. Biophys.,* 247, 294, 1986.

35. **Ohnishi, S. T.,** Effects of halothane, caffeine, dantrolene and tetracaine on the calcium permeability of skeletal sarcoplasmic reticulum of malignant hyperthermic pigs, *Biochim. Biophys. Acta,* 897, 261, 1987.

36. **Cheah, K. S.,** Skeletal-muscle mitochondria and phospholipase A_2 in malignant hyperthermia, *Biochem. Soc. Trans.,* 12, 358, 1983.

37. **Sessler, D. I.,** Malignant hyperthermia, *J. Pediatr.* 109, 9, 1986.

38. **Braughler, J. M.,** Calcium and lipid peroxidation, in *Oxygen Radicals and Tissue Injury,* B. Halliwell, Ed., FASEB, Maryland, 1988, 99.

39. **O'Brien, P. J., Forsyth, D. W., Olexson, H. S., Thatte, K. S., and Addis, P. B.,** Canine malignant hyperthermia susceptibility: erythrocyte defects-osmotic fragility, glucose-6-phosphate dehydrogenase deficiency and abnormal Ca^{2+} homeostasis, *Can. J. Comp. Med.,* 48, 381, 1984.

40. **Schanus, E. G., Lovrien, R. E., and Taylor, C. A.,** Malignant hyperthermia (MH) in humans: deficiencies in the protective systems for oxidative damage, *Prog. Clin. Biol. Res.,* 97, 95, 1982.

41. **Schanus, E. G., Schendel, F., Lovrien, R. E., Rempel, W. E., and McGrath, C.,** Malignant hyperthermia (MH): porcine erythrocyte damage from oxidation and glutathione peroxidase deficiency, in *The Red Cell: Fifth Ann Abor Conf.,* G. J. Brewer, Ed., Alan R. Liss, New York, 1981, 323.
42. **Younker, D., DeVore, M., and Hartlage, P.,** Malignant hyperthermia and glucose-6-phosphate deficiency, *Anesthesiology,* 60, 601, 1984.

APPENDIX:
ERYTHROCYTE LIPID PEROXIDATION AS A DIAGNOSTIC TEST FOR MH

Blood is withdrawn from the jugular vein of each pig into evacuated heparinized tubes. Aliqots (0.25 ml) of the blood are washed twice with 2 ml of saline solution (0.9% sodium chloride) and are finally resuspended in 1.5 ml of saline solution. Hydrogen peroxide (H_2O_2, 30% w/v) solution is added to give a final volume of 2.7 ml and concentrations of 0, 0.3, 0.9, and 1.5%. Solutions of hydrogen peroxide are prepared as follows:

Solution (%)	Volume H_2O_2 (ml)	Volume 0.9% NaCl (ml)
0	0	10
1	0.333	9.667
3	1	9
5	1.670	8.330

At these concentrations, frothing is slight and the addition of a catalase inhibitor such as sodium azide is not required. The cells are incubated at 37°C for 90 min in a shaking water bath. Reactions are then stopped by the addition of 0.5 ml of 10% trichloroacetic acid. After centrifugation (10 min at 1500 × g), the supernatant is passed through filter paper (Whatman No. 1 or equivalent) and 0.75 ml of 0.67% thiobarbituric acid is added to 0.5 ml of the filtrate. Samples are then incubated at 100°C for 20 min and, after cooling to room temperature, are read spectrophotometrically at 535 or 540 nm against a saline blank.

This method provides complete discrimination between genetically well-identified MH-susceptible and -resistant pigs homozygous for the presence or absence of the halothane gene. Further development is required to assess the effects of age and intercurrent disease and whether the test can identify heterozygote-resistant pigs that carry the MH trait. In addition, because vitamin E and selenium deficiencies also increase erythrocyte peroxidation, trials with large numbers of pigs are required to assess whether the method gives clear discrimination in the field. It is not known whether the test is clinically applicable for identification of MH in the human. Results of the method are described in Reference 27.

Part IV
Diagnosis of
Malignant Hyperthermia

Chapter 13

THE NORTH AMERICAN PROTOCOL FOR THE CAFFEINE HALOTHANE CONTRACTURE TEST IN THE DIAGNOSIS OF MALIGNANT HYPERTHERMIA

Beverley A. Britt

TABLE OF CONTENTS

I.   Introduction 172

II.   Selection of Patients 172

III.   Time of Testing and Associated Microscopy 172

IV.   Anesthesia 173

V.   Selection of Muscle 173

VI.   Surgical Excision of Muscle 173

VII.   Transport of Muscle from Operating Room
        to Laboratory 174

VIII.   Subdivision of the Fascicles in the Laboratory 176

IX.   Mounting of Muscle Strips 176

X.   Stimulation of the Muscle Strips 177

XI.   Drug Additions to Muscle Strips 178

XII.   Termination of the Test 179

XIII.   Effect of Halothane on Muscle Strips 180

XIV.   Effect of Caffeine on Muscle Strips 180

XV.   Effect of Caffeine Plus 1% Halothane on Muscle Strips 185

XVI.   Influence of Temperature on the CHC Test 186

XVII.   Effect of Other Drugs on Contractures 188

XVIII. Conclusions...193

References..194

I. INTRODUCTION

The caffeine halothane contracture (CHC) test is now used as the main method of diagnosing malignant hyperthermia (MH) in many laboratories in North America, Iceland, Europe, Australia, New Zealand, and South Africa.[1-69] In an attempt to overcome the considerable methodological variations that have existed among the various laboratories, thereby making comparisons in results between laboratories difficult, attempts have been made to introduce international standards. Standards common to all laboratories in North America were agreed upon at a meeting on November 11, 1987, at Lake Bluff, IL. These standards have since been updated at two further meetings, the last of which was held on June 4, 1990, in Hershey, PA. The European protocol is somewhat different from the North American protocol and is described in References 25 through 51. Still another protocol is used in Australia.[70,71] This paper describes the North American protocol.

II. SELECTION OF PATIENTS

Patients should weigh at least 20 kg. If the first parent biopsied is found to be nonsusceptible to MH, then the second parent should also be biopsied. All patients with an unequivocal clinical history of an MH reaction and all patients who have experienced a clinical episode that is possibly MH (including masseter muscle rigidity) are to be biopsied. Optionally, patients who have had a combination of muscle pain and an elevated creatine kinase (CK), an episode of acute rhabdomyolysis, central core disease, muscle dystrophy or other myopathies, apparent stress-induced MH reactions, sudden infant death syndrome (SIDS), and neuroleptic malignant syndrome may also be biopsied.

III. TIME OF TESTING AND ASSOCIATED MICROSCOPY

Whenever possible a period of at least two or three months should elapse between a fulminant MH reaction or an episode of rhabdomyolysis and performance of the CHC test. If the test must be done within a shorter time, a histological examination must also be carried out and should reveal no significant evidence of muscle destruction for the CHC test results to be valid. Additionally histological and histochemical examination of muscle from all patients undergoing the CHC test is strongly recommended.

IV. ANESTHESIA

For control patients, anesthesia may be any triggering or nontriggering anesthetic agent, and for patients possibly susceptible to MH, anesthesia must be a nontriggering agent. The technique may be regional, conduction, or general anesthesia. Local anesthesia should not be used. Within each test center a standard anesthetic regimen is encouraged in order to avoid possible pharmacological effects. No dantrolene should be given before or during a muscle biopsy unless an inadvertent MH reaction commences.

V. SELECTION OF MUSCLE

The muscle for the CHC test may be excised from the vastus lateralis, rectus abdominis, or other large mixed type I/II muscle, for example, the gracilis, pectoralis major, obliquus externis abdominis, or the paravertebral muscles. The deltoid and gluteal muscles should not be used as they do not yield reproducible results nor do they give good diagnostic discrimination. Brownell[68] has shown that in rats type I (red) fibers develop contractures at lower concentrations of caffeine or caffeine plus halothane than do type II (white) fibers. Most information about the CHC test in humans has been obtained from the vastus lateralis, a muscle composed of about one third type I fibers and two thirds type II fibers. Therefore, when using a muscle other than the vastus lateralis for the CHC test, one should choose a muscle with approximately the same type I/II fiber ratio as the vastus lateralis. The gracilis, rectus abdominis, pectoralis major, and obliquus externis abdominis all have type I/II fiber ratios that are similar to that of the vastus lateralis. Most other muscle types remain to be assessed.

VI. SURGICAL EXCISION OF MUSCLE

Prior to dissection, each end of the fascicle may be clamped (Figures 1A and B) or may be secured with black silk sutures onto a balsa wood stick (Figure 2). With the muscle now maintained at a constant tension either through being clamped or through being tied to the balsa wood stick, the fascicle is dissected from its surrounding muscle belly in such a manner as to preserve it free from artifactual stretching or contracture. Additionally, the muscle specimen should be handled as little as possible to avoid damage to the muscle. A third, less desirable, alternative is to neither clamp the muscle nor tie it to a stick, in which case the muscle ends should be tied at each end

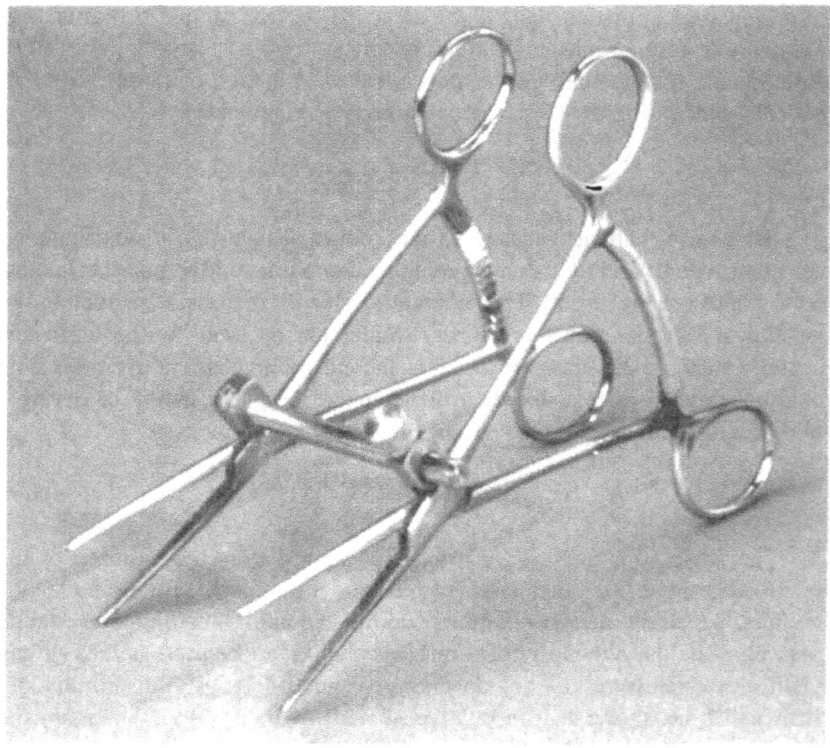

FIGURE 1.   (A) A new clamp.

with black silk sutures to prevent leakage of intracellular fluid out of the muscle cells. Great care must be taken to make the long cuts parallel to the long sides of the muscle cells (Figure 2).

VII. TRANSPORT OF MUSCLE FROM OPERATING ROOM TO LABORATORY

Once excised the muscle specimens are transported immediately to the laboratory in Krebs Ringer solution pregassed in carbogen (95% oxygen and 5% carbon dioxide) at 22°C and pH 7.4 (Tables 1A and B). The temperature of the muscle during transportation is of some importance. Muscle transported at 4°C stays suboptimally reactive for several hours. On the other hand, muscle transported at 37°C is, upon being placed in the electrolyte bath, immediately optimally reactive but fatigues more rapidly than does muscle transported at 22°C. Furthermore, MH-susceptible (MHS) but not control muscle transported at 2°C but measured at 37°C may develop a spontaneous contracture when first lowered into the 37°C Krebs Ringer bath.[6] This initial spontaneous contracture does not occur in muscle transported at 37°C.[13,14]

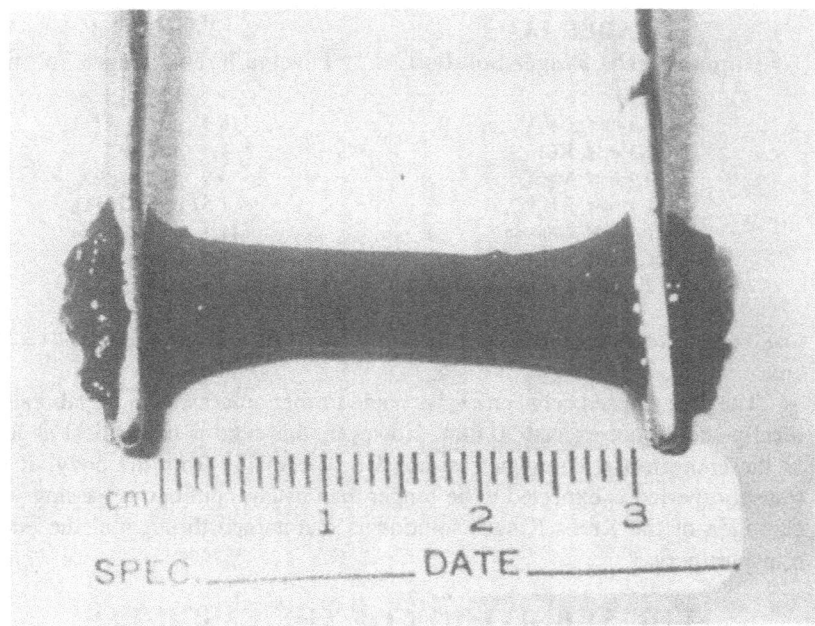

FIGURE 1. (B) Fascicle clamp.

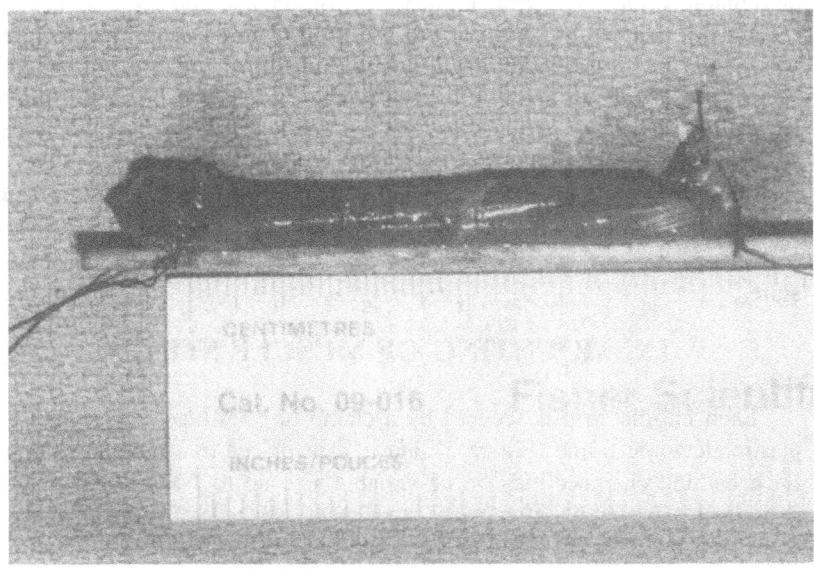

FIGURE 2. Fully dissected skeletal muscle fascicle is about 6 cm long. (From Britt, B. A., Ed., *Malignant Hyperthermia*, Martinus Nijhoff Publishing, Boston, 1987, 198. With permission.)

TABLE 1A	TABLE 1B
Human Krebs Ringer Solution	Porcine Krebs Ringer Solution

118.4 mM NaCl	118.4 mM NaCl
3.3 mM KCl	3.3 mM KCl
0.9 mM MgSO$_4$	0.9 mM MgSO$_4$
1.1 mM KH$_2$PO$_4$	1.57 mM KH$_2$PO$_4$
11.1 mM Glucose	11.1 mM Glucose
24.9 mM NaHCO$_3$	35.9 mM NaHCO$_3$
2.5 mM CaCl$_2$	2.5 mM CaCl$_2$

Note: pH of medium adjusted to 7.4 at 37°C.   *Note:* pH of medium adjusted to 7.4 at 37°C.

The time elapsed between excision and further processing in the laboratory ideally should not exceed 30 min. However, this time is not critical as long as the entire test is completed within 5 h of excision from the body. If the transport period is expected to be longer than usual, continuous gassing with carbogen of the Krebs Ringer solution is maintained throughout the entire transport period.

VIII. SUBDIVISION OF THE FASCICLES IN THE LABORATORY

In the laboratory, the muscle samples are trimmed free of any irregularities or remaining fat. To permit replicate measurements and measurements of several different drugs, drug doses, and drug combinations, the fascicle is subdivided into several strips each about 1–2 cm long and 0.1 to 0.5 cm wide. These samples weigh about 100 to 300 mg. Throughout the dissection the muscle is kept immersed in a Krebs Ringer solution that is being continuously bubbled with carbogen. Before mounting, each muscle strip should be examined through either a very powerful magnifying glass or a low-power microscope. All strips marred by nicks should be discarded. Prior to use, extra strips are kept in carbogenated Krebs Ringer solution at room temperature.

IX. MOUNTING OF MUSCLE STRIPS

Each muscle strip is secured by a clamp or by a black silk suture to a plastic electrode frame (Figure 3) and is then placed in a bathing chamber. Each bathing chamber may be of variable size up to 100 ml and must be periodically (preferably after every experiment) washed with acid or detergent and extensively rinsed prior to use. The bathing chambers are filled with Krebs Ringer solution maintained at 37°C and pH 7.4 ± 0.1. The pH of the Krebs Ringer solution should be rechecked daily. The bathing solution is aerated with 95% O$_2$ and 5% CO$_2$ at 20 ml/min. All tubing used in the carbogen/carbogen plus halothane lines must be made of Teflon® to reduce

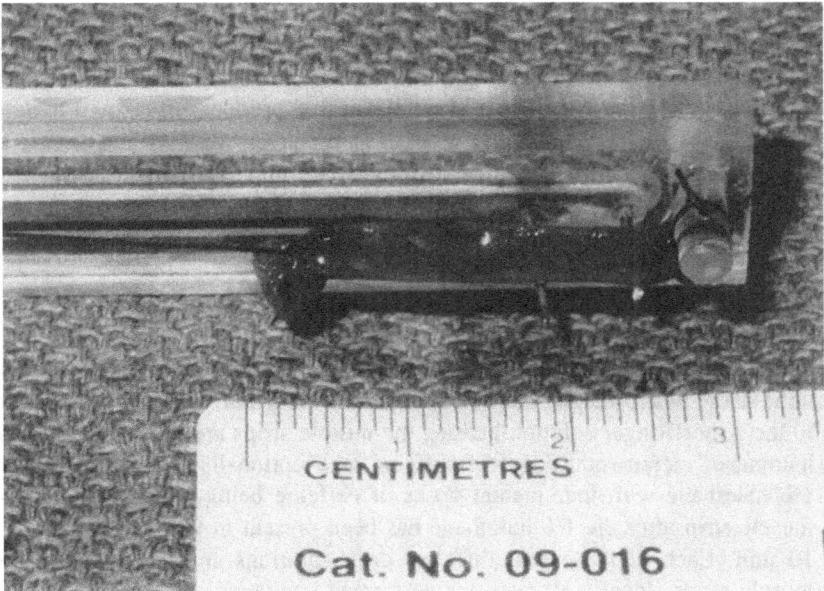

FIGURE 3. Subdivided skeletal muscle strip tied at each end with black silk sutures mounted on electrode housing and ready for placement in Krebs Ringer solution.

the amount of anesthetic adsorption unless the carbogen plus halothane line is totally separate from the carbogen line. In the latter case Tygon tubing may be substituted. The gas mixture enters the bottom of the chamber through a scintered porous ceramic or glass disk. This disk breaks the gas into very small bubbles, thereby increasing the area of surface contact between gas and muscle. All muscle testing should be done in a fume hood so that the anesthetic gases may be scavenged. Gloves are worn when coming into contact with the muscle because it is potentially infectious.

The upper end of the muscle strip is connected via a second black silk suture to a model FT.03 Grass force displacement transducer or a similar substitute. Linear calibration of the force displacement transducer with a known gram weight is done and shown on the polygraph record prior to attaching the muscle to the transducer. The polygraph used to record muscle tension may be any suitable model, for example, a Grass model 7 or a Gould Brush 2200.

X. STIMULATION OF THE MUSCLE STRIPS

To enable assessment of viability, triplicate muscle fascicles are stimulated every 5 to 10 s with a pulse duration of 1 to 5 ms to confirm muscle viability via platinum plate or prong electrodes. If a prong is used, it should be 0.5 to 1.0 mm in diameter. Each electrode is connected to a stimulator that is set to deliver impulses of 2 to 5 m in duration. Good twitch viability in each specimen should be demonstrated prior to testing. The stimulator should produce sufficient voltage and current to permit the attainment of supramaximal voltage (110% of the voltage that produces maximum twitch) in all tested fibers. The initial tension is set at an optimal length that is determined by first reversing polarity to obtain maximal response, then increasing the voltage to maximal twitch tension, and finally stretching the muscle strip to achieve absolute supramaximal twitch tension.

XI. DRUG ADDITIONS TO MUSCLE STRIPS

Before commencing drug additions, at least 15 min is allowed to elapse until stable twitch height and twitch baselines are achieved. The drugs added to the Krebs Ringer solution bathing the muscle strips are the following: 3% halothane, incremental doses of caffeine, and optionally 2% halothane and 1% halothane with incremental doses of caffeine being added to the same muscle strip after the 1% halothane has been present in the bath for at least 10 min. Each of these four different drug additions are made to separate muscle strips. Ideally all tests are performed simultaneously. If insufficient chambers are available, tests can be done sequentially, but at least three chambers should be used so that each test can be done in triplicate simultaneously.

The duration of exposure to 3% halothane is 10 min. The concentration of halothane in the gas line just before entry to the bathing chamber is measured daily. The most commonly used and least expensive device for doing this is a hand-held Riken portable anesthetic gas indicator, Model 18. The halothane line is also checked daily for back pressure that if present must be eliminated prior to its entrance into the bathing solution either by inserting a roller pump into the halothane line or by opening up an exit port from the halothane line to room air. At least once every 6 months (ideally more frequently) the concentration of halothane in the gas phase should be correlated with the concentration of halothane in the liquid Krebs Ringer solution. Serial measurements need to be made every 30 s or so until the halothane has achieved equilibrium in the bathing solution. The range of acceptable halothane concentrations is 2.7 to 3.3% (21 to 25 torr partial pressure). For the 3% halothane addition, the parameter measured is the amplitude of contracture, i.e., the distance from the lowest point to peak contracture. A contracture of greater than 0.2 to 0.7 g is defined as normal.

Caffeine alone is added to triplicate muscle strips. This drug is used because it is known to accelerate release of calcium from the sarcoplasmic reticulum (SR).[19,72-76] When preparing caffeine solutions, free-base caffeine is completely dissolved in a carbogenated human Krebs Ringer solution that is maintained at a pH of 7.4 ± 0.1 and a temperature of 37°C. Caffeine may be added either incrementally using a concentrated stock solution without draining the previous dose of caffeine from the bath or by fully draining the bath contents before replacement with the next highest concentration using a solution at a final concentration. The doses added are: 0.5, 1.0, 2.0, 4.0, (8.0 mM if the response at 4.0 mM is <1.0 g), and 32 mM. Each muscle strip is exposed to every concentration, except 32 mM, for at least 4 min or until a contracture plateau has been achieved, whichever is longer. Each strip is exposed to 32-mM caffeine solution for at least 10 min or until a double peak has been observed, whichever is longer.

The parameters measured for caffeine alone are the contractures noted 4 min after the addition of each caffeine dose, expressed as grams of tension. The values are then plotted on a semi-log graph and the concentration of caffeine needed to elevate the resting tension by 1.0 g is calculated. This concentration is termed the caffeine-specific concentration (CSC). Values in different laboratories of 2.0 to 4.0 mM are considered to be normal. Also reported is the amplitude of grams tension observed after the addition of 2.0 mM caffeine and the percent maximal tension achieved at 2.0 mM caffeine, i.e., 100 × tension at 2 mM concentration — tension before adding caffeine/total tension at 32 mM — tension before adding caffeine. For the former parameter the reference point ranges from 0.2 to 0.5 g and for the latter parameter the reference point is set between 1 and 7%, depending on the laboratory.

Optionally separate triplicate muscle fascicles are equilibrated for 15 min with 1.0 vol% halothane via the carbogen line. The functionality of the halothane vaporizer should be checked as described above. Caffeine is then added as previously described but in increments ascending from 0.25 mM. A smaller starting dose is used because of the potentiating effect of halothane on the caffeine contractures. The gram tension increase for each dose of caffeine plus 1% halothane is measured in the same manner as the fascicles equilibrated without halothane.

For caffeine plus 1% halothane, the parameters measured and the calculations made are the same as for caffeine alone. The reference point for the various laboratories in the North American group ranges from 0.3 to 1.0 mM caffeine. For caffeine plus halothane the CSC is termed the CSC-H.

Addition of 2% halothane to triplicate muscle strips is another separate and optional test. The testing conditions and the parameters reported are identical to those for 1 and 3% halothane alone. However, the reference point for 2% halothane has not yet been decided by the North American MH Registry.

XII. TERMINATION OF THE TEST

At the end of the contracture test, while the specimens are still mounted between the clamps or silk ties, each bath is drained and the dimensions of its fascicle are measured. The weight of the muscle is determined after cutting the muscle ends off within the silk ties or clamp and blotting the muscle dry on filter paper. Then the cross-sectional area (CSA) of each strip is calculated as follows: CSA = weight (g)/1.06 × length (cm), where 1.06 = the density of the muscle.

XIII. EFFECT OF HALOTHANE ON MUSCLE STRIPS

With the North American method of measurement, either 1 or 3% halothane alone produces contractures in the muscle from severely afflicted MHS individuals that are significantly bigger than those seen in control muscle (Tables 2 and 3 and Figure 4).[5,8,9,12,13,67,76-79] Efficiency, specificity, and sensitivity obtained with 3% halothane are somewhat greater than with 1% halothane. Sensitivity is low compared to specificity; however, it must be noted that sensitivity is probably falsely low for all parameters of the CHC test because the data in Table 4 include a number of individuals whose clinical reactions have been only possibly and not certainly due to MH. Furthermore, unlike MHS pigs, humans suspected of having MH cannot have the diagnosis clinically confirmed by deliberate challenge with halothane and succinylcholine under controlled laboratory conditions as such a procedure would be clearly highly unethical.

XIV. EFFECT OF CAFFEINE ON MUSCLE STRIPS

Several aspects of the caffeine-contracture and caffeine-twitch curves differ between MHS and normal muscle (Table 5, Figures 5 and 6A,B). At low concentrations of caffeine, twitches are higher in MHS than in control muscle, while at high concentrations twitches may be lower in MHS muscle because of earlier fatigue of the MHS than of the control muscle. Hence, in control muscle twitches continue to increase as the dose of caffeine rises, while in MHS muscle the twitches first increase sharply at low caffeine doses and then decline at high caffeine concentrations.

In control muscle the caffeine contracture, once developed, persists for some time at a level close to the peak, while in MHS muscle the contracture generally subsides substantially from its initial peak (Figure 5). This fatigue effect becomes more marked as the caffeine dose increases. The concentration of caffeine required to induce a threshold contracture is smaller in MHS than in control muscle (Figures 5 and 6B). The caffeine-contracture curve, however, is rather flat at low doses, especially in control muscle (Figure 6B). This makes determination of the threshold contracture quite difficult in some cases. Just below a 1-g tension the caffeine-contracture curve usually becomes much steeper (Figure 6). Therefore, a point on the curve at 1 g of tension is much easier to determine than that of a threshold contracture where the slope may be so flat as to be almost indistinguishable from the horizontal axis (Figure 6B). The CSC for MHS muscle is significantly lower than the CSC for control patients (Table 5).[80,81] Similarly the amplitude of contracture at 2 mM caffeine is significantly greater in MHS than in normal muscle (Table 6).

TABLE 2
1% Halothane Contractures in MHS and
Control Patients

Patient status	1% halothane contractures	t (MHS vs. Control)	p
MHS patients			
$\bar{x}$	0.850		
SE	0.203		
SD	2.140		
N	111		
		3.852	<0.0002
Control patients			
$\bar{x}$	0.063		
SE	0.024		
SD	0.153		
N	40		

Note: $\bar{x}$ = amplitude of halothane induced contracture in grams; SE = standard error; SD = standard deviation; N = sample size; MHS patients = all individuals described in Section II; and control patients = all individuals who have had no MH reaction or clinical anomalies associated with the MHS trait and who have no relatives who have had such a reaction.

TABLE 3
3% Halothane Contractures in MHS and
Control Patients

Patient status	3% halothane contractures	t (MHS vs. Control)	p
MHS patients			
$\bar{x}$	1.661		
SE	0.229		
SD	2.419		
N	111		
		6.330	<0.0001
Control patients			
$\bar{x}$	0.192		
SE	0.034		
SD	0.209		
N	39		

Note: $\bar{x}$ = amplitude of halothane induced contracture in grams; SE = standard error; SD = standard deviation; N = sample size; MHS patients = all individuals described in Section II; and control patients = all individuals who have had no MH reaction or clinical anomalies associated with the MHS trait and who have no relatives who have had such a reaction.

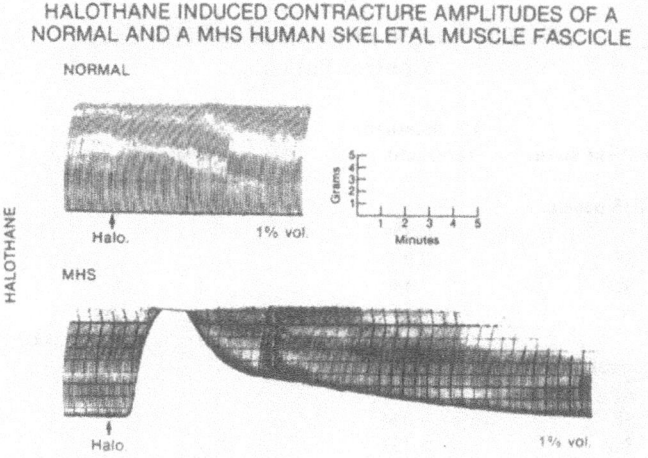

FIGURE 4. Halothane-induced contracture amplitudes of a normal and MHS human skeletal muscle fascicle. (From Britt, B. A., Ed., *Malignant Hyperthermia*, Martinus Nijhoff Publishing, Boston, 1987, 195. With permission.)

TABLE 4
Efficiency, Specificity, and Sensitivity of the Caffeine Halothane Contracture Test in MHS Probands and Controls

	EFFIC.	SPEC.	SENS.	TN	FP	TP	FN
1% halothane contractures ($\leq$0.3 g)	50.00	90.62	34.15	29	3	28	54
3% halothane contractures ($\leq$0.7 g)	55.86	96.88	39.24	31	1	31	48
CSC ($\geq$4.0 mM)	59.65	93.75	46.34	30	2	38	44
CSC–H ($\geq$0.35 mM)	55.26	93.75	40.24	30	2	33	49
2 mM caffeine contractures ($\geq$0.2 g)	47.62	96.88	26.03	31	1	19	54
2/32 mM caffeine contractures ($\geq$0.7%)	52.38	93.75	34.25	30	2	25	48

Note: EFFIC = efficiency = $\dfrac{TP + TN}{TP + FN + FP + FN}$;

SPEC = specificity = $\dfrac{TN}{TN + FP}$;

SENS = sensitivity = $\dfrac{TP}{TP + FN}$;

TN = true negative; FP = false positive; TP = true positive; and FN = false negative.

TABLE 5
Caffeine-Specific Concentrations (CSC) in MHS and Control Patients

Patient status	CSC	t (MHS vs. Control)	p
MHS patients			
$\bar{x}$	3.497		
SE	0.152		
SD	1.597		
N	41		
		−4.903	<0.0001
Control patients			
$\bar{x}$	4.698		
SE	0.192		
SD	1.232		
N	41		

Note: $\bar{x}$ = mean value of CSC (caffeine-specific concentration), i.e., dose of caffeine required to raise resting tension of a skeletal muscle fascicle by 1.0 g in absence of halothane. SE = standard error; SD = standard deviation; N = sample size; MHS patients = all individuals described in Section II; and control patients = all individuals who have had no MH reaction or clinical anomalies associated with the MHS trait and who have no relatives who have had such a reaction.

CAFFEINE DOSE — CONTRACTURE GRAPHS FOR A NORMAL AND
A MHS HUMAN SKELETAL MUSCLE FASCICLE
IN THE ABSENCE OF HALOTHANE

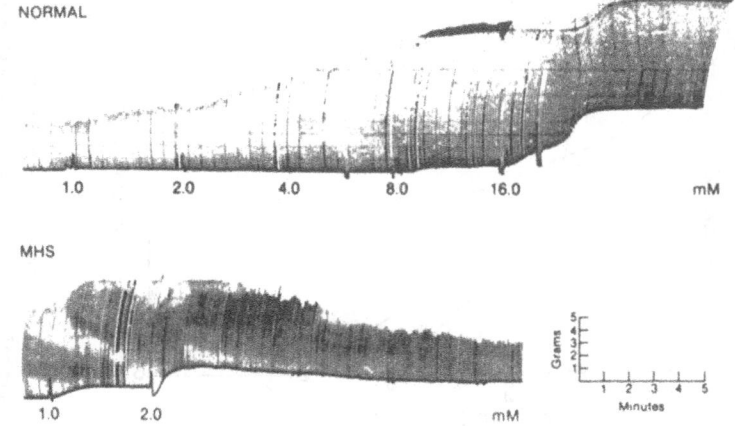

FIGURE 5. Caffeine dose — contracture graphs for a normal and a MHS skeletal muscle fascicle in the absence of halothane. (From Britt, B. A., Ed., *Malignant Hyperthermia*, Martinus Nijhoff Publishing, Boston, 1987, 194. With permission.)

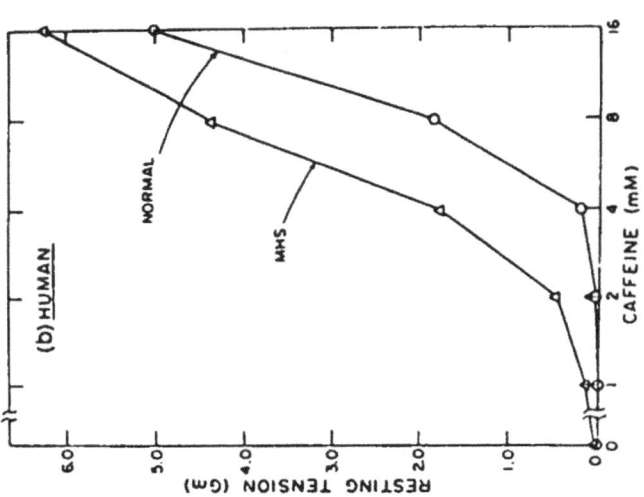

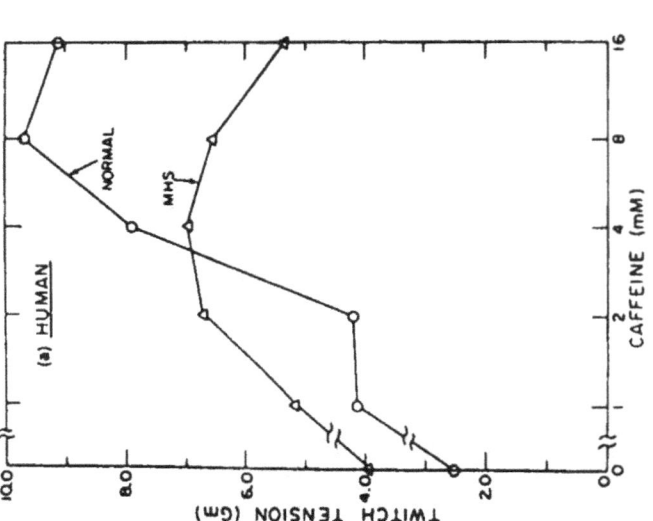

FIGURE 6. Effect of incremental doses of caffeine on (a) twitch and (b) resting tension; studies were done on human skeletal muscle. Horizontal axis shows cumulative doses of caffeine (in m*M*) added to each skeletal muscle fascicle. Thus, comparisons among these caffeine doses are within fascicles. Vertical axis shows mean (a) twitch and (b) resting tension (in gms) of the skeletal muscle fascicles. Two plots are shown: normal with caffeine and MHS with caffeine; comparisons between plots are between fascicles. (From Britt, B. A., et al., *Can. Anaesth. Soc. J.*, 31, 130, 1984. With permission.)

Finally, the percent tension increase (tension at 2 mM caffeine/tension at 32 mM caffeine) is greater in MHS than in normal muscle (Table 7).

XV. EFFECT OF CAFFEINE PLUS 1% HALOTHANE ON MUSCLE STRIPS

A left shift of the caffeine-contracture curve is obtained by adding halothane and caffeine together to the same muscle strip (Table 8, Figure 7).[80,81] This potentiating influence of halothane is particularly marked in MHS muscle strips. The CSC-H is the most sensitive of the various parameters measured in the CHC test (Table 4). On the other hand, normal values for the CSC but abnormal or borderline CSC-H values have been noted in a few healthy control subjects. In a previously reported series,[80] one such deviant value has been found among 35 control patients. There are four such values in a second and independent series of 34 controls;[81] therefore, it could be that a common, possibly recessive, genetic variant that may affect as much as 3 to 10% of the population is associated with positive CSC-H values but normal CSC values and normal halothane contractures. Such a variant could be responsible for mild MH reactions such as masseter muscle rigidity only (known to occur in 1:125 of halothane-succinylcholine pediatric anesthetics in the U.S.[82]). The coincidence of these masseter muscle rigidity reactions in pediatric patients based on *in vitro* testing by the CHC test ranges from about 50 to

TABLE 6
Contractures in Grams at 2 mM Caffeine in MHS and Control Patients

Patient status	Contractures at 2 mM caffeine	t (MHS vs. Control)	p
MHS patients			
$\bar{x}$	0.432		
SE	0.105		
SD	1.106		
N	111		
		2.890	0.0044
Control patients			
$\bar{x}$	0.086		
SE	0.057		
SD	0.362		
N	40		

Note: $\bar{x}$ = Contractures recorded after the addition of 2 mM caffeine, expressed as grams of tension. SE = standard error; SD = standard deviation; N = sample size; MHS patients = all individuals described in Section II; and control patients = all individuals who have had no MH reaction or clinical anomalies associated with the MHS trait and who have no relatives who have had such a reaction.

TABLE 7

Ratio of Contractures at 2 m*M* Caffeine Divided by
Tension at 32 m*M* Caffeine

Patient status	2/32 caffeine contractures	t (MHS vs. Control)	p
MHS patients			
$\bar{x}$	2.071		
SE	0.409		
SD	4.112		
N	101		
		4.781	<0.0001
Control patients			
$\bar{x}$	0.097		
SE	0.054		
SD	0.339		
N	40		

Note: $\bar{x}$ = Percent tension (tension at 2 m*M* caffeine) over tension at 32
m*M* caffeine; SE = standard error; SD = standard deviation; N =
sample size; MHS patients = all individuals described in Section II;
and control patients = all individuals who have had no MH reaction
or clinical anomalies associated with the MHS trait and who have
no relatives who have had such a reaction.

100%.[82-85] It might also be that a rare, probably dominant variant causes
fulminant MH reactions (occurring in about 1:15,000 to 1:150,000 anesthetics)
and positive halothane contractures and CSC values (unpublished postulation
by Dr. M. A. Rockoff).

XVI. INFLUENCE OF TEMPERATURE ON THE CHC TEST

CHC test results using halothane, caffeine, and 1% halothane plus caffeine
as the stimulating agents have been reported at both 22 and at 37°C (Tables
9 through 11).[12,86] We have observed that contractures induced by halothane
are not significantly less at 37 than at 22°C (Table 9); however, we have also
noted that diagnostic discrimination between normal and MHS halothane
contractures is greater at 37 than at 22°C. CSCs are significantly less at 37
than at 22°C (Table 10) because of greater contractures induced by caffeine
at 37 than at 22°C. In the presence of halothane CSC-Hs of MHS muscle but
not of control muscle are also significantly greater than those obtained at
22°C (Table 11). Sullivan and Denborough[86] have reported that raising the
temperature from 5 to 20°C markedly lowers caffeine contractures of both
MHS and control muscle strips, while further elevating the temperature to
37°C moderately enhances caffeine contractures of MHS but not of control
muscle. Therefore, in the laboratory of Sullivan and Denborough,[86] diagnostic

TABLE 8
Caffeine-Specific Concentrations in the Presence of Halothane (CSC–H) in MHS and Control Patients

Patient status	CSC–H	t (MHS vs. Control)	p
MHS patients			
$\bar{x}$	0.418		
SE	0.029		
SD	0.306		
N	111		
		−4.281	<0.0001
Control patients			
$\bar{x}$	0.786		
SE	0.081		
SD	0.511		
N	40		

Note: $\bar{x}$ = Mean value of CSC (caffeine-specific concentration), i.e., dose of caffeine required to raise resting tension of a skeletal muscle fascicle by 1.0 g in the presence of halothane. SE = standard error; SD = standard deviation; N = sample size; MHS patients = all individuals described in Section II; and control patients = all individuals who have had no MH reaction or clinical anomalies associated with the MHS trait and who have no relatives who have had such a reaction.

CAFFEINE DOSE — CONTRACTURE GRAPHS FOR A NORMAL AND A MHS HUMAN SKELETAL FASCICLE IN THE PRESENCE OF HALOTHANE

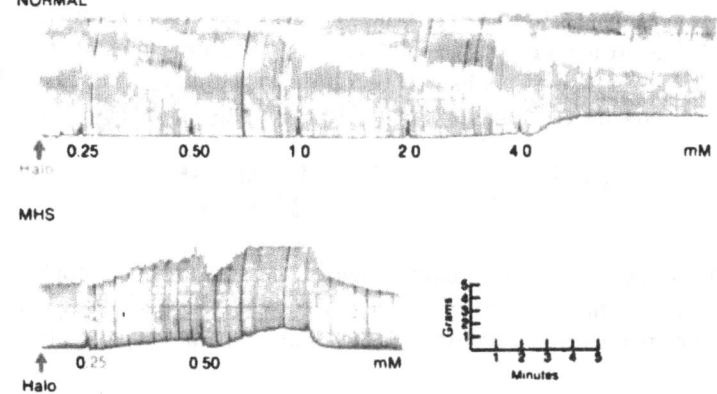

FIGURE 7. Caffeine-contracture graphs for a normal and a MHS human skeletal fascicle in the presence of halothane. (From Britt, B. A., in *Malignant Hyperthermia Current Concepts*, Nalda Felipe, M. A., Gottman, S., and Khambatta, H. J., Eds., Normed Verlag, Bad Hornburg, 1989, 62. With permission.)

TABLE 9
Effect of Temperature on Halothane-Induced
Muscle Contractures

Patient status	22°C	37°C	p[a]	Z (22 vs. 37)[b]
MHS patients				
$\bar{x}$	0.53	0.47	n.s.	n.s.
SE	0.19	0.16		
N	32	32		
Control patients				
$\bar{x}$	0.12	0.01	n.s.	n.s.
SE	0.06	0.01		
N	20	20		
p[a] (nonparametric)	n.s.	—		

Note: $\bar{x}$ = average contracture in grams, SE = standard error,
N = sample size, t = t test, p = probability.

[a] Probability levels of nonparametric test statistics based on the
sign test for paired observations and the Mann-Whitney test for
unpaired readings.
[b] Standardized normal variable comparing, under two conditions,
proportions of subjects having nonzero contractures.

From Britt, B. A. et al., *Can. Anaesth. Soc. J.*, 27, 1, 1980. With
permission.

discrimination between MHS and control muscle is better at 37 than at 22°C.
Because the CHC test can be performed considerably more rapidly at 37 than
at 22°C due to the steeper rate of ascent of the contractures at the former
temperature, most workers have chosen to measure human muscle at 37°C,
and this is now the temperature required by the North American MH Registry.

XVII. EFFECT OF OTHER DRUGS ON CONTRACTURES

The response of isometrically mounted muscle strips to theophylline is
qualitatively similar to that of caffeine, except that quantitatively the contracture responses are weaker in both the absence and in the presence of 1.0%
halothane.[88]

Nelson[88] has demonstrated that reduction of calcium in the bathing solution lowers caffeine-induced contractures of both control and MHS muscle
and, when bathing calcium is below 1.0 mM, the abnormal contracture responses of MHS muscle are eliminated. In MHS, but not in control, muscle
raising the concentration of potassium in the bathing solution (to 80 mM KCl)

TABLE 10

**Relationship between Caffeine-Specific Concentrations (CSC)
and Temperature in Control and MHS Patients**

Patient status	CSC in absence of halothane		Ratio 22/37	t (22 vs. 37)	p
	22°C	37°C			
MHS patients					
$\bar{x}$	4.78	2.92	1.64	3.87	—
SE	0.40	0.26			
N	15	15			
Control patients					
$\bar{x}$	16.85	7.33	2.30	4.85	—
SE	1.87	0.59			
N	13	13			
Statistics					
t (MHS vs. normal)	6.74	7.15			
p (MHS vs. normal)	—	—			

Note: $\bar{x}$ = CSC (caffeine-specific concentration), i.e., dose of caffeine required to raise the resting tension of skeletal muscle fascicle by 1.0 g in the absence of halothane; SE = standard error; N = sample size; t = t test; p = probability.

From Britt, B. A. et al., *Can. Anaesth. Soc. J.*, 27, 1, 1980. With permission.

induces (without other additives) a contracture but eliminates twitch tensions of MHS muscles but not of control muscles.[89]

Rosenberg,[90] following a suggestion made several years ago by Moulds,[91] has shown that the combined use of halothane and succinylcholine (50 mM) provides greater diagnostic differentiation than does the use of halothane, or caffeine, or succinylcholine alone when the succinylcholine is added to the bathing chamber after commencement of the halothane. Values noted in our laboratory are in agreement with these findings (Table 12, Figure 8). It is of interest that the sequential use of halothane followed by succinylcholine seems to correlate well with the combined use of halothane and caffeine. Consequently, individuals whose muscle fails to develop a contracture when exposed to halothane alone and demonstrates normal CSC levels but lower than normal CSC-H levels tend to be the same people whose muscle exhibits no contractures in the presence of succinylcholine alone but does so when exposed first to halothane and then to succinylcholine (50 mM).

We have compared the effects of halothane, enflurane, isoflurane, and methoxyflurane on MHS and control human muscle strips (Table 13).[13] Halothane exhibits the greatest ability to potentiate caffeine contractures, with enflurane and isoflurane following and methoxyflurane showing the least

TABLE 11
Relationship between Caffeine Plus Halothane-Specific Concentrations (CSC–H) and Temperature in Control and MHS Patients

Patient status	CSC in presence of halothane		Ratio	t	
	22°C	37°C	22/37	(22 vs. 37)	p
MHS patients					
x̄	0.54	0.88	0.62	2.76	—
SE	0.07	0.10			
N	15	15			
Control patients					
x̄	1.96	2.52	0.77	1.67	n.s.
SE	0.24	0.24			
N	13	13			
Statistics					
t (MHS vs. control)	6.08	6.68			
p (MHS vs. control)	—	—			

Note: x̄ = CSC-H (caffeine-specific concentration), i.e., dose of caffeine required to raise the resting tension of skeletal muscle fascicle by 1.0 g in the presence of halothane; SE = standard error; N = sample size; t = t test; p = probability.

From Britt, B. A. et al., *Can. Anaesth. Soc. J.*, 27, 1, 1980. With permission.

ability. The best diagnostic discrimination between the MHS and the control muscles is provided by halothane (Table 13). These *in vitro* findings are in agreement with the *in vivo* results reported by McGrath et al.[92]

Ryanodine, an alkaloid extracted from *Ryania speciosa*, has been suggested as an alternative to caffeine as a test drug for the diagnosis of MH[93] (P. Adnet, unpublished data). As ryanodine is freer than caffeine of actions on structures other than the SR and because of its effect on the foot plate, which links the transverse tubules to the SR, is more potent than that of caffeine, ryanodine should be preferred as a test drug to caffeine. This is especially so as it has recently been postulated that the site of the MH defect is this linking foot plate, which is now known as the ryanodine receptor.[94-97] On the other hand, contractures induced by ryanodine take a very long time to develop — upward of 30 min — and this problem may make the use of ryanodine as a test drug in the diagnosis of MH impractical.

In vivo pretreatment with dantrolene may make MHS skeletal muscle fascicles behave like normal skeletal muscle fascicles.[11,98,99] Thus, CSC values may rise into the normal range while halothane contractures are inhibited. *In vitro* treatment with dantrolene inhibits both twitch and resting tensions of normal and MHS muscle strips (Figures 9 and 10).

TABLE 12
Comparison of Succinylcholine and Halothane Plus Succinylcholine Contractures — MHS Patients and Their Relatives vs. Unrelated Control Patients: According to Type of CHC Test Result

	MHS patients and their relatives				
	All type H tests (HCK,HK,HC,H)	All type C tests (HCK,CK,HC,C)	All type K tests	Negative	Control patients
Succinylcholine					
$\bar{x}$	0.35	0.25	0.02	0.00	0.00
SE	0.18	0.10	0.01	0.00	0.00
N	27	49	78	31	10
T	0.89	0.82	0.84	0.00	—
p	n.s.	n.s.	n.s.	n.s.	—
Halothane + succinylcholine					
$\bar{x}$	1.53	0.14	0.39	0.08	0.16
SE	0.26	0.16	0.04	0.14	0.12
N	28	51	83	30	9
T	2.21	1.90	1.31	1.08	—
p	—	—	n.s.	n.s.	—

Note: $\bar{x}$ = arithmetic mean of contracture amplitudes of skeletal muscle fascicles, SE = standard error, N = sample size, T = MHS group compared to controls, p = probability.

From Britt, B. A., Ed., *Malignant Hyperthermia*, Martinus Nijhoff, Boston, 1987, 224. With permission.

EFFECT OF SUCCINYLCHOLINE ON MUSCLE CONTRACTURE OF NORMAL AND MHS PATIENTS IN THE PRESENCE OF HALOTHANE

NORMAL PATIENT

MHS PATIENT

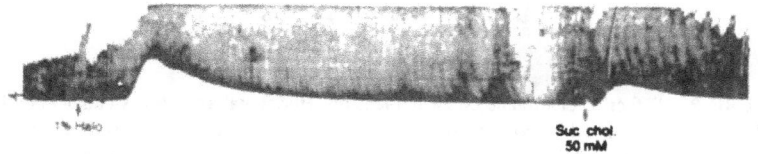

FIGURE 8. Effect of succinylcholine on contractures of normal and MHS human skeletal muscle fascicles in the presence of halothane. (From Britt, B. A., Ed., *Malignant Hyperthermia*, Martinus Nijhoff Publishing, Boston, 1987, 195. With permission.)

TABLE 13
Mean Caffeine-Specific Concentrations[a] in the Presence and Absence of Anaesthetics

Patient	Caffeine with			
status	Methoxyflurane	Enflurane	Isoflurane	Halothane
Control patients	5.04 ± 0.41[b] (19)[c]	3.69 ± 0.55 (16)	3.24 ± 0.75 (10)	1.92 ± 0.13 (31)
MHS patients	1.82 ± 0.28 (11)	1.49 ± 0.32 (9)	1.23 ± 0.32 (11)	0.62 ± 0.09 (20)
Ratio t[d]	2.77 ± 0.45 6.82***	2.48 ± 0.66 3.85**	2.64 ± 0.97 3.80*	3.12 ± 0.44 8.72***

[a]   The concentration required to raise the resting skeletal muscle tension by 1 g.
[b]   Geometric mean ± its standard error.
[c]   Number of subjects.
[d] t statistic comparing caffeine-specific concentrations of patients and controls. The levels of statistical significance are based on Duncan's multiple range test: *($p \leq 0.05$); **($p \leq 0.01$); ***($p \leq 0.005$).

From Britt, B. A. et al., *Can. Anaesth. Soc. J.*, 27, 12, 1980. With permission.

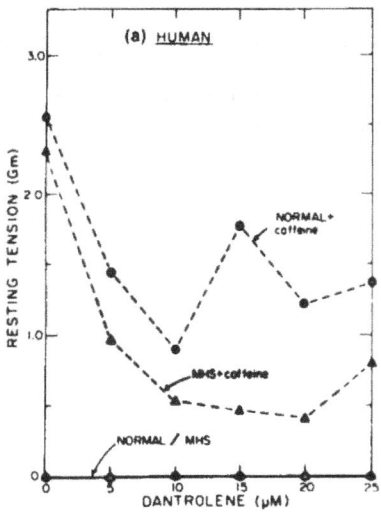

FIGURE 9. Effect of dantrolene on twitch tension: Horizontal axis shows cumulative doses of dantrolene (in μM) added to each skeletal muscle fascicle; thus, comparisons among these dantrolene doses are within fascicles. Vertical axis shows mean twitch tension (in gms) of the fascicles in the presence of various dose combinations of danitrolene and caffeine. Four plots are shown: (1) normal without caffeine; (2) normal with caffeine CSC × 2; (3) MHS without caffeine; (4) MHS with caffeine CSC × 2. Thus, comparisons between plots are between fascicles. (From Britt, B. A., et al., *Can. Anaesth. Soc. J.*, 31, 132, 1984. With permission.)

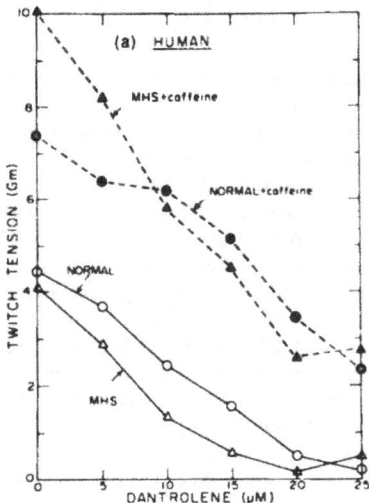

FIGURE 10. Effect of dantrolene on resting tension: Horizontal axis shows cumulative doses of dantrolene (in μ*M*) added to each skeletal muscle fascicle; thus, comparisons among these danitrolene doses are within fascicles. Vertical axis shows mean twitch tension (in gms) of the fascicles in the presence of various dose combinations of danitrolene and caffeine. Four plots are shown: (1) normal without caffeine; (2) normal with caffeine CSC × 2; (3) MHS without caffeine; (4) MHS with caffeine CSC × 2. Thus, comparisons between plots are between fascicles. (From Britt, B. A., et al., *Can. Anaesth. Soc. J.*, 31, 143, 1984. With permission.)

XVIII. CONCLUSIONS

To conclude, over 20 years of experience have shown the CHC test to be both a sensitive and a specific means of diagnosing MH because: (1) it provides several parameters in which MHS muscle differs from normal muscle and (2) there is little overlapping between the MHS and the normal muscle.

REFERENCES

1. **Britt, B. A.,** Malignant hyperthermia — an investigation of three patients, *Ann. R. Coll. Surg. Engl.,* 48, 73, 1971.
2. **Harrison, G. G.,** Recent advances in the understanding of anaesthetic-induced malignant hyperpyrexia, *Anaesthesist,* 22, 373, 1973.
3. **Anderson, I. L. and Jones, E. W.,** Dantrolene sodium in porcine MH: studies on isolated muscle strips, in *Second Int. Symp. Malignant Hyperthermia,* J. A. Aldrete and B. A. Britt, Eds., New York, Grune & Stratton, 1978, 509.
4. **Britt, B. A., Kalow, W., and Endrenyi, L.,** Malignant hyperthermia — pattern of inheritance in swine, in *Second Int. Symp. Hyperthermia,* J. A. Aldrete and B. A. Britt, Eds., New York, Grune & Stratton, 1978, 195.
5. **Britt, B. A., Endrenyi, L., Kalow, W., and Peters, P. L.,** The adenosine triphosphate depletion test: comparison with the caffeine contracture test as a method of diagnosing malignant hyperthermia susceptibility, *Can. Anaesth. Soc. J.,* 23, 624, 1976.
6. **Moulds, R. F. W. and Denborough, M. A.,** Biochemical basis of malignant hyperpyrexia, *Br. Med. J.,* ii, 241, 1974.
7. **Nelson, T. E.,** Excitation-contraction coupling: a common etiologic pathway for malignant hyperthermia susceptible muscle, in *Second Int. Symp. Malignant Hyperthermia,* J. A. Aldrete and B. A. Britt, Eds., New York, Grune & Stratton, 1978, 23.
8. **Britt, B. A., McComas, A. J., Endrenyi, L., and Kalow, W.,** Motor unit counting and the caffeine contracture test in malignant hyperthermia, *Anesthesiology,* 47, 490, 1977.
9. **Britt, B. A.,** Preanaesthetic diagnosis of malignant hyperthermia, *Int. Anesthesiol. Clin.,* 17, 62, 1979.
10. **Britt, B. A., Endrenyi, L., Peters, P. L. et al.,** Screening of malignant hyperthermic susceptible families by CPK measurement and other clinical investigation, *Can. Anaesth. Soc. J.,* 23, 263, 1976.
11. **Nelson, T. E. and Flewellen, E. H.,** Does prior dantrolene affect the *in vitro* diagnosis of malignant hyperthermia susceptibility?, *Can. Anaesth. Soc. J.,* 26, 484, 1979.
12. **Britt, B. A., Endrenyi, L., Scott, E., and Frodis, W.,** The effect of temperature, time and fascicle size on the caffeine contracture test, *Can. Anaesth. Soc. J.,* 27, 1, 1980.
13. **Britt, B. A., Endrenyi, L., Frodis, W. et al.,** Comparison of effects of several inhalation anaesthetics on caffeine-induced contractures of normal and malignant hyperthermic skeletal muscle, *Can. Anaesth. Soc. J.,* 27, 12, 1980.
14. **Ellis, F. R., Harriman, D. G. F., Kyei-Mensa, K. et al.,** Halothane-induced muscle contracture as a cause of hyperpyrexia, *Br. J. Anaesth.,* 43, 721, 1971.
15. **Anderson, I. L. and Jones, E. W.,** Porcine malignant hyperthermia: effect of dantrolene sodium on *in vitro* halothane-induced contraction of susceptible muscle, *Anesthesiology,* 44, 57, 1976.
16. **Anderson, I. L., Rawstron, R. E., and Dunlop, D. L.,** Screening for malignant hyperthermia susceptibility, *N. Z. Med. J.,* 91, 417, 1980.
17. **Nelson, T. E., Bedell, D. M., and Jones, E. W.,** Porcine malignant hyperthermia: effects of temperature and extracellular calcium concentration on halothane-induced contracture of susceptible skeletal muscle, *Anesthesiology,* 42, 301, 1975.
18. **Harriman, D. G. F. and Ellis, F. R.,** Structural and neuropharmacological aspects of malignant hyperpyrexia, *J. Pathol.,* 107, 9, 1972.
19. **Gutmann, E. and Sandow, A.,** Caffeine-induced contracture and potentiation of contraction in normal and denervated rat muscle, *Life Sciences,* 4, 1149, 1965.
20. **Rosenberg, J. and Reed, S.,** *In vitro* contracture tests for susceptibility to malignant hyperthermia, *Anesth. Analg.,* 62, 415, 1983.
21. **Iwatsuki, N., Koga, Y., and Amaha, K.,** Responses of *in vitro* muscle susceptible to malignant hyperthermia to caffeine, halothane, enflurane, succinylcholine and diltiazem, *Hiroshima J. Anaesth.,* 19, 68, 1983.

22. **Britt, B. A.**, Muscle assessment of malignant hyperthermia susceptible patients, in *Malignant Hyperthermia*, B. A. Britt, Ed., Martinus Nijhoff, Boston, 1987, 269.

23. **Ording, H.**, The European MH group: protocol for *in vitro* diagnosis of susceptibility to MH and preliminary results, in *Malignant Hyperthermia*, B. A. Britt, Ed., Martinus Nijhoff, Boston, 1987, 269.

24. **Gallant, E. M. and Rempel, W. E.**, Porcine malignant hyperthermia: false negatives in the halothane test, *Am. J. Vet. Res.*, 48, 488, 1987.

25. **Ording, H., Ranklev, E., and Fletcher, R.**, Investigation of malignant hyperthermia in Denmark and Sweden, *Br. J. Anaesth.*, 56, 1138, 1984.

26. **Ording, H. and Skovgaard, L. T.**, *In vitro* diagnosis of susceptibility to malignant hyperthermia: comparison between dynamic and static halothane and caffeine tests, *Acta Anaesth. Scand.*, 31, 458, 1987.

27. **Ording, H. and Skovgaard, L. T.**, *In vitro* diagnosis of susceptibility to malignant hyperthermia: evaluation of tests with halothane-caffeine, potassium chloride, suxamethonium and caffeine-suxamethonium, *Acta Anaesth. Scand.*, 31, 462, 1987.

28. **Ranklev, E. and Fletcher, R.**, Investigation of malignant hyperthermia in Sweden, *Acta Anaesth. Scand.*, 31, 462, 1987.

29. **Ranklev, E., Fletcher, R., and Bloomquist, S.**, Static v. Dynamic tests in the *in vitro* diagnosis of malignant hyperthermia susceptibility, *Br. J. Anaesth.*, 58, 646, 1986.

30. **Mauritz, W., Sporn, P., and Steinbereithner, K.**, Epidemiological and clinical aspects of 65 cases of malignant hyperthermia (MH) in Austria, *Anaesthesist*, 35, 639, 1986.

31. **Krivosic-Horber, R., Theunynck, D., Krivosic, I. et al.**, Exploration de la famille d'un sujet sensible a l'hyperthermie maligne anesthesique, *Ann. Fr. Anesth. Reanim.*, 5, 326, 1986.

32. **Kozak-Reiss, G., Gascared, J. P., and Redouane-Benicou, K.**, Depistage de l'hyperthermie maligne anesthesique par les tests de contracture musculaire et par la spectroscopie RMN, *Ann. Fr. Anesth. Renanim.*, 5, 584, 1986.

33. **Klein, W., Spiess-Kiefer, C., Kuther, G. et al.**, Diagnose der Anlage zu maligner Hyperthermie mit Hilfe des vitro-Kontrakturtests, *Anaesthesist*, 36, 685, 1987.

34. **Ellis, F. R.**, Laboratory diagnosis of malignant hyperpyrexia susceptibility, *Br. J. Anaesth.*, 57, 1038, 1985.

35. **Ellis, F. R., Halsall, P. J., and Harriman, D. G. F.**, The work of the Leeds malignant hyperpyrexia unit, 1971–1984, *Anaesthesia*, 41, 809, 1986.

36. **Krovosic-Horber, R., Adnet, P., Krivosic, I. et al.**, Tests de contracture et sensibilte a l'hyperthermie anesthesique chez vingt-sept sujets suspects, *Ann. Fr. Anesth. Reanim.*, 7, 132, 1988.

37. **Ording, H.**, Diagnosis of susceptibility to malignant hyperthermia in man, *Br. J. Anaesth.*, 60, 287, 1988.

38. **Ording, H. and Nielsen, V. G.**, Atracurium and its antagonism by neostigmine (plus glycopyrrolate) in patients susceptible to malignant hyperthermia, *Br. J. Anaesth.*, 58, 1001, 1986.

39. **Ording, H., Hansen, U., and Skovgaard, T.**, Age, fiber type composition and *in vitro* contracture responses in human malignant hyperthermia, *Acta Anaesth. Scand.*, 32, 121, 1988.

40. **European MH Group**, A protocol for the investigation of malignant hyperpyrexia (MH) susceptibility, *Br. J. Anaesth.*, 56, 1267, 1984.

41. **Benedetti, A., Bresadola, F., Welber, D.**, Ipertermia maligna, *Minn. Anesthesiol.*, 55, 287, 1989.

42. **Hackl, W., Winkler, M., Mauritz, W., and Steinbereithner, K.**, Die Wirkung von Ketamin auf das muskulare Kontraktionsverhalten: in vitro Studien an der muskulatur von Anlagetragern der Malignen Hyperthermi (MH), *Anaesthesist*, 38, 681, 1989.

43. **Adnet, P. J., Krivosic-Horber, R. M., Adamantidis, M. M., Haudecoeur, G., Reyfort, G. H., and Dupuis, B. A.**, Clinical concentrations of verapamil affect the *in vitro* diagnosis of susceptibility to malignant hyperpyrexia, *Br. J. Anaesth.*, 64, 64, 1990.

44. Ording, H., Influence of propranolol on the *in vitro* response to caffeine and halothane in malignant hyperthermia-susceptible muscle, *Acta Anaesthesiol. Scand.*, 33, 405, 1989.
45. Meier-Hellmann, A., Romer, M., Hannemann, L., Kersting, T., and Reinhart, K., Fruherkennung einer malignen Hyperthermie durch Capnometrie, *Anaesthesist*, 39, 41, 1990.
46. Krivosic-Horber, R. and Krivosic, I., Myopathie a axe central (central core disease) associee a une sensibilite a l'hyperthermie maligne, *La Presse Medicale*, 18, 828, 1989.
47. Jacquot, C., Stieglitz, P., Kozak-Reiss, G., Krivosic-Horber, R., Laxenaire, M. C., Lienhart, A., and Nivoche, Y., *Ann. Fr. Anesth. Reanim.*, 7, 524, 1988.
48. Iaizzo, P. A. and Lehmann-Horn, F., The *in vitro* determination of susceptibility to malignant hyperthermia, *Muscle Nerve*, 12, 184, 1989.
49. Heiman-Patterson, T., Fletcher, J. E., Rosenberg, H., and Tahmoush, A. J., No relationship between fiber type and halothane contracture test results in malignant hyperthermia, *Anesthesiology*, 67, 82, 1987.
50. Heiman-Patterson, T., Martino, C., Rosenberg, H., Fletcher, J., and Tahmoush, A., Malignant hyperthermia in myotonia congenita, *Neurology*, 38, 810, 1988.
51. Backman, E., Lennmarken, C., Rutberg, H., and Henriksson, K. G., Skeletal muscle contraction characteristics *in vivo* in malignant hyperthermia susceptible subjects, *Acta Neurol. Scand.*, 77, 278, 1988.
52. Allen, G. C. and Rosenberg, H., Malignant hyperthermia susceptibility in adult patients with masseter muscle rigidity, *Can. J. Anaesth.*, 37, 31, 1990.
53. Fletcher, J. E. and Rosenberg, H., *In vitro* muscle contractures induced by halothane and suxamethonium. II. Human skeletal muscle from normal and malignant hyperthermia susceptible patients, *Br. J. Anaesth.*, 58, 1433, 1986.
54. Gallant, E. M. and Rempel, W. E., Porcine malignant hyperthermia: false negatives in the halothane test, *Am. J. Vet. Res.*, 48, 488, 1987.
55. Gallant, E. M., Fletcher, T. F., Goettl, V. M., and Rempel, W. E., *Muscle Nerve*, 9, 174, 1986.
56. Fletcher, J. E., Rosenberg, H., and Lizzo, F. H., Effects of droperidol, haloperidol and ketamine on halothane, succinylcholine and caffeine contractures: implications for malignant hyperthermia, *Acta Anaesthesiol. Scand.*, 33, 187, 1989.
57. Ervasti, J. M., Mickelson, J. R., and Louis, C. F., Transverse tubule calcium regulation in malignant hyperthermia, *Arch. Biochem. Biophys.*, 269, 497, 1989.
58. Ervasti, J. M., Claessens, M. T., Mickelson, J. R., and Louis, C. F., Altered transverse tubule dihydropyridine receptor binding in malignant hyperthermia, *J. Biol. Chem.*, 264, 2711, 1989.
59. O'Brien, P. J., Klip, A., Britt, B. A., and Kalow, B. I., Malignant hyperthermia susceptibility: biochemical basis for pathogenesis and diagnosis, *Can. J. Vet. Res.*, 54, 83, 1990.
60. Allen, G. and Rosenberg, H., Muscle biopsy: testing for malignant hyperthermia, *Plast. Reconstr. Surg.*, 84, 373, 1989.
61. Larach, M. G., Standardization of the caffeine halothane muscle contracture test, *Anesth. Analg.*, 69, 511, 1989.
62. Melton, A. T., Martucci, R. W., Kien, N. D., and Gronert, G. A., Malignant hyperthermia in humans — standardization of contracture testing protocol, *Anesth. Analg.*, 69, 437, 1989.
63. Allen, G. C., Fletcher, J. E., Huggins, F. J., Conti, P. A., and Rosenberg, H., Caffeine and halothane contracture testing in swine using the recommendations of the North American malignant hyperthermia group, *Anesthesiology*, 72, 71, 1990.
64. Klip, A., Mills, G. B., Britt, B. A., and Elliott, M. E., Halothane-dependent release of intracellular Ca^{2+} in blood cells in malignant hyperthermia, *Am. J. Physiol.*, 258 (*Cell Physiol.* 27), C495, 1990.
65. Wieland, S. J., Fletcher, J. E., Rosenberg, H., and Gong, Q. H., Malignant hyperthermia: slow sodium current in cultured human muscle cells, *Am. J. Physiol.*, 257 (*Cell Physiol.* 26), C759, 1989.

66. **Britt, B. A.**, Elective diagnosis of malignant hyperthermia — review, in *Malignant Hyperthermia, Proc. Sixth Myology Colloquium*, J. G. Hofmann and A. Schmidt, Eds., Berlin: VEB Verlag Volk und Gesundheit, 1988, 42–90.

67. **Britt, B. A.**, The North American caffeine halothane contracture test, in *Malignant Hyperthermia Current Concepts, International Course*, Barcelona, Spain, Sept. 15–17, 1988, M. A. Nalda Felipe, S. Gottmann, and H. J. Khambatta, Eds., Normed Verlag, Bad Homburg, 1989, 53.

68. **Brownell, A. K. W. and Szabo, M.**, The *in vitro* caffeine contracture test: influence of the muscle histochemical profile on test results, *Can. Anaesth. Soc. J.*, 29, 218, 1982.

69. **Frank, G. B. and Buss, W. C.**, Caffeine-induced contractures in mammalian skeletal muscle, *Arch. Int. Pharmacodyn.*, 170, 343, 1967.

70. **Collins, S. P., White, M. D., and Denborough, M. A.**, Calmodulin-antagonist drugs and porcine malignant hyperpyrexia, *Clin. Exp. Pharmacol. Physiol.*, 15, 473, 1988.

71. **Foster, P. S., Hopkinson, K. C., and Denborough, M. A.**, Effect of diltiazem, verapamil and dantrolene on the contractility of isolated malignant hyperpyrexia-susceptible human skeletal muscle, *Clin. Exp. Pharmacol. Physiol.*, 16, 799, 1989.

72. **Caputo, C.**, Caffeine- and potassium-induced contractures of frog striated muscle fibers in hypertonic solutions, *J. Gen. Physiol.*, 50, 129, 1966.

73. **Weber, A.**, The mechanism of the action of caffeine on sarcoplasmic reticulum, *J. Gen. Physiol.*, 52, 760, 1968.

74. **Weber, A. and Herz, R.**, The relationship between caffeine contracture of intact muscle and the effect of caffeine on reticulum, *J. Gen. Physiol.*, 52, 750, 1968.

75. **Lin, W. and Bittar, E.**, Some observations on caffeine-induced contracture of barnacle muscle fibers, *Life Sci.*, 15, 1611, 1975.

76. **Britt, B. A.**, Malignant hyperthermia, in *Complications in Anesthesiology*, F. K. Orkin and L. H. Cooperman, Eds., Lippincott, Philadelphia, 1982, 291.

77. **Nelson, T. E. and Schochet, S. S., Jr.**, Malignant hyperthermia: a disease of specific myofiber type?, *Can. Anaesth. Soc. J.*, 29, 163, 1982.

78. **Ellis, F. R.**, Malignant hyperpyrexia, *Br. Med. J.*, i, 249, 1973.

79. **Britt, B. A., Frodis, W., Scott, E. et al.**, Comparison of the caffeine skinned fibre tension (CSFB) test with the caffeine-halothane contracture (CHC) test in the diagnosis of malignant hyperthermia, *Can. Anaesth. Soc. J.*, 29, 550, 1982.

80. **Kalow, W., Britt, B. A., and Richter, A.**, The caffeine test of isolated human muscle in relation to malignant hyperthermia, *Can. Anaesth. Soc. J.*, 24, 678, 1977.

81. **Britt, B. A.**, Malignant hyperthermia: a review, in *Handbook of Experimental Pharmacology*, A. S. Milton, Ed., Berlin, Springer-Verlag, 60, 1982, 547.

82. **Schwartz, L., Koka, B. V., and Rockoff, M. A.**, Masseter spasm after halothane and succinylcholine: incidence and implications, *Anesthesiology*, 59, A438, 1983.

83. **Rosenberg, H. and Reed, S.**, *In vitro* contracture tests for susceptibility to malignant hyperthermia, *Anesth. Analg.*, 72, 415, 1983.

84. **Ellis, D. R. and Halsall, P. J.**, Suxamethonium spasm: a differential diagnostic conundrum, *Br. J. Anaesth.*, 56, 381, 1984.

85. **Rosenberg, H. and Fletcher, J. E.**, More about masseter spasm and malignant hyperthermia, *Anesthesiology*, 62, 212, 1985.

86. **Sullivan, J. S. and Denborough, M. A.**, Temperature dependence of muscle function in malignant hyperpyrexia-susceptible swine, *Br. J. Anaesth.*, 53, 1217, 1981.

87. **Sullivan, J. S. and Denborough, M. A.**, Is theophylline, aminophylline or caffeine (methylxanthines) contraindicated in malignant hyperthermia susceptible patients?, *Anesth. Analg.*, 62, 115, 1983.

88. **Nelson, T. E.**, Abnormality in calcium release from skeletal sarcoplasmic reticulum of pigs susceptible to malignant hyperthermia, *J. Clin. Invest.*, 72, 862, 1983.

89. **Moulds, R. F. W., Denborough, M. A., Anderson, R. M., and Dennett, X.**, Studies on muscle in malignant hyperpyrexia, *Aust. N.Z. J. Med.*, iv, 106, 1974.

90. **Rosenberg, H.**, Masseter muscle rigidity, presented at the 4th *Int.* Malignant Hyperpyrexia Workshop, York, England, September 1986.

91. **Moulds, F. R. W.**, The site of the abnormality in MH muscle: a comparison of MH muscle and denervated muscle, in *Second Int. Symp. Malignant Hyperthermia,* J. A. Aldrete and B. A. Britt, Eds., Grune & Stratton, New York, 1978, 49.

92. **McGrath, C. J., Rempel, W. E., Addis, P. B., and Crimi, A. J.**, Acepromazine and droperidol inhibition of halothane-induced malignant hyperthermia (porcine stress syndrome) swine, *Am. J. Vet. Res.,* 42, 195, 1981.

93. **Casson, H. and Downes, J.**, Ryanodine toxicity as a model of malignant hyperthermia, in *Second Int. Symp. Malignant Hyperthermia,* J. A. Aldrete and B. A. Britt, Eds., Grune & Stratton, New York, 1978, 3.

94. **MacLennan, D. H., Duff, C., Zorzato, F., Fujii, J., Phillips, M., Korneluk, R. G., Frodis, W., Britt, B. A., and Worton, R. G.**, Ryanodine receptor gene is a candidate for predisposition to malignant hyperthermia, *Nature,* 342, 559, 1990.

95. **McCarthy, T. V., Healy, J. M. S., Heffron, J. J. A., Deufel, T., Lehmann-Horn, F., Farrell, M., and Johnson, K.**, Localization of the malignant hyperthermia susceptibility locus to human chromosome 19q 12–13.2, *Nature,* 343, 562, 1990.

96. **Fill, M., Coronado, R., Mickelson, J. R., Vilven, J., Ma, J., Jacobson, B. A., and Louis, C. F.**, Abnormal ryanodine receptor channels in malignant hyperthermia, *Biophys. J.,* 50, 471, 1990.

97. **Nelson, T. E.**, Ryanodine: antithetical calcium channel effects in skeletal muscle sarcoplasmic reticulum, *J. Pharmacol. Exp. Ther.,* 242, 56, 1987.

98. **Lambert, W.**, Dantrolene and caffeine contracture test, *Can. Anaesth. Soc. J.,* 27, 304, 1980.

99. **Paasuke, R. T. and Brownell, A. K. W.**, Dantrolene and *in vitro* contracture testing, presented at the 4th Int. Malignant Hyperpyrexia Workshop, York, England, September 1986.

Chapter 14

MEASUREMENT OF CALCIUM-INDUCED CALCIUM RELEASE ACTIVITY IN THE SARCOPLASMIC RETICULUM MEMBRANE WITH SPECIAL REFERENCE TO DIAGNOSIS OF MALIGNANT HYPERTHERMIA

Makoto Endo

TABLE OF CONTENTS

I. Introduction 200

II. General Consideration for CICR Activity Determination 201

III. Preparation of Skinned Fibers 201

IV. Ca^{2+} Measurements 202

References 210

0-8493-8093-6/94/$0.00 + $.50
© 1994 by CRC Press, Inc.

I. INTRODUCTION

The membrane of the sarcoplasmic reticulum (SR) has at least two physiological functions, Ca^{2+} uptake and Ca^{2+} release. Responsible for Ca^{2+} uptake is the Ca^{2+} pump protein (Ca^{2+}-Mg^{2+}-ATPase), which is densely packed in most parts of the SR membrane. On the other hand, physiological Ca^{2+} release is caused by an opening of Ca^{2+} release channels that are located at a specialized part of the SR opposite the T-tubule membrane. The physiological signal to open these Ca^{2+} release channels is considered to be mediated on T-tubule depolarization through some protein-protein interaction between the T-tubule voltage sensor and the channel protein (Ebashi, 1991). These Ca^{2+} release channels can also be opened in an entirely different mode by raising the cytoplasmic Ca^{2+} concentration. This mode of channel opening, Ca^{2+}-induced Ca^{2+} release (CICR), was discovered in about 1970 in skinned fibers (Ford and Podolsky, 1970; Endo et al., 1970), long before channel protein isolation. The CICR mode of channel opening is not physiological, however, as the physiological signal mediator is something other than Ca^{2+} as mentioned above. This mode operates under the action of drugs such as caffeine or halothane. Caffeine, a well-known contraction-inducing alkaloid, increases the Ca^{2+} sensitivity of CICR so much that the resting Ca^{2+} concentration could evoke Ca^{2+} release and hence muscle contraction (Endo, 1985).

CICR is also important pathophysiologically. Malignant hyperthermia (MH) is a hereditary disease in which an extremely high fever is developed during inhalation anesthesia without any obvious causes (Denborough and Lovell, 1960). The most plausible theory for the etiology of MH is accelerated CICR. CICR of muscles in MH patients or animals has a higher Ca^{2+} sensitivity and greater opening probability at a given Ca^{2+} concentration than that of normal muscle (Endo et al., 1983; Ohta et al., 1989). Abnormal CICR from the fragmented SR of MH pigs has also been reported by several groups (Kawana et al., 1992). As halothane and other usual inhalation anesthetics increase the Ca^{2+} sensitivity of CICR (Matsui and Endo, 1986), CICR in MH muscle (but not in normal muscle) is so sensitized under anesthetics that the resting Ca^{2+} concentration causes Ca^{2+} release from the SR to evoke contraction, which in turn produces heat for the extreme fever. Therefore, determination of Ca^{2+} sensitivity of CICR is expected to have a diagnostic value, and indeed we have shown that this is the case (for references, see Kawana et al., 1992): a point mutation in the CICR channel protein (ryanodine receptor) in porcine MH was recently reported (Fujii et al., 1991). In this chapter, the method of determining the activity of the CICR of skeletal muscle by using the skinned fiber preparation will be described.

II. GENERAL CONSIDERATION FOR CICR ACTIVITY DETERMINATION

In this chapter, description of the method of determining CICR activity is confined to using skinned fiber preparation. Vesicles of fragmented SR constitute a purer system, but skinned fibers have the following advantages over fragmented SR:

1. Skinned fibers are more physiological and less susceptible to possible denaturation during preparation procedure.
2. Exchange of environmental solutions could be made very rapidly in skinned fibers, while in fragmented SR it must be either slow because filtration or centrifugation is necessary or less precise as in the case of dilution.
3. In fragmented SR, vesicles could be heterogeneous and some vesicles may not have CICR channels; therefore, a simple exponential Ca^{2+} release cannot be expected even in an ideal experimental condition. In skinned fibers, on the other hand, Ca^{2+} release follows an exponential time course if proper care as described below is taken, probably because the system is uniform and large with the continuous lumen.
4. Volume of muscle necessary for the determination is much smaller in the experiments with skinned fibers than with fragmented SR.

During Ca^{2+} release experiments using skinned fibers, the facts depicted in Figure 1 must be taken into account: (1) the SR has a strong Ca^{2+}-uptake activity and unless the Ca^{2+} pump is properly inhibited released Ca^{2+} stimulates the pump as well and is partly taken up again, which obscures the release process (negative feedback), and (2) in CICR Ca^{2+} released secondarily stimulates further release of Ca^{2+} (positive feedback); therefore, it is difficult to interpret how much Ca^{2+} is released by Ca^{2+} initially applied externally and how much is released secondarily. For this reason, simple monitoring of extra SR Ca^{2+} concentrations is not suitable for analyzing CICR activity, but Ca^{2+} concentrations in the medium during the release process should be fixed as far as possible by the use of a strong Ca^{2+} buffer. In this case, the Ca^{2+} release can be estimated by the time course of decrease in the amount of Ca^{2+} in the SR.

III. PREPARATION OF SKINNED FIBERS

A small muscle bundle about 5 mm in width and 15 to 20 mm in length is excised from each patient or animal. Both ends should be tied to a plastic

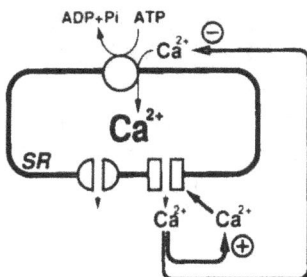

FIGURE 1. A scheme showing feedback mechanisms in the process of Ca^{2+} release from the SR. Positive feedback through the CICR and negative feedback through the Ca^{2+} pump are shown. For further explanation, see text. A Ca^{2+} release channel of the SR other than CICR channel is depicted to indicate the complexity of the preparation.

or stainless steel bar to avoid shortening. The samples should be kept in an ice-cooled relaxing solution for transportation to the laboratory. If they are frozen, the SR membrane might be destroyed functionally.

The biopsied muscles are divided in a relaxing solution into thin bundles. They are then treated with saponin (50 μg/ml) for 1 h to render the surface membrane permeable (chemical skinning). Saponin makes big holes in the membrane by acting on cholesterol molecules (Ohtsuki et al., 1978), and because the cholesterol content of the surface membrane is much higher than that of the SR membrane (Martonosi, 1968), it specifically perforates the surface membrane without affecting the SR functions (Endo and Iino, 1980).

A segment of either a single fiber or a sufficiently thin bundle of fibers (75 to 100 μm in width and 1.5 to 3 mm in length) is isolated from saponin-treated bundles. All the manipulations are made under a stereomicroscope of 40 to 80× magnification, with the aid of forceps and small scissors, knives, or needles. The tips of these instruments should be sharpened on an oil stone. In order to secure the quality of the preparation it is recommended to examine it before use under a microscope of a sufficient power to determine if it has uniform striations.

IV. Ca^{2+} MEASUREMENTS

As described in Section II, measurement of Ca^{2+} release should be made by determining the time course of decrease in the amount of Ca^{2+} in the SR at a fixed Ca^{2+} concentration to avoid the secondary CICR. Measurement of the amount of Ca^{2+} in the SR can be made by discharging all of its Ca^{2+} and measuring the amount discharged. A high concentration of caffeine under appropriate conditions reversibly discharges Ca^{2+} in the SR almost completely, and by utilizing this caffeine action one can repeatedly load and discharge and thus determine many time courses using only one skinned fiber. Direct measurement by using $^{45}Ca^{2+}$ is theoretically possible, but it would be cumbersome because a large number of skinned fibers are required to obtain a single time course. It would be possible to continuously monitor the amount of $^{45}Ca^{2+}$ in skinned fibers if extremely high specific activity $^{45}Ca^{2+}$ and very careful experimental apparatus and design are employed, but this is impractical.

The amount of Ca^{2+} discharged from the SR in a skinned fiber preparation can be determined either by using the size of contracture of the preparation (bioassay of Ca^{2+} utilizing the contractile reaction of skinned fiber as Ca^{2+} indicator) or by using other Ca^{2+} indicators. In the following only the method of bioassay will be described.

Both ends of a skinned fiber preparation are tied with a single silk thread to hooks, one of which is connected to a strain-gauge transducer (AE801; Akers, Norway) and the other to a micromanipulator to adjust the length of the skinned fiber. The length of the skinned fiber is set at about 130% of the slack length, because rundown of the fiber is slower when the fiber is lightly stretched. After amplification by a carrier amplifier (DSA-601B; NMB, Japan), the tension signal is either directly recorded on a pen recorder (Recticorder; NihonKohden, Japan) or digitized at 10 Hz using an A/D converter board in a microcomputer (PC9801 VM2; NEC, Japan) and stored on floppy disks.

To exchange solutions, a volume of desired solutions, which is several times that of the experimental trough, is rapidly injected from a reservoir through a thin, short tubing and the overflow is aspirated. The injection could be made manually or by a computer-operated pump and valve system. Alternatively, the method depicted in Figure 2 originally devised by Horiuti (1988) may be used. Solutions are placed in small wells (about 0.5 ml in volume), which are drilled in aluminum or plastic plate and resin-coated in such a way that the surface of the solution is protuberant about 2 to 3 mm above the plate surface. The skinned fiber is set horizontally in the protuberant part of the solution, and by moving the plate horizontally the fiber could be transferred from one solution to another.

If a temperature other than room temperature is to be used, the temperature of solutions is kept at the desired level by circulating water of an appropriate temperature just underneath the trough or the plate as well as the surroundings of the reservoir. The uniformity of temperature of the solution could be secured by means of a small magnetic bar in the solution and a magnetic stirrer placed under the stage holding the trough or plate (Figure 2).

Protocols for the measurement of Ca^{2+} release essentially consist of three steps (Figure 3).

1. Ca^{2+} loading — the SR is loaded with a fixed amount of Ca^{2+} by immersing the skinned fiber with empty SR in a medium containing a fixed concentration of Ca^{2+} as well as MgATP for a fixed period of time to allow the SR to accumulate Ca^{2+} by Ca^{2+} pump ATPase.

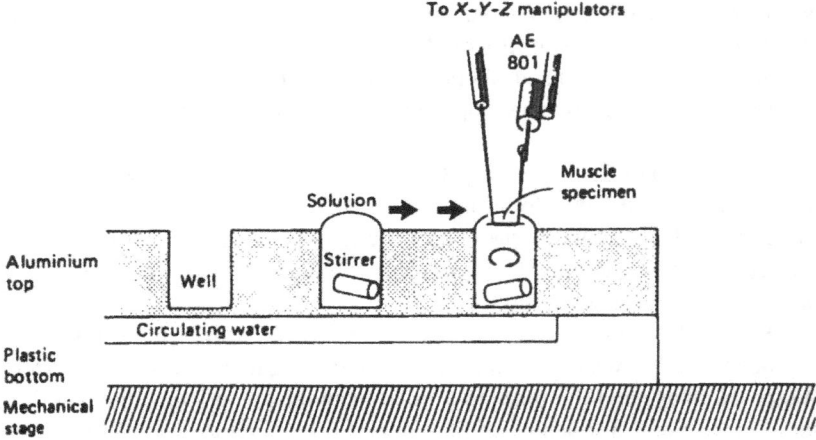

FIGURE 2. Experimental apparatus for skinned fiber experiments in which a series of solution exchanges can easily be made. For further explanation, see text. (From Horiuti, K., *J. Physiol.*, 398, 131, 1988. With permission.)

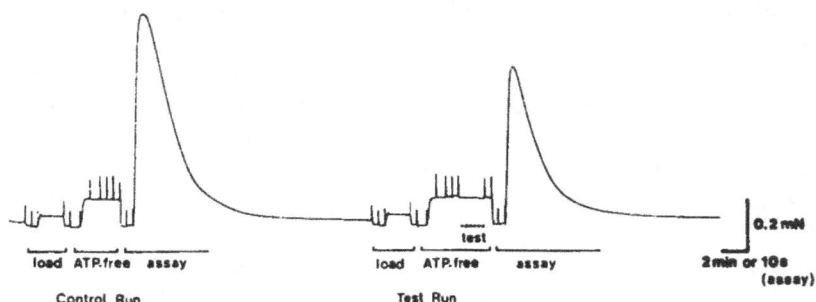

FIGURE 3. A part of a typical record of skinned fiber experiments to determine the activity of the CICR. Shown are the control run (left) and test run (right), each consisting of three steps: load, test (ATP-free), and assay. Artifacts in each tension record indicate the solution change. For detailed explanations for all of the solution changes, see text. The difference in the size of caffeine contracture between control and test runs represents the amount of Ca^{2+} released during the test period. (From Kawana et al., *Biomed. Res.*, 13, 287, 1992. With permission.)

2. Test — Ca^{2+} is applied for an appropriate period of time to induce CICR. As already mentioned, secondary CICR and simultaneous Ca^{2+} uptake during CICR should be avoided.

3. Assay — Ca^{2+} remaining in the SR after the test is assayed by thoroughly discharging it with a high concentration of caffeine.

    The amount of Ca^{2+} released during the test period is estimated by comparing the amount of Ca^{2+} remaining in the SR in the test run with that of a control run in which no test solution is applied.

Figure 3 also shows a typical tension record in the control and test run. Here the runs start with the empty SR since the assay step immediately preceding the runs should have discharged all of the Ca^{2+} in the SR. The assay solution is replaced by G2 relaxing solution (Table 1); to secure the washout of caffeine applied in the previous assay step, a new G2 relaxing solution is given once again. Then Ca^{2+} loading starts by applying the loading solution (Table 1), in which Ca^{2+} is buffered with a high concentration of a Ca^{2+} buffer. After an appropriate period of time, the loading solution is replaced by G10 relaxing solution to stop the loading immediately. The reason for using the G2 relaxing solution instead of the G10 relaxing solution immediately before loading is to shorten the delay of the start of Ca^{2+} loading due to diffusion as far as possible. Ca^{2+} concentration in the loading solution and length of the loading period could be adjusted to obtain a proper level of loading. With excessive loading Ca^{2+} tends to be released very easily or even spontaneously. On the other hand, with a too low level of loading, accurate determination of the time course of Ca^{2+} release may be difficult.

Before the real test period, ATP should be removed to stop the Ca^{2+} pump. The washout of ATP takes a rather long time because of its slow apparent diffusion due to the presence of concentrated ATP-binding sites in the fiber. In the example in Figure 3, the first application of rigor solution (Table 1) did not cause development of rigor tension, but the second application of the same solution did. To secure the removal of ATP, another application of the same rigor solution as done in Figure 3 is recommended. Prereleasing solution (Table 1), which is the same as releasing solution except

TABLE 1
Important Constituents of the Solutions used for Measurement of CICR Activity in Skinned Fiber

	Mg^{2+} (mM)	MgATP^{2-} (mM)	EGTA total (mM)	Ca^{2+} (M)	Caffeine (mM)	Procaine (mM)
G2 relaxing solution	1	4	2	0	0	0
Loading solution	1	4	10	2×10^{-7}	0	0
G10 relaxing solution	1	4	10	0	0	0
Rigor solution	1	0	2	0	0	0
Pre-releasing solution	0	0	2	0	0	0
Releasing solution	0	0	10	Variable	0	0
Stopping solution	10	0	10	0	0	10
Preassay solution	1	4	0.1	0	0	5
Assay solution	0.02	1	0.1	0	50	0

Note: All solutions contain 20 mM PIPES [piperazine-*N*-*N'*-bis(2-ethanesulfonic acid)], and pH is adjusted to 7.0 at 20°C with KOH. EGTA stands for ethylene glycol bis(β-aminoethylether)-*N,N,N',N'*-tetra-acetic acid. In assay solution total ATP is nearly 5 mM. For further information, see Endo and Iino (1988).

that it does not contain Ca^{2+}, is then applied. In this example, Mg^{2+} is removed in this procedure. Again to secure the removal of Mg^{2+}, application of prereleasing solution is repeated in this example. Then releasing solution (Table 1) is applied to cause CICR for a predetermined period of time. This test (CICR) period is terminated by applying stopping solution (Table 1), which is not only devoid of Ca^{2+} but also contains inhibitors of CICR, Mg^{2+} and procaine. This is to shut off the CICR as quickly as possible, because the duration of stimulation given should be accurate. Care is taken for the rapid initiation of the stimulation period as well, by using a low concentration of EGTA in the prereleasing solution and a high concentration of Ca^{2+} buffer in the releasing solution.

Before the application of assay solution (Table 1) containing 50 mM caffeine, the skinned fiber is washed with preassay solution (Table 1) twice, in order to make the composition of the solution closer to that of the assay solution. Thus, Mg-ATP is reintroduced and EGTA concentration is reduced. However, when the skinned fiber is kept in a relaxing solution containing such a low concentration of EGTA with minimal buffering capacity, CICR may be spontaneously evoked before the assay is made by Ca^{2+} leaking out of the SR which is not effectively buffered in this condition. To avoid this, a higher Mg^{2+} concentration is used in the preassay solution than in the assay solution and, furthermore, procaine is added. As a result, in the assay the decrease in Mg^{2+} and procaine is not immediate. Unlike the test period, however, what is important here is not the immediate initial rise in Ca^{2+} release activity but constancy of the condition at every application of the assay solution.

Experiments as shown in Figure 3 are repeated by changing the Ca^{2+} concentration and the duration of the test period. To account for a slow run down of the skinned fiber, control runs are inserted after every 4 to 6 test runs. The relation between duration of Ca^{2+} stimulation (test period) and relative amount of Ca^{2+} remaining in the SR is given in Figure 4. As is seen in the figure, time courses of decrease of Ca^{2+} in SR is almost exponential with the duration of Ca^{2+} stimulation. Therefore, the rate of CICR can be calculated from the result of one test period for each Ca^{2+} concentration by assuming single exponential decay during the test period and expressed by a rate constant with the dimension of min^{-1}. Recommended Ca^{2+} concentrations for test runs for the diagnosis of MH are 0, 0.3, 1, 3, and 10 μM in the absence of Mg^{2+} and the test period of 5 to 360 s at room temperature.

The amount of Ca^{2+} remaining in the SR after the test step is estimated by the tension time integral of the caffeine contracture due to assay solution. For the rationale of this caffeine contracture bioassay method in general, including the use of the tension time integral, see Endo and Iino (1988).

The use of caffeine in this method has an entirely different meaning from that in the halothane-caffeine test for MH diagnosis based on the original finding by Kalow et al. (1970). In the latter case, caffeine or halothane

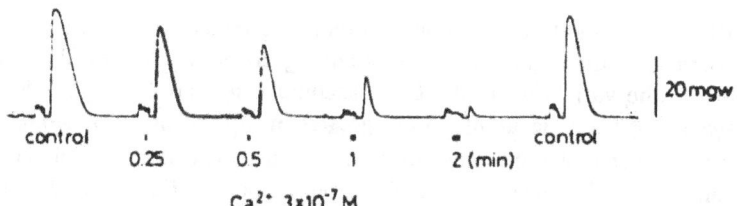

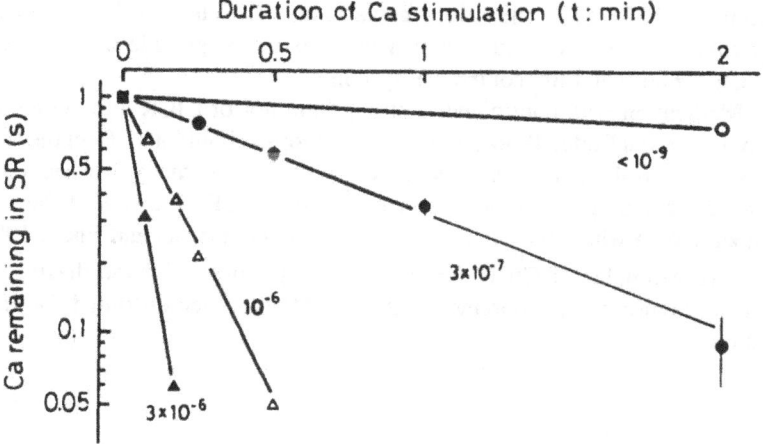

FIGURE 4. Relation between the duration of Ca^{2+} stimulation (test period) and relative amount of Ca^{2+} remaining in the SR, showing an exponential decrease in the remaining Ca^{2+} during test period. (Top): actual chart record of a CICR experiment; four test runs of different test periods with 3×10^{-7} M Ca^{2+} are bracketed by control runs. (Bottom): relation between duration of Ca^{2+} stimulation (t) and logarithm of relative amount of Ca^{2+} remaining in the SR (s). Each point and vertical line shows the mean $\pm$ SE (n = 4). (From Ohta et al., *Am. J. Physiol.*, 256, C358, 1989. With permission.)

concentration is raised in a stepwise fashion to find the "threshold" concentration for contracture. The rationale is that because both caffeine and halothane produce contractures by enhancing CICR, the threshold concentrations should be lower in MH with already hereditarily enhanced CICR. On the other hand, in the method described in this chapter, the magnitude of CICR in the absence of caffeine and halothane (test period) is directly determined and caffeine is used only to discharge completely the Ca^{2+} remaining in the SR after the test period, and for this purpose a single dose of a very high concentration of caffeine is used.

Although contracture of the skinned fibers is used for the bioassay in the present method, variations in the contractile activity among different skinned fibers do not matter, because in this method, not the absolute but the relative magnitude of contracture is used; whatever the magnitude of activity, if it is constant, it is sufficient for this purpose. On the other hand, in halothane-caffeine test, the threshold concentration is directly affected by the possible variations in the contractile activity among different samples. The same applies to the variability in the Ca^{2+} accumulating capacity of the SR. If the capacity of Ca^{2+} accumulation is greater in a preparation, it would tend to give a lower threshold concentration, because with the same magnitude of opening of Ca^{2+} release channels a larger amount of Ca^{2+} would be released from more heavily loaded SR. This again does not matter in the present method for exactly the same reason. In other words, the present method purely examines CICR, while the halothane-caffeine test examines the overall ease of evoking CICR contracture, which includes the magnitude of activities of the Ca^{2+} pump and the contractile system.

Medication with dantrolene, a strong inhibitor of CICR at body temperature (Ohta and Endo, 1986), at the time of biopsy should not affect the CICR activity determinations described here, because it is easily washed out of skinned fiber preparation and its effect on the CICR is absent at the room temperature at which the determination is carried out (Ohta and Endo, 1986).

Two examples of CICR determination experiments for the diagnosis of human (Figure 5) and porcine (Figure 6) MH are demonstrated for information.

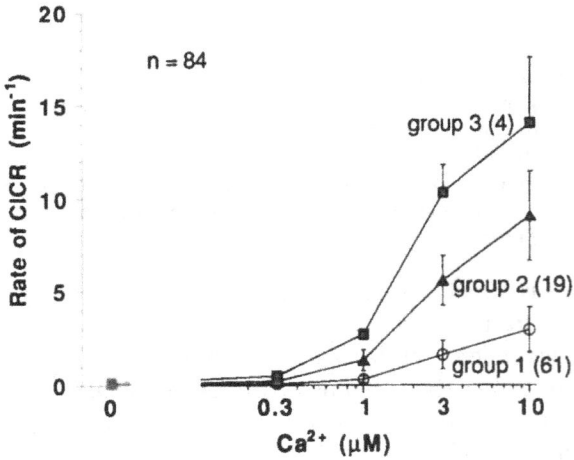

FIGURE 5. Mean rates of CICR in skinned fibers from three groups of human samples. All of the average CICR data (4 to 7 skinned fibers from each individual) of 84 people are objectively classified into three groups by a cluster analysis, samples from definitely normal individuals being unavailable. (Group 1): CICR unaccelerated; (group 2): CICR moderately accelerated; (group 3): CICR highly accelerated. Correlation between the grouping and clinical signs of MH are excellent, group 1 being normal, groups 2 and 3 MH. (From Kawana et al., *Biomed. Res.*, 13, 287, 1992. With permission.)

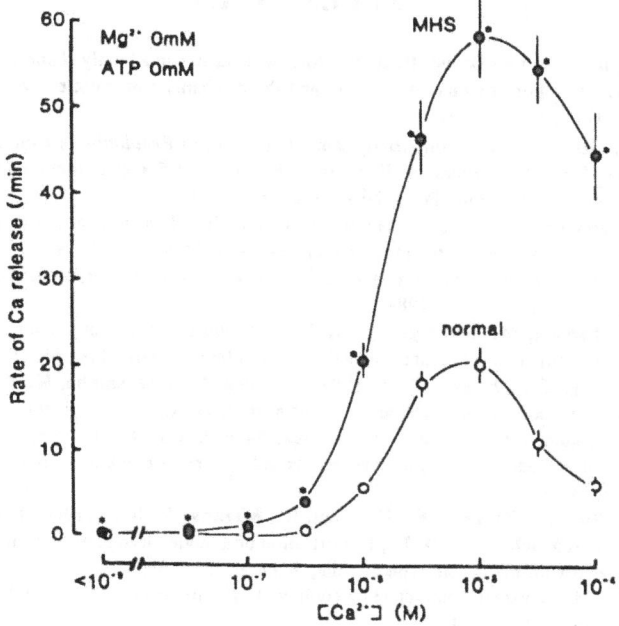

FIGURE 6. Rates of CICR in skinned fibers from MH-susceptible (MHS) and normal pig muscles. (From Ohta et al., *Am. J. Physiol.*, 256, C358, 1989. With permission.)

REFERENCES

Denborough, M. A. and Lovell, R. R. H., Anesthetic deaths in a family, *Lancet*, II, 45, 1960.

Ebashi, S., Excitation-contraction coupling and the mechanism of muscle contraction, *Annu. Rev. Physiol.*, 53, 1, 1991.

Endo, M., Calcium release from sarcoplasmic reticulum, in *Regulation of Calcium Transport across Muscle Membranes*, A. E. Shamoo, Ed., Current Topics in Membranes and Transport, Vol. 25, Academic Press, New York, 1985, 181.

Endo, M. and Iino, M., Specific perforation of muscle cell membranes with preserved SR functions by saponin treatment, *J. Muscle Res. Cell Motil.*, 1, 89, 1980.

Endo, M. and Iino, M., Measurement of Ca^{2+} release in skinned fibers from skeletal muscle, *Meth. Enzymol.*, 157, 12, 1988.

Endo, M., Tanaka, M., and Ogawa, Y., Calcium-induced release of calcium from the sarcoplasmic reticulum of skinned skeletal muscle fibres, *Nature*, 228, 34, 1970.

Endo, M., Yagi, S., Ishizuka, T., Horiuti, K., Koga, Y., and Amaha, K., Changes in the calcium-induced calcium release mechanism in the sarcoplasmic reticulum of the muscle from a patient with malignant hyperthermia, *Biomed. Res.*, 4, 83, 1983.

Ford, L. E. and Podolsky, R. J., Regenerative calcium release within muscle cells, *Science*, 167, 58, 1970.

Fujii, J., Otsu, K., Zorzato, E., De Leon, S., Khanna, V. K., Weiler, J. E., O'Brien, P. J., and MacLennan, D. H., Identification of a mutation in porcine ryanodine receptor associated with malignant hyperthermia, *Science*, 253, 448, 1991.

Horiuti, K., Mechanism of contracture on cooling of caffeine-treated frog skeletal muscle fibres, *J. Physiol.*, 398, 131, 1988.

Kalow, W., Britt, B. A., Terreau, M. E., and Haist, C., Metabolic error of muscle metabolism after recovery from malignant hyperthermia, *Lancet*, II, 895, 1970.

Kawana, Y., Iino, M., Horiuti, K., Matsumura, N., Ohta, T., Matsui, K., and Endo, M., Acceleration in calcium-induced calcium release in the biopsied muscle fibers from patients with malignant hyperthermia, *Biomed. Res.*, 13, 287, 1992.

Martonosi, A., Sarcoplasmic reticulum. V. The structure of sarcoplasmic reticulum membranes, *Biochim. Biophys. Acta*, 150, 694, 1968.

Matsui, K. and Endo, M., Effect of inhalation anesthetics on the rate of Ca release from the sarcoplasmic reticulum of skeletal muscle in the guinea pig, *Jpn. J. Pharmacol.*, 40, Suppl. 245P, 1986.

Ohta, T. and Endo, M., Inhibition of calcium-induced calcium release by dantrolene at mammalian body temperature, *Proc. Jpn. Acad.*, 62, 329, 1986.

Ohta, T., Endo, M., Nakano, T., Morohoshi, Y., Wanikawa, K., and Ohga, A., Ca-induced Ca release in malignant hyperthermia-susceptible pig skeletal muscle, *Am. J. Physiol.*, 256, C358, 1989.

Ohtsuki, I., Manzi, R. M., Palade, G. E., and Jamieson, J. D., Entry of macromolecular tracers into cells fixed with low concentrations of aldehydes, *Biol. Cell.*, 31, 119, 1978.

Chapter 15

MEASUREMENT OF CALCIUM ACCUMULATION BY SARCOPLASMIC RETICULUM IN WHOLE HOMOGENATE — A POTENTIAL DIAGNOSTIC TEST FOR MALIGNANT HYPERTHERMIA SUSCEPTIBILITY

Khay S. Cheah, A. M. Cheah, J. E. Fletcher, and H. Rosenberg

TABLE OF CONTENTS

I.   Abstract..212

II.   Introduction...212

III.   Experimental Procedures...213

IV.   Results...214

V.   Discussion 220

Acknowledgments...221

References...222

I. ABSTRACT

A diagnostic test for MH susceptibility was developed using measurements of Ca^{2+} accumulation by sarcoplasmic reticulum (SR) in whole muscle homogenate preparations with a Ca^{2+} electrode at 35°C. The Ca^{2+} accumulation test requires a small amount of material and does not rely on the integrity of the biopsy muscle samples. This offers a less invasive diagnosis for MH susceptibility, as it might be possible for the test to be performed on needle biopsy samples.

The Ca^{2+} accumulation test is based on the greater instability of the Ca^{2+} accumulating capacity of the SR in whole muscle homogenate preparations of MH-susceptible individuals. The SR from these individuals showed a significant (p <0.001) loss in Ca^{2+} accumulating capacity after prolonged aging in ice and can be differentiated from normal by using a demarcation value of 50% reduction in Ca^{2+} accumulation. In parallel studies with the conventional contracture tests conducted on muscle biopsy strips of vastus lateralis with 3% halothane at 37°C, the Ca^{2+}-accumulation test appears to give only one false-positive result in 29 patients diagnosed as MH$^-$, and no false-negatives in patients diagnosed as MH$^+$ when the aging period of the whole muscle homogenate preparations was extended from 22 to 48 h. The Ca^{2+} accumulation test does not give any false-negatives or -positives with genetically selected MH$^+$ and MH$^-$ British Landrace pigs, which are generally used as an experimental model for studies of human malignant hyperthermia.

II. INTRODUCTION

Malignant hyperthermia (MH) is a genetically inherited and potentially fatal disorder affecting primarily the skeletal muscle (see References 1 through 4). The syndrome can be induced in MH-susceptible humans and pigs by halothane and other halogenated hydrocarbon anesthetics. Once initiated, the classical symptoms of the syndrome are gross muscular rigidity, a rapid rise in body temperature, hyperventilation, severe metabolic acidosis, and elevated levels of serum metabolites,[1-4] and if uncontrolled with dantrolene, death occurs. The incidence of MH in apparently healthy patients is about 1 in 15,000[5] and can be as high as 88% in stress-susceptible pigs.[6]

The current diagnostic test for MH susceptibility in humans is based on the magnitude of contracture induced by halothane and/or caffeine in muscle biopsy strips at 37°C.[7] In pigs, MH susceptibility is identified by anesthetizing the pigs with a mixture of oxygen and halothane (2 to 4%) supplied through a face mask for 2 to 5 min.[8,9] Pigs are classified as MH-susceptible if they exhibit rigidity in the hind legs and those that do not are designated as nonsusceptible. Various other pilot diagnostic tests have been developed for detecting MH susceptibility in both humans[3] and pigs (for reviews, see

References 8, 10, and 11), but none were found to be either practical or completely reliable for general application. In pigs, blood testing based on osmotic fragility of erythrocytes[12,13] and specific blood groups[14] and recently based on ionized Ca^{2+} in lymphocytes[15] and spin-label technique on red blood cells[16] offer some potential but have not yet been adopted for screening purposes. In humans, recent reports of a noninvasive nuclear magnetic resonance spectroscopy on the value of the P_i/PCr ratio[17] and halothane-induced increase in ionized Ca^{2+} in blood mononuclear cells[18] and spin-label technique on red blood cells[19] for detecting MH susceptibility have yet to be fully evaluated.

In this paper, we report the measurement of Ca^{2+} accumulation in whole muscle homogenate preparations as a potential diagnostic test for MH susceptibility. Calcium accumulation is measured with a Ca^{2+} selective electrode, and MH susceptibility is characterized by the instability of the SR following prolonged aging of the whole muscle homogenate preparations in ice.

III. EXPERIMENTAL PROCEDURES

Vastus lateralis muscle biopsies were obtained from patients referred to the Department of Anesthesiology, Hahnemann University, for diagnosis of MH susceptibility. The open surgical biopsies were performed under femoral and lateral femoral cutaneous nerve blocks. The muscle biopsies were taken from the operating room at room temperature in Krebs Ringer solution (pH 7.4) to the laboratory. The procedure for obtaining the muscle biopsies and for the classification of positive (MH^+) and negative (MH^-) patients by the contracture test with 3% halothane at 37°C has been described previously by Fletcher and Rosenberg.[20] Patients were classified as MH^+ if 3% halothane induced a tension ≥ 0.7 g in any of the 6 to 8 muscle strips tested.[20] Approval was obtained from the Hahnemann University Human Studies Committee for the studies on human patients. Genetically selected British Landrace pigs for MH susceptibility (MH^+) and nonsusceptibility (MH^-) were obtained from the Agricultural and Food Research Council, Institute of Genetics and Physiology, Edinburgh. The pigs were classified by halothane testing with 4% halothane via face masks for up to 3 min[9] by Dr. A. J. Webb, and all experiments were conducted without prior knowledge of the identity of the pigs.

Ten percent muscle homogenates were prepared by mincing muscles with a pair of scissors in a medium (pH 7.4) containing 300 mM sucrose and 10 mM Tris-HCl in ice and then homogenizing the muscles with three passes of the Teflon® pestle in a Thomas glass homogenizer (size B) in a cold room (4°C). The muscle homogenate preparations were then kept in ice for 2 h (control) before being used for the Ca^{2+} accumulation experiments. Human biopsy samples of vastus lateralis, kept at 21°C in Krebs Ringer solution (pH 7.4) and continuously bubbled with a mixture of O_2 (95%) and CO_2 (5%), were used for the muscle homogenate preparations within 30 min of obtaining the samples from the operating room. Postmortem samples of longissimus dorsi were used within 3 min of obtaining the muscle samples.

Calcium accumulation by the 10% muscle homogenate preparations were determined using a Radiometer calcium ion electrode (F2212Ca) and an Orion single junction reference electrode connected to a Radiometer (Model PHM 84) and a recorder with a variable voltage range. The voltage range required on the recorder depends on the output voltage of the pH meter used. The total millivolt change during the course of an experiment is approximately 25, and the initial reading before Ca^{2+} addition is normally about 50. The Ca^{2+} electrode performance is checked at the beginning of each day by measuring the difference in potential between measurements in 100 mM and 1 mM CaCl$_2$ in 300 mM KCl. The potential difference should be at least 55 mV and is usually 59 to 60 mV when the electrode is in good working order. The reaction medium (pH 7.4) contained 100 mM KCl, 5 mM MgCl$_2$, 20 mM imidazole chloride, 5 mM NaN$_3$, 2 µg oligomycin, 2 µM rotenone and 1 µg antimycin A in a total volume of 5.80 ml. After equilibration at 35°C in a temperature-controlled and magnetically stirred vessel, 5 mM ATP and 45 mM P$_i$ were added, followed by small additions of exogenous stock solution of 25 mM CaCl$_2$ (a total of 198 µM for humans and 153 µM for pigs) prior to starting the reaction with the addition of either the human (900 µl) or the pig (250 µl) muscle homogenate preparations. Calcium accumulation by the SR was recorded until completion as illustrated in Figure 1. The amount of Ca^{2+} accumulated by the SR was determined from the calibration curve constructed from each experiment as shown in Figure 2 by plotting the millivoltage against the exogenous Ca^{2+} added on the semi-logarithmic scale. The experiment was designed so that the total Ca^{2+} accumulated, recorded as millivolts in the tracing (see Figure 1), occurred only on the linear portion of the calibration curve as illustrated in Figure 2. In all these experiments the contribution of Ca^{2+} uptake by the mitochondria and sarcolemma was eliminated using the inhibitors, antimycin A and NaN$_3$

IV. RESULTS

Calcium accumulation by SR can be measured in a whole muscle homogenate preparation with a Ca^{2+} electrode.[21,22] Figure 3 illustrates typical tracings obtained with the Ca^{2+} electrode showing Ca^{2+} accumulation by SR in whole muscle homogenate preparations of MH$^-$ (A) and MH$^+$ (B) patients after aging in ice for 2 h (control, —) and 22 h (----). Table 1 summarizes the comparative study of Ca^{2+} accumulation by the SR between these two groups of patients as described in Figure 3. A significant (p <0.001) reduction in Ca^{2+} accumulation was only observed with the MH$^+$ patients following aging of the whole muscle homogenate preparations in ice for 22 h. Calcium accumulation of MH$^+$ patients at 22 h of aging showed a loss of 74% against a reduction of only 20% in the MH$^-$ patients when compared with the control

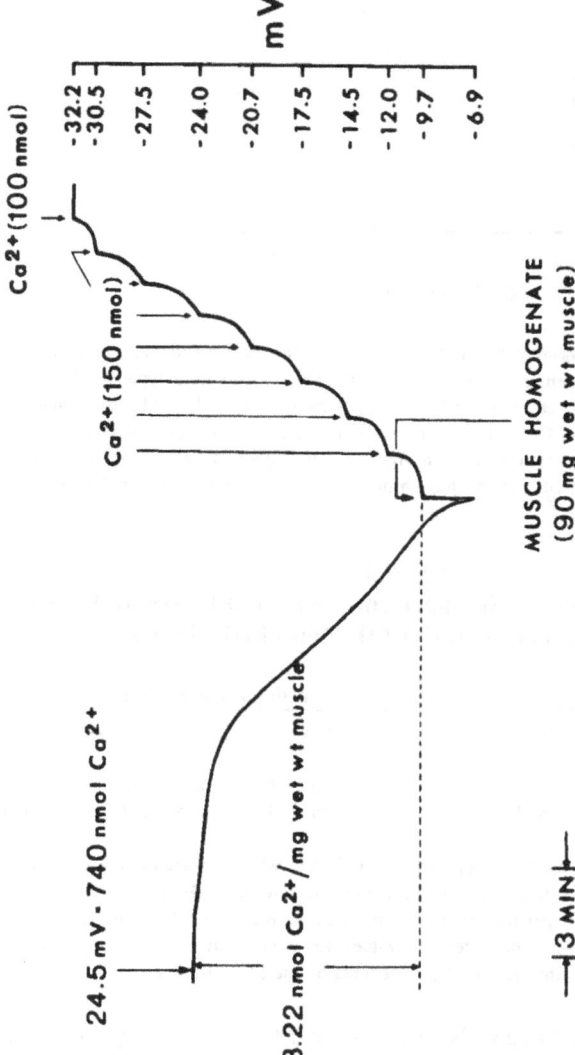

FIGURE 1. Calcium accumulation by SR in a whole muscle homogenate preparation at 35°C: This figure illustrates a typical Ca²⁺ accumulation by the SR in a whole homogenate preparation of human vastus lateralis aged for 2 h in ice (control experiment). The maximum Ca²⁺ uptake, recorded as millivolts in the trace, was converted to nanomoles of Ca²⁺ by using the linear portion of the calibration curve (450 to 1150 nmol Ca²⁺) of Figure 2, which was constructed for the experiment represented by this figure.

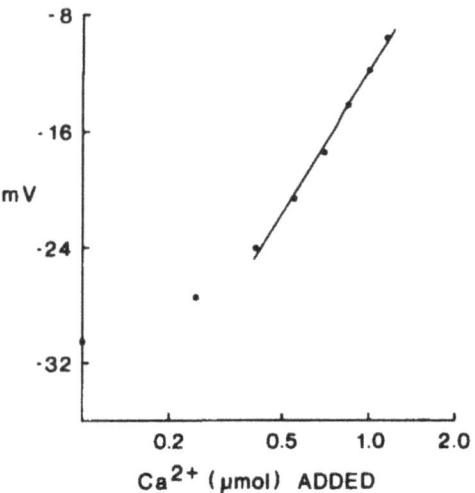

FIGURE 2.   A calibration curve of the Radiometer Ca^{2+} electrode for Ca^{2+} accumulation by SR in a whole muscle homogenate preparation at 35°C: This represents a typical calibration curve obtained by plotting the potential (mV) measured by the Ca^{2+} electrode following the various additions of exogenous Ca^{2+} shown in the abscissa prior to the addition of the whole muscle homogenate preparation as illustrated in Figure 1. This figure is the calibration curve of the control experiment conducted with the human muscle homogenate preparation described in Figure 1.

TABLE 1
Calcium Accumulation by Sarcoplasmic Reticulum in Whole Muscle Homogenate Preparations of MH^+ and MH^- Patients

| Patients | 3% Halothane-induced tension (g) at 37°C | Calcium accumulation | |
		2 h aging	22 h aging
MH^+	2.21 ± 1.59 (n = 8)*	8.74 ± 0.55 (n = 8)	2.32 ± 1.25 (n = 8)*
MH^-	0.35 ± 0.21 (n = 18)	8.23 ± 0.81 (n = 18)	6.60 ± 1.00 (n = 18)

Note: Calcium accumulation by the sarcoplasmic reticulum in whole muscle homogenate preparations was measured with a Radiometer calcium-selective electrode at 35°C. The results, expressed in nmol Ca^{2+} per mg wet weight muscle, are means ± SD for the number of patients in parentheses. * indicates the values for MH^+ patients were significantly ($p < 0.001$) different from those of MH^- patients by the Student *t* test.

values obtained at 2 h of aging. No significant difference was observed in the Ca^{2+} accumulating capacity of the SR between the MH^+ and MH^- patients at 2 h of aging (control experiments) of the whole muscle homogenate preparations.

The diminished Ca^{2+} accumulating capacity of the SR in whole muscle homogenate preparations of MH^+ patients in our experimental protocol could be used for differentiating MH^+ and MH^- patients. Figure 4 illustrates the

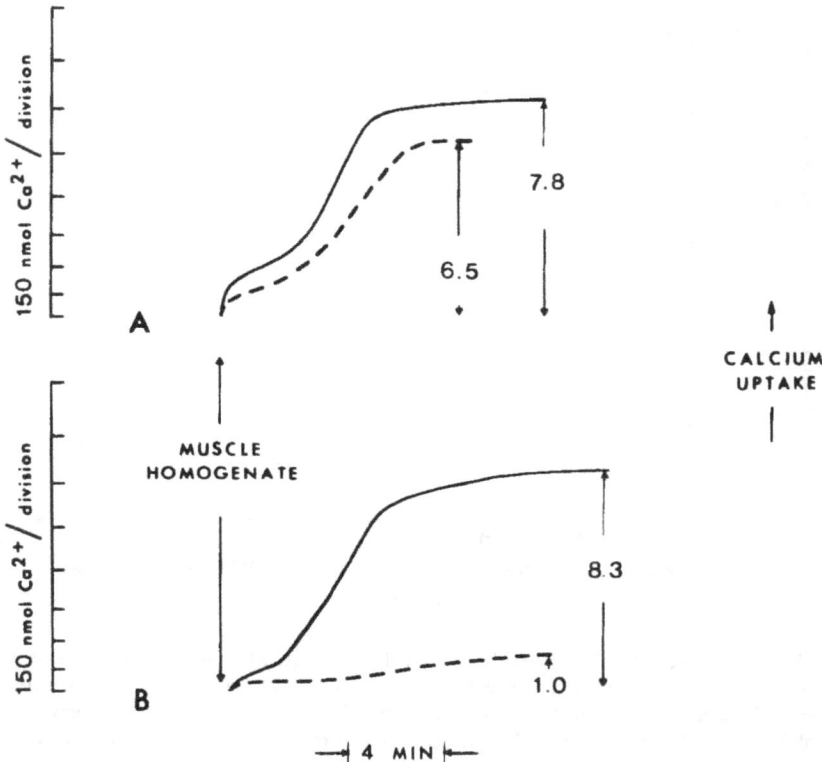

FIGURE 3. Calcium electrode tracings showing Ca^{2+} accumulation by SR in whole muscle homogenate preparations of MH$^-$ (A) and MH$^+$ (B) patients aged in ice for 2 h (—, control) and 22 h (----, test).

relationship between Ca^{2+} accumulation by the SR aged for 22 h in ice against the maximal tension induced by 3% halothane in biopsy muscle strips of vastus lateralis at 37°C. The data suggest that MH$^+$ patients (■) could be identified from MH$^-$ patients (●) by using a value of 50% reduction in Ca^{2+} accumulation. Figure 4 also illustrates four patients (two adults and two children) classified as MH$^+$ by the 3% halothane-induced contracture test showed normal stability in Ca^{2+} accumulation by the SR. The muscle biopsy strips showing a maximal tension of 2.6 g (■, A) were from a 59-year-old man with no family history of MH susceptibility and had no problems in four previous exposures to general anesthetics. The muscle biopsy strips showing a maximal tension of 0.8 g (■, B) were from a 22-year-old man with a history of two episodes of hyperthermia during general anesthesia for jaw surgery. The two young patients, a 5-year-old boy and an 8-year-old girl, had a history of masseter muscle rigidity and were identified as MH$^+$ by the 3% halothane-induced contracture test. Muscle biopsy strips from the 5-year-old boy showed a maximal tension of 1.0 g (■, C) and the 8-year-old girl a maximal tension

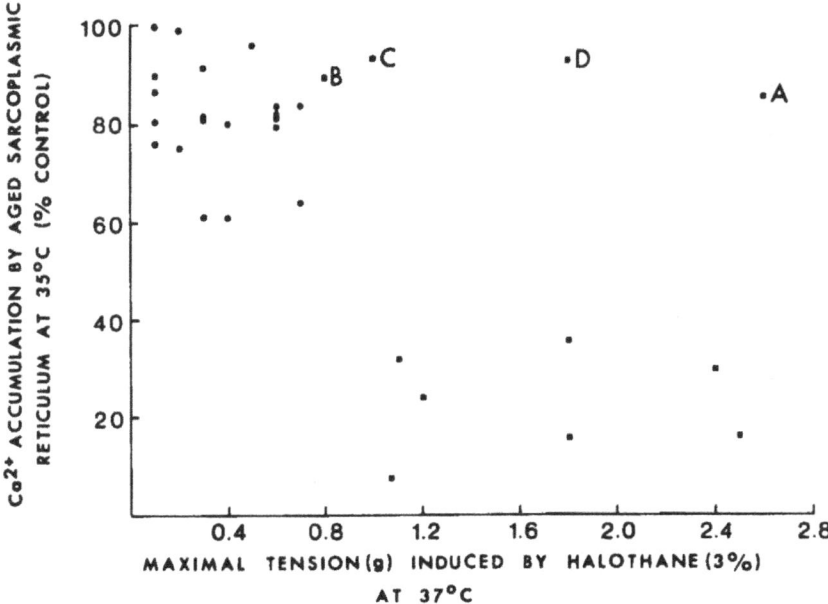

FIGURE 4. Relationship between Ca^{2+} accumulation by aged SR in whole muscle homogenate preparations and the maximal tension induced by 3% halothane in muscle biopsy strips of patients at 37°C. Calcium accumulation of SR was measured in the whole muscle homogenate preparations of 20 MH$^-$ (●) and 11 MH$^+$ (■) patients identified by 3% halothane-induced contractures tests.[20] Other details concerning the discrepancies between the Ca^{2+} accumulation and the halothane-induced contracture tests are described in Section IV.

of 1.8 g (■, D), but in both of these patients a decrease of only 15% was observed in Ca^{2+} accumulation by the SR in the whole muscle homogenate preparations after aging for 22 h in ice. These four discrepancies could be prevented by increasing the sensitivity of the Ca^{2+} accumulation test.

The sensitivity of the Ca^{2+} accumulation test was improved by prolonging the aging of the whole muscle homogenate preparations from 22 to 48 h in ice. Table 2 summarizes the results conducted on the whole muscle homogenate preparations aged up to 48 h in ice, and it shows that the false-negatives provided by the Ca^{2+} accumulation test (see Figure 4) probably would not have occurred had the tests been performed at 48 instead of 22 h. Only 1 out of 11 whole muscle homogenate preparations of MH$^-$ patients (including one of control patient) showed a further significant reduction in Ca^{2+} accumulation. This patient would have been classified MH$^-$ by the Ca^{2+} accumulation test at 22 h of aging, in agreement with the 3% halothane-induced contracture test, but MH$^+$ at 48 h of aging. Muscle biopsy strips from this 19-year-old man showed a maximal tension of 0.4 g by the 3% halothane-induced contracture test. Hyperthermia was observed with this patient during a hernia operation and he was treated with dantrolene. With the MH$^+$ patients, however,

TABLE 2
Calcium Accumulation by Aged SR in Whole Muscle Homogenate Preparations at 35°C

Patients	3% Halothane-induced tension (g) at 37°C	Ca^{2+} accumulation (% control)	
		22 h aging	48 h aging
MH⁻ patients			
1 (18 years, F)	0.6	69	70
2 (19 years, M)	0.4	93	33*
3 (8 years, F)	0.6	85	85
4 (12 years, F)	0.3	97	96
5 (25 years, M)	0.4	91	90
6 (37 years, M)	0.5	85	73
7 (75 years, M)	0.4	84	80
8 (12 years, F)	0.4	97	88
9 (6 years, F)	0.0	100	83
10 (29 years, F)	0.2	98	83
11 (72 years, M)**	0.0	83	74
MH⁺ patients			
1 (28 years, F)	1.0	46*	6*
2 (20 years, M)	1.2	81	38*
3 (70 years, M)	0.7	76	37*
4 (43 years, F)	6.0	67	27*
5 (33 years, F)	0.9	0*	0*

Note: Calcium accumulation is expressed as a percent of the control value. The (3%) halothane-induced tension refers to the maximal tension observed in any one of the 6 to 8 muscle biopsy strips at 37°C.[20] Patients were classified as MH⁺ (*) by the Ca^{2+} accumulation test if the aged SR retained less than 50% of the control value. ** = control patient; F = female; M = male.

a significant reduction in Ca^{2+} accumulation was observed by extending the aging period to 48 h. Three out of five patients identified as MH⁺ by the 3% halothane-induced contracture test would have been classified as MH⁻ by the Ca^{2+} accumulation test at 22 h of aging but MH⁺ at 48 h of aging. The results presented in Table 2 probably account for the four false-negatives (Figure 4) when the Ca^{2+} accumulation tests were conducted on the whole preparations aged for 22 h in ice. Thus, the discrepancy in the false-negatives would probably not have occurred if the Ca^{2+} accumulation tests had been conducted in the first place on the whole muscle homogenate preparations aged for 48 instead of 22 h.

In MH research, pigs are widely used as excellent experimental models for investigating the human MH syndrome, because they also develop MH when treated with halothane.[1-3] With the British Landrace pigs, genetically selected either for susceptibility or resistance to MH by halothane,[9] a clear differentiation was also obtained for MH⁺ and MH⁻ animals when the Ca^{2+}

accumulation tests were performed on the whole muscle homogenate preparations. Longissimus dorsi, a predominantly white skeletal muscle, was used for the pig studies instead of the red vastus lateralis in humans. With pigs, a smaller volume (250 μl) of muscle homogenate preparation, equivalent to 25 mg wet weight muscle, and a maximum aging period of 7 h were employed instead of 900 μl (90 mg wet weight muscle) and 22 and 48 h of aging for humans. At 7 h of aging, Ca^{2+} accumulation by the SR of MH^+ pigs was significantly (p <0.001) lower than MH^- pigs (Table 3). A reduction of 96% in Ca^{2+} accumulation was observed at 7 h of aging as against a loss of only 41% in the MH^- pigs. With the British Landrace pigs, the Ca^{2+} accumulation tests did not give any false results.

V. DISCUSSION

Calcium accumulation by the SR in whole muscle homogenate preparations was significantly reduced in MH^+ humans and pigs following prolonged aging in ice when compared with MH^- individuals. The Ca^{2+}-accumulation tests were performed on muscle homogenates prepared from a small amount of skeletal muscle (200 to 300 mg for humans and 70 mg for pigs). Two estimations of Ca^{2+} accumulation were required for predicting MH susceptibility, one at 2 h (control values for humans and pigs) and the other (test value) at 22 or 48 h for humans and 7 h for pigs. The data presented suggest that measurements of the instability of Ca^{2+} accumulation by the SR in whole muscle homogenates provides a potentially good diagnostic method for MH susceptibility in humans and pigs. For humans, it is recommended that the second Ca^{2+} accumulation test should be conducted with whole muscle homogenate preparations aged for 48 h in order to prevent false-negative results. Out of the 28 MH^- patients, only one false-positive was given by the Ca^{2+} accumulation test.

TABLE 3
Calcium Accumulation by SR in Whole Muscle
Homogenate Preparations of Halothane-Sensitive (MH*)
and Halothane-Insensitive (MH⁻) British Landrace Pigs

British Landrace pigs	Calcium accumulation	
	2 h aging	7 h aging
MH⁺	24.9 ± 6.1 (n = 12)	1.1 ± 1.5 (n = 12)*
MH⁻	28.8 ± 5.9 (n = 8)	17.1 ± 8.0 (n = 6)

Note: Experimental details are described in section III and in Table 1. The results, expressed in nmol Ca^{2+} per mg wet weight of muscle at 35°C, are means ± SD for the number of pigs in parentheses. * indicates the values for MH^+ pigs were significantly (p <0.001) different from those of MH^- pigs by the Student *t* test.

The diagnostic test based on Ca^{2+} accumulation by the SR in whole muscle homogenate preparations has several advantages against the current diagnostic test for MH susceptibility based on drug-induced contracture in biopsy muscle strips. First, a maximal total wet weight of 300 mg of muscle is sufficient compared to a maximum of about 2 g recommended for achieving reliable diagnostic information for humans.[7] Second, the test is simple to perform. Third, it might be possible for the test to be conducted with needle muscle biopsy samples because it does not rely on the integrity of the muscle samples.

The Ca^{2+} accumulation diagnostic test was devised on the basis of the earlier report[22] that the Ca^{2+} transport system of the SR in whole muscle homogenate preparations of MH^+ pigs deteriorated considerably faster than those of MH^- pigs. The cause of the instability was postulated to be due to an excess of free, long-chain unsaturated fatty acids liberated by an enhanced phospholipase A_2 activity.[20,21] This hypothesis was substantiated by the inhibition of Ca^{2+} accumulation of isolated SR by the byproducts (arachidonic, oleic, and linoleic acids) of phospholipase A_2.[21,22] In addition, muscle homogenate preparations of MH^+ pigs produced 2.5 times more fatty acids than those of MH^- pigs following incubation for 40 min at 35°C (K. S. Cheah and A. M. Cheah, unpublished data). MH^+ patients had also been shown to produce 2.5 times more free fatty acids than MH^- patients following incubation of the muscle homogenates for 3 h at 37°C.[23] Excess liberation of fatty acids was also postulated by these authors to be responsible for the greater than normal halothane-induced contracture in muscle biopsy strips of MH^+ patients.[23]

In conclusion, our data support that we have developed a simple test that is of potential value for diagnosis of MH susceptibility in humans and that the test could be refined further using needle biopsy samples. The Ca^{2+} accumulation test gives only 1 false-positive result out of 28 MH^- patients when compared to the halothane-induced contracture test. By improving the diagnostic test through extending the aging period of the whole muscle homogenate preparations to 48 h, the incidence of false-negatives appears to be eliminated. The validity of the Ca^{2+} accumulation test was supported by results obtained with the British Landrace pigs genetically selected for susceptibility and nonsusceptibility to MH. However, the Ca^{2+} accumulation test needs further corroboration before it could be recommended as a diagnostic test for MH susceptibility in humans.

ACKNOWLEDGMENTS

The research was initiated with genetically selected British Landrace pigs while the authors, K. S. Cheah (Principal Scientific Officer and Head of Cell Biology Section) and A. M. Cheah (Senior Scientific Officer), were employed at the Agricultural and Food Research Council, Food Research Institute — Bristol Laboratory, Langford, U.K. The authors are grateful to Mrs. F. Lizzo for conducting the halothane-induced contracture tests on human biopsy samples. The research on human patients was supported by the Hahnemann Anesthesia Research Foundation and U.S. NIH Grant GM 34872.

REFERENCES

1. **Gronert, G. A.**, Malignant hyperthermia, *Anesthesiology*, 53, 395, 1980.
2. **Cheah, K. S. and Cheah, A. M.**, Malignant hyperthermia: molecular defects in membrane permeability, *Experientia*, 41, 656, 1985.
3. **Ellis, F. R. and Heffron, J. J. A.**, Clinical and biochemical aspects of malignant hyperthermia, in *Recent Advances in Anaesthesia and Analgesia* R. S. Atkinson and A. P. Adams, Eds., Churchill Livingstone, Edinburgh, 1985, 173.
4. **Rosenberg, H. and Fletcher, J. E.**, Malignant hyperthermia, in *Muscle Relaxants: Side Effects and a Rational Approach to Selection*, I. Azar, Ed., Marcel Dekker, New York, 1987, 115.
5. **Britt, B. A. and Kalow, W.**, Malignant hyperthermia: statistical review, *Can. Anaesth. Soc.*, 17, 293, 1970.
6. **Webb, A. J.**, The incidence of halothane sensitivity in British pigs, *Anim. Prod.*, 31, 101, 1980.
7. **Britt, B. A.**, Muscle assessment of malignant hyperthermia patients, in *Malignant Hyperthermia*, B. A. Britt, Ed., Martinus Nijhoff, Boston, 1987, 193.
8. **Sybesma, W. and Eikelenboom, G.**, Methods of predicting pale, soft and exudative pork and their application in breeding programmes — a review, *Meat Sci.*, 31, 101, 1980.
9. **Webb, A. J. and Jordan, C. H. C.**, Halothane sensitivity as a field test for stress susceptibility in the pig, *Anim. Prod.*, 26, 157, 1978.
10. **Cheah, K. S. and Cheah A. M.**, Mitochondrial calcium efflux and porcine stress susceptibility, *Experientia*, 35, 1001, 1979.
11. **Allen, W. M., Cheah, K. S., Imlah, P., Lister, D., Steane, D. E., and Webb, A. J.**, Testing methods for PSE syndrome: current research in the U. K., *Livestock Prod. Sci.*, 7, 305, 1980.
12. **Harrison, G. G. and Verburg, C.**, Erythrocyte osmotic fragility in hyperthermic susceptible swine, *Br. J. Anaesth.*, 45, 131, 1973.
13. **Cheah, K. S. and Cheah, A. M.**, Membrane permeability in porcine malignant hyperthermia, in *Membrane Fluidity*, M. Kates and A. Kuksis, Eds., Humana Press, NJ, 1980, 141.
14. **Imlah, P.**, Linkage studies between halothane (Hal), phosphohexose isomerase (PHi) and the S(A-O) and H red blood cell loci of Pietrain/Hampshire and Landrace pigs, *Anim. Blood Groups Biochem. Genet.*, 13, 245, 1982.
15. **Klip, A., Ramlal, T., Walker, D., Britt, B. A., and Elliot, M. S.**, Selective increase in cytoplasmic calcium by anesthetic in lymphocytes from malignant hyperthermic-susceptible pigs, *Anesth. Analg.*, 66, 381, 1987.
16. **Ohnishi, S. T., Katagi, H., Ohnishi, T., and Brownell, A. K. W.**, Detection of malignant hyperthermia susceptibility using a spin label technique on red blood cells, *Br. J. Anaesth.*, 61, 565, 1988.
17. **Olgin, J., Argove, Z., Rosenberg, H., Tuchler, M., and Chance, B.**, Non-invasive evaluation of malignant hyperthermia susceptibility with phosphorus nuclear magnetic resonance spectroscopy, *Anesthesiology*, 68, 507, 1988.

18. **Klip, A., Elliott, M. E., Frodis, W., Britt, B. A., Pegg, W., and Scott, E.**, Anaesthetic-induced increase in ionized calcium in blood mononuclear cells from malignant hyperthermia patients, *Lancet*, 1, 463, 1987.
19. **Ohnishi, S. T. and Ohnishi, T.**, Halothane induced disorders of red cell membranes of subjects susceptible to malignant hyperthermia, *Cell Biochem. Funct.*, 6, 257, 1988.
20. **Fletcher, J. E. and Rosenberg, H.**, *In vitro* interaction between halothane and succinylcholine in human skeletal muscle: implications for malignant hyperthermia and masseter rigidity, *Anesthesiology*, 63, 190, 1985.
21. **Cheah, A. M.**, Effect of long chain unsaturated fatty acids on the calcium transport of sarcoplasmic reticulum, *Biochim. Biophys. Acta*, 648, 113, 1981.
22. **Cheah, K. S. and Cheah, A. M.**, Skeletal muscle mitochondrial phospholipase A_2 and the interaction of mitochondria and sarcoplasmic reticulum, *Biochim. Biophys. Acta*, 638, 40, 1981.
23. **Fletcher, J. E. and Rosenberg, H.**, *In vitro* muscle contractures induced by halothane and suxamethonium. II, Human skeletal muscle from normal and malignant hyperthermia-susceptible patients, *Br. J. Anaesth.*, 58, 1433, 1986.

Chapter 16

NONINVASIVE SCREENING FOR MALIGNANT HYPERTHERMIA BY MEANS OF THE LYMPHOCYTE TEST

Beverley A. Britt, Amira Klip,
Peter J. O'Brien, and Barbara I. Kalow

TABLE OF CONTENTS

I.   Introduction 226

II. Results using Single Wavelength Spectrofluorometry
     and Quin 2 229

III. Results using Single Wavelength Spectrofluorometry
     and Indo 1 232

IV. Results using Single Wavelength Spectrophotometry and
     Fura 2 235

V.   Results using Dual Wavelength Spectrophotometry and
     Indo 1 237

VI. Concluding Remarks 247

References 247

I. INTRODUCTION

Until now, accurate diagnosis of malignant hyperthermia (MH), a pharmacogenetic muscle disorder, has been possible only by means of the caffeine halothane contracture (CHC) test.[1-16] This test, unfortunately, requires a large volume of muscle, several hours of a highly trained technician's time, and a large amount of expensive equipment. It is, therefore, complex, costly, and time consuming. Moreover, the patient is left with a large, permanent, and unsightly scar. A less invasive test is urgently needed.

MH is thought to be a widespread membrane disorder involving not just membranes within skeletal muscle cells but also membranes within other cell types including those in the blood.[9] The defect in the skeletal muscle cells is now known to be due to an error of calcium distribution.[9,17-33] Thus, excessive amounts of calcium, in the presence of triggering drugs such as halothane or succinylcholine, are released from the sarcoplasmic reticulum (SR)[22,23,25,27,29-33] due to a defect in the ryanodine receptor,[34] which is the site of the calcium release channel. As a result, the concentration of calcium in the cytoplasm of malignant hyperthermic-susceptible (MHS) individuals is greater than normal.[35,36] It might be possible, in cells more accessible than skeletal muscle cells, to devise a screening or diagnostic test based on this error of calcium metabolism.

The advent of calcium indicators such as Quin 2 and Indo 1 has enabled just such a test using lymphocytes. Lymphocytes have been used because of their easy availability, simplicity of isolation, long *in vitro* half life, and the familiarity of most hospital laboratories with the isolation procedure. The lymphocyte test[37-40] uses the cytoplasmic calcium assay of Tsien et al.[41] and is based on the premise that the uncharged precursors Quin 2-acetoxy methyl ester or Indo 1-acetoxy methyl ester, after permeating into the lymphocyte cytoplasm, are cleaved by cytosolic esterases to form formaldehyde and acetic acid and negatively charged Quin 2 or Indo 1 in their free acid forms. Both Quin 2 and Indo 1 are repelled from the negatively charged inner surface of the cell membrane and thus are unable to leave the interior of the lymphocyte. They also bind exclusively with positively charged calcium; the Quin 2-calcium or Indo 1-calcium product is fluorescent so it can be quantitatively measured in a spectrofluorometer. Because the K_d of the Quin 2-Ca^{2+} complex is 115 nm and that of the Indo 1-Ca^{2+} complex is 240 nm, the fluorophors are efficient indicators of free calcium concentrations in the 10^{-7} to 10^{-6} M range, which is similar to that existing in the cytoplasm of the majority of mammalian cells.

Patients and pigs are selected for the lymphocyte studies in the following way. *Malignant hyperthermic susceptible (MHS) humans and pigs* are those who have had an MH reaction or who have had a family history of an MH reaction and who have also had a CHC test positive for MH.[16] *Normal humans and pigs* are those who have never had an MH reaction, have no family history of MH reactions, and whose CHC tests are negative for MH.[16]

The lymphocyte assay is performed as follows.[37-40] First, 10 ml of blood are taken via a Vacutainer® into a heparinized glass tube. The blood is diluted 1:1 with Roswell Park Memorial Institute 1640 (RPMI) culture medium, which is a basic Ringer's solution containing glutamine plus a phenol red dye indicator. Each tube is gently inverted two or three times. Then 10 ml of this diluted blood are layered on top of 3 ml of Ficoll-Paque. The resulting mixture is spun at 1500 rpm in a bench-top centrifuge at room temperature for 30 min to produce a layer of lymphocytes, monocytes, and platelets between lighter RPMI above and heavier Ficoll-Paque below and still heavier red blood cells and neutrophils at the very bottom. After this first centrifugation the lymphocytes and platelets are collected with a plastic Pasteur pipette and are then diluted with 10 ml of RPMI medium. During this collection, care must be taken not to excessively contaminate the lymphocyte-platelet layer with the Ficoll-Paque layer. The diluted preparation is centrifuged at 1200 rpm for 10 min. At the end of centrifugation, the lymphocytes and monocytes are collected into a pellet at the bottom of the tube. The platelet-rich supernatant is, therefore, discarded and the lymphocyte-rich pellet is resuspended in 0.5 ml of RPMI and is again spun at 750 rpm for 5 min. Once more the supernatant is discarded and the lymphocyte pellet is suspended in 0.5 ml of bicarbonate-free RPMI modified with 5 mM of HEPES, pH 7.4 (HPMI). This fraction contains approximately 80% lymphocytes and 20% monocytes and is commonly referred to as either "lymphocytes" or "mononuclear cells".

The lymphocyte-HPMI mixture is loaded with 100 μM Quin 2-AM or with 2 μM Indo 1-AM. The mixture containing Quin 2 is incubated in the dark at 37°C for 30 min while the mixture containing Indo 1 is incubated also in the dark at 37°C but for 60 min. Then the lymphocyte-HPMI-indicator mixture is centrifuged for 5 min at 750 rpm. The cell pellet is suspended in 0.5 ml HPMI, respun for 5 min at 750 rpm, and resuspended in 0.1 ml of HPMI to produce the final preparation. The above two spinnings remove the remaining acetoxy methyl ester.

Fluorescent assay buffer is composed of 10 mM HEPES, 10 mM glucose, 140 mM NaCl, 3 mM KCl, and 1 mM MgCl$_2$, pH 7.3. This solution is passed through a filter with a 0.22-μm pore diameter to remove any particulate matter that might interfere with fluorescence determinations. Following this, 5 mM TPEN, a heavy metal chelator, is added to the buffer. This addition has been made only in studies utilizing Indo 1, but could also be employed if Quin 2 is utilized as the fluorescent indicator. Measurements of the buffer, when using Quin 2, are made at a wavelength of 339 nm for excitation (3 nm-slit width) and 485 nm for emission (15-nm slit width). When using Indo 1, measurements are made at a wavelength of 331 nm for excitation (3-nm slit width) and 485 nm for emission (15-nm slit width). All measurements are carried out at room temperature. To calibrate the baseline, fluorescence is read first in the presence of the buffer alone in a fluorescence quartz (not plastic) cuvette placed over a specially adapted constant magnetic stirrer within the spectrofluorometer. Then 20 μl of the indicator-loaded lymphocytes are

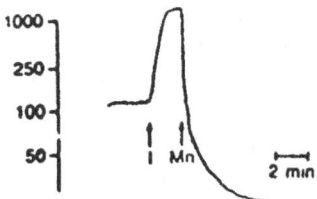

FIGURE 1. Fluorescence tracings in units of $[Ca^{2+}]$ in Quin2-loaded blood mononuclear cells (calibration): Quin2-loaded blood mononuclear cells were suspended in isotonic saline solution containing 1 mmol/l $CaCl_2$ and fluorescence was recorded and calibrated. The traces show the effect of addition of the ionophore ionomycin (I), which increases $[Ca^{2+}]_i$, and of Mn, which displaces calcium ions from Quin2. (From Klip, A., et al., *Lancet*, 28, 463, 1987. With permission.)

added to 1.0 ml of the assay buffer and the fluorescence measurement is repeated. $CaCl_2$ 1.0 *M* is added to the mixture and fluorescence is also measured at this time to make certain that the lymphocytes are not leaky. A small increase in fluorescence (about 10%) is expected under these conditions.

Next, various doses of halothane are added to the cuvette and fluorescence measurements (F) are made. The halothane is prepared by dilution in dimethylsulfoxide 10 times to produce 0.5 mmol/l increments of halothane. All transfers of halothane are made in a Drummond model 210 syringe. These halothane additions can be added either to separate lymphocyte samples or can be added cumulatively to a single lymphocyte sample. The latter is preferable as it requires fewer lymphocytes and less time to produce more accurate results. If using the latter, care must be taken not to perturb the preparation.

Finally, the maximum possible rise in cytoplasmic calcium (F_{max}) is determined by adding 0.5 m*M* of ionomycin, a nonfluorescent calcium ionophore and measuring fluorescence (Figure 1). Cell autofluorescence (AF) is determined by adding 3 μl of 1.0 *M* of manganese chloride (final concentration = 3 m*M*) and measuring fluorescence (Figure 1).

The results are calculated as follows:

$$F\ min = AF\ + \frac{(F_{max} - AF)^{41,42}}{N}$$

where N = the ratio of fluorescence for the complexed to uncomplexed form of the indicator and is 6 for Quin 2 and 12 for Indo 1 based on values determined in our laboratory. F_{min} is the minimum fluorescence of the uncomplexed indicator.

Then $(Ca^{2+})_i$ is calculated from the above as:

$$(Ca^{2+})_i = \frac{K_d(F - F_{min})}{F_{max} - F}$$

115 being the apparent Kd for Ca^{2+}/Quin 2 at 37°C and 240 being the apparent Kd For Ca^{2+}/Indo 1 at 37°C.[41-42] In the laboratory of Dr. A. Klip, independent determinations at room temperature of the K_d value in KCl solution mimicking the cytosolic composition yields a value of 175 nM for the Indo 1 K_d.[40] This latter value is used for calculating Klip's data. By the above equation, measurements are independent of the concentration of indicator and of the number of cells in the cuvette since they are calibrated within each sample.

Every 30 min the cells loaded with fluorescent indicator should be centrifuged prior to sampling in order to remove any leaked dye. In addition, following halothane additions the measurements should be completed within 5 min to obtain maximum diagnostic discrimination. Other nondiagnostic studies should be completed ideally within 30 to 60 min and at most within 120 min. It may be that in the diagnostic test halothane damage is responsible for the reduction in the time of viability of the cells.

II. RESULTS USING SINGLE WAVELENGTH SPECTROFLUOROMETRY AND QUIN 2

Values obtained in the laboratory of Dr. B. A. Britt for human normal and MHS patients are shown in Table 1.[9] Values from the laboratory of Dr. A. Klip[37-39] for human normal and MHS patients are shown in Table 2 and an example is given in Figure 2A and B. In both laboratories halothane produces a rise in the concentration of cytoplasmic calcium of normal and MHS human lymphocytes.[9,37-39] In the presence of halothane, cytoplasmic calcium is significantly greater in MHS than in normal lymphocytes. It is certain that this rise in the concentration of free calcium in the lymphocyte cytoplasm cannot be due to a reduction of cell volume because measurements

TABLE 1
Effect of Halothane on $[Ca^{2+}]_i$ of Lymphocytes with a Calcium Indicator

$[Ca^{2+}]$ nM		Quin 2 Halothane (−)	Quin 2 Halothane (+)	Indo 1 Halothane (−)	Indo 1 Halothane (+)	$T_{Quin\ 2}$	vs.	Indo 1
NORMAL	x	105.10	167.60	227.50	421.90	−7.39***		− halo
	SE	8.09	13.10	14.60	41.50	−5.86***		+ halo
T − vs. + halo		−4.07 ***		−4.60***				
MHS	x	118.70	286.80	176.00	1426.00	−2.11*		− halo
	SE	16.00	83.00	22.70	458.00	−2.64*		+ halo
T − vs. + halo		−1.99*		−2.72***				
T N vs. MHS		−0.85	−1.85	2.00	3.28			
		n.s.	*	*	***			

Note: $\bar{x}$ = sample size — 13 normal and 6 MHS patients, SE = standard error, halo = halothane, * = $p < 0.05$, ** = $p < 0.01$, *** = $p < 0.001$.

TABLE 2
Effect of Halothane on [Ca²⁺]ᵢ of Lymphocytes using Quin 2

	Patients		Pigs	
	Normal	MH	Normal	MH
− Halothane	149 ± 15(12)	141 ± 12(14)	152 ± 14(8)	153 ± 10(17)
+ Halothane	173 ± 16(12)	253 ± 33(14)	183 ± 14(8)	267 ± 27(17)
p	>>0.05	<0.01	>>0.05	<0.001

Note: The cytoplasmic free Ca²⁺ concentration (nM) was determined in Quin 2-loaded
cells suspended in isotonic saline solution containing 1 mM CaCl₂. Two to four
determinations were made with each cell sample. Results are the mean ± SE
of (n) patients or pigs. The p value of (two-tail) for the comparison of + v.s. −
halothane is indicated.

From Klip, A., Britt, B. A., Elliott, M. E. et al., *Biochem. Cell Biol.,* 64, 1184,
1986. With permission.

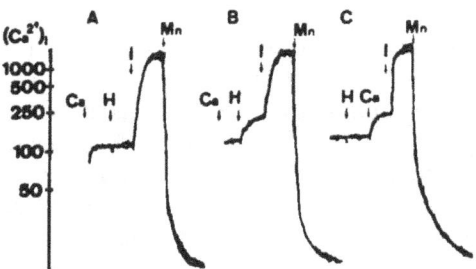

FIGURE 2.   Determination of the cytoplasmic free Ca²⁺ concentration in human lymphocytes.
Ca²⁺ (final concentration 1 mM) or 4 μl halothane (H)/ml was added where indicated. The
fluorescence was calibrated as described in Materials and Methods by permeabilization to Ca²⁺
with 0.5 μM ionomycin (I), followed by addition of 3 mM MnCl₂ (Mn). (A) Effect of halothane
in cells from a normal patient (R.C.) in the presence of extracellular Ca²⁺. (B) Effect of halothane
in cells from a malignant hyperthermia-susceptible patient (M.T.) in the presence of extracellular
Ca²⁺. (C) Effect of halothane in fells from the malignant hyperthermia-susceptible patient in
experiment B, in the absence of extracellular Ca²⁺. (From Klip, A., et al., *Biochem. Cell Biol.,*
64, 1184, 1986. With permission.)

by Klip et al.[38] have shown that the addition of halothane to MHS lymphocytes
does not change their cell volume.

The above work has been performed using 4 μl/ml or 38 mM of halothane.
Because the concentration of halothane in clinically anesthetized rats is calculated to be only 3.34 mM,[43] it might be argued that 38 mM halothane is
high enough to damage the cells in some nonspecific way. However, Klip et
al.[38] have shown that this is not true because viability studies revealed no
abnormality produced by halothane. For example, the lactic dehydrogenase
content of the lymphocytes and viability determined by exclusion of Trypan

blue in the absence and in the presence of halothane does not differ.[37] Furthermore, when halothane is diluted in dimethyl sulfoxide concentrations as low as 5.4 mM of halothane, it still causes an increase in free calcium in cells from MHS pigs while dimethoxysulfoxide alone does not cause any measurable change in the cytoplasmic calcium of pig lymphocytes.[37]

Using this indicator the halothane-induced rise in $(Ca^{2+})_i$ occurs only in the presence of exogenous calcium.[37-39] Thus, addition of halothane to lymphocytes suspended in a calcium-free solution does not cause a rise in the concentration of cytoplasmic calcium of both human and pig MHS lymphocytes (Figure 2C).[37,39] Addition of calcium after the halothane, however, restores the rise in the cytoplasmic free calcium concentration (Figure 2C).[39] This effect of calcium after the addition of halothane is larger than the increase in cytoplasmic calcium after the addition of extracellular calcium in the absence of halothane (compare Figures 2(B) and (C)).[39] These results suggest, therefore, that halothane may increase the permeability of the lympholemma to calcium ions and that the source of the excess calcium is extracellular fluid calcium transported across the lympholemma, perhaps through voltage-sensitive channels.

It should be realized, however, that the above observations do not rule out an intracellular source for the increased $(Ca^{2+})_i$ in addition to the extracellular site. This second possibility has also been tested by Klip and her fellow workers.[37] First, the intracellular concentration of Quin 2 is determined by loading the cells with (3H) Quin 2 tetra-acetoxy methyl ester. The radioactivity trapped by the cells, the number of cells, and the correction for osmotically active space are used to calculate the cytoplasmic concentration of the Quin 2. Using this value, with the peak cytoplasmic free calcium caused by the ionomycin, and with the dissociation constant of the Quin 2/Ca^{2+} complex, the amount of calcium released from intracellular stores per cell can be calculated. All these measurements are made in Ca^{2+} free medium containing 0.5 mM EGTA. It is then possible to determine the amount of halothane-induced calcium released from intracellular stores by calculating the ratio of the effect of ionomycin on release of free calcium after addition of halothane to its effect before the addition of halothane. This ratio is known as "releasable calcium".

In these experiments it has again been found that halothane does not produce a measurable increase in $(Ca^{2+})_i$ in cells suspended in calcium-free medium. This finding is consistent with either a lack of effect of halothane on the calcium from the intracellular stores or, alternatively, with a flux of calcium from the stores into the cytoplasm and then out of the cell that is too fast to be measurable. To test the latter possibility, halothane is added to MHS and normal human lymphocytes immediately before ionomycin. In normal lymphocytes, ionomycin produces a calcium release that is nearly (although not quite) as great as that seen with ionomycin addition alone (Figure 3).[37] In MHS lymphocytes ionomycin causes only a very small calcium release

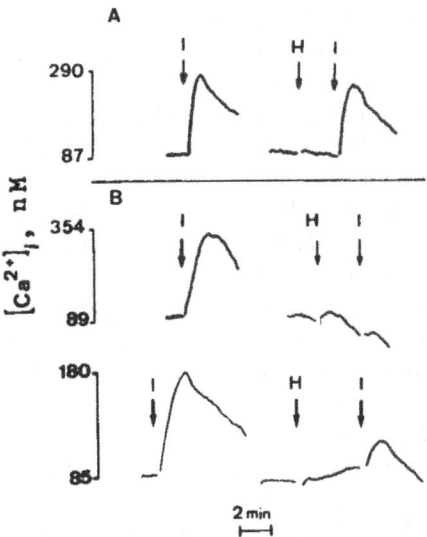

FIGURE 3.   Effect of ionomycin and halothane on the releasable Ca^{2+} from intracellular stores. Quin2-loaded human lymphocytes were suspended in Ca^{2+}-free solution (containing 0.5 mM EGTA). Ionomycin (I) (0.5 mM) and 4 μl halothane (H)/ml were added where indicated. (A) Lymphocytes from a normal patient (F.C.). (B and C) Lymphocytes from two malignant hyperthermia-susceptible patients (H.T. and B.C., respectively). (From Klip, A., et al., *Biochem. Cell Biol.*, 64, 1184, 1986. With permission.)

or no calcium release at all.[37] These data suggest that there is less releasable Ca^{2+} available to ionomycin after halothane additions (Table 3). Therefore, it is conceivable that halothane releases Ca^{2+} from intracellular stores (in addition to inducing increased transport of extracellular Ca^{2+} into the cytoplasm), but that this Ca^{2+} is lost from the cytoplasm to the extracellular fluid so rapidly that it cannot be measured by direct means.[36] Moreover, this halothane-dependent release of intracellular Ca^{2+} is higher in MHS cells than in normal cells. The transience in $(Ca^{2+})_i$ caused by halothane may have been buffered by the high concentration of intracellular Quin 2 that has been used for these fluorescent studies. Indeed, this concentration reaches the millimolar range, and in cells suspended in Ca^{2+}-free medium (as required for these experiments) this may effectively chelate $(Ca^{2+})_i$ sufficiently to prevent the detection of small and rapid changes in this parameter.[40]

III. RESULTS USING SINGLE WAVELENGTH SPECTROFLUOROMETRY AND INDO 1

This potentiality has been resolved in studies using Indo 1 as the fluorescent indicator, since much lower intracellular concentrations of this indicator are required to obtain measurable fluorescence readings (see below).

TABLE 3
Fraction of Releasable Ca^{2+} from Intracellular Stores after Exposure to Halothane using Quin 2

Patients		Pigs	
Normal	MH	Normal	MH
0.71 ± 9.07^{10}	$0.49 \pm 0.10^{9\,a}$	0.75 ± 0.15^{6}	$0.42 \pm 0.05^{6\,a}$

Note: Releasable Ca^{2+} is defined as the Ca^{2+} released by ionomycin (0.5 μM) into the cytoplasm in cells suspended in Ca^{2+} free medium. The data represent the ratio of the effect of ionomycin after addition of halothane to before halothane (4 μl/ml for 60 s) and are expressed as the mean $\pm$ SE of (n) patients or pigs.

a $p < 0.05$ for malignant hyperthermia vs. normal.

From Klip, A., Britt, B. A., Elliott, M. E. et al., *Biochem. Cell Biol.,* 64, 1186, 1986. With permission.

When human lymphocytes are loaded with Indo 1, in the laboratory of Dr. Britt, the basal $(Ca^{2+})_i$ (in the absence of halothane) is slightly but significantly lower in cells from MHS patients than from normal patients (Table 1).[9] In the laboratory of Dr. Klip, on the other hand, the reverse has been found (Table 4).[40] The addition of halothane (38 mM) in the laboratory of Dr. Britt and clinical concentrations of 2.5 to 5.8 mM in the laboratory of Dr. Klip elevate $(Ca^{2+})_i$ in both groups of cells, but the effect is much higher in the MHS group (Tables 1 and 4). Similar differences have been observed between cells of MHS pigs relative to normal pigs (Table 5).[40] Using 38 mM

TABLE 4
Effect of Halothane on $[Ca^{2+}]_i$ in Lymphocytes from Normal and MHS Humans using Indo 1

Halothane concentration (mmol/l)	Normal			MHS		
	0	2.85	5.7	0	2.85	5.7
nM $[Ca^{2+}]_i$	146 ± 14	205 ± 21	187 ± 32	198 ± 18	342 ± 43	461 ± 73
p ($-$H vs. $+$H)	—	<0.0025	>0.025	—	<0.005	<0.001
p (N vs. MHS)	—	—	—	<0.025	<0.005	<0.005

Note: Lymphocytes were suspended in solution 1 containing 1 mM $CaCl_2$. Results are the mean $\pm$ S.E. of (n) individual patients. N = Normal; MHS = malignant hyperthermia susceptible; H = halothane concentration. Statistical parameters correspond to Student t test.

From Klip, A., Mills, G. B., Britt, B. A., and Elliott, M. E., *Am. J. Physiol.,* 258, (*Cell Physiol.,* 27), C495, 1990. With permission.

TABLE 5
Effect of Halothane on $[Ca^{2+}]_i$ in Lymphocytes from Normal and MHS Pigs using Indo 1

Halothane concentration (mmol/l)	Normal		MHS		
	0	5.7	0	2.85	5.7
nM $[Ca^{2+}]_i$	279 ± 64	340 ± 44	301 ± 21	462 ± 53	530 ± 75
p (−H vs. +H)	—	>0.05	—	<0.005	<0.005
p (N vs. MHS)	—	—	>0.05	—	<0.05

Note: Lymphocytes were suspended in solution 1 containing 1 mM CaCl$_2$. Results are the mean ± S.E. of (n) individual patients. N = normal; MHS = malignant hyperthermia susceptible; H = halothane concentration. Statistical parameters correspond to Student t test.

From Klip, A., Mills, G. B., Britt, B. A., and Elliott, M. E., *Am. J. Physiol.*, 258, (*Cell Physiol.*, 27), C495, 1990. With permission.

halothane, the differences noted in Indo 1-loaded cells are much more marked than in Quin 2-loaded cells (Table 1).[9,40] Using 2.85 or 5.7 mM halothane, the increase in $(Ca^{2+})_i$ is still significantly different in cells from MHS patients than from normal individuals (Tables 4 and 5).[40]

Measurements performed in Indo 1-loaded lymphocytes, suspended in a Ca^{2+}-free medium, reveal that, unlike Quin 2-loaded lymphocytes, halothane does increase $(Ca^{2+})_i$ in lymphocytes suspended in Ca^{2+}-free medium, although the absolute increase is lower than in the extracellular presence of the cation (Table 6).[40] To test whether the observations of lack of response to halothane in $(Ca^{2+})_i$ in Quin 2-loaded lymphocytes in the absence of extracellular Ca^{2+} have been due to buffering of the cytoplasmic cation, experiments have been performed with Indo 1-loaded lymphocytes containing cytoplasmically trapped BAPTA, a Ca^{2+} chelator.[40] The results indicate that under these conditions, which mimic the situation in Quin 2-loaded lymphocytes, the effect of halothane on $(Ca^{2+})_i$ is abolished (Table 6). This confirms that the anesthetic does induce the release of Ca^{2+} from intracellular stores and that this is better detected by Indo 1 than by Quin 2 by virtue of the lower concentration required of the former indicator, which causes significantly less chelation and buffering of $(Ca^{2+})_i$ transients. However, the full response to the anesthetic has been observed in the presence of extracellular Ca^{2+}, suggesting that the latter is required either to replenish the intracellular Ca^{2+} stores or to allow a permissive amount of Ca^{2+} to enter the lymphocytes which magnifies the halothane-induced release of intracellular Ca^{2+}.

In this regard it is interesting to note that removing the calcium from the Krebs Ringer solution normalizes the CHC test (Figure 4)[44] which indicates that the elevated cytoplasmic calcium of MHS muscle cells also has more than one source — extracellular fluid as well as SR. It may be, therefore, that within a given cell type more than one membrane is involved. In muscle,

TABLE 6
Role of Extracellular Ca²⁺ in the Response
of [Ca²⁺]ᵢ to Halothane in Lymphocytes
from MHS Patients using Indo 1

Extracellular Ca²⁺	Halothane	[Ca²⁺]ᵢ (nM)	[Ca²⁺]ᵢ (nM)
+	−	137 ± 12	
+	+	281 ± 38	145
−	−	81 ± 14	
−	+	158 ± 28	77

Measurements in BAPTA-loaded lymphocytes

+	−	214 ± 41	
+	+	316 ± 104	104
−	−	100 ± 15	
−	+	99 ± 16	−1

Note: Values represent the mean ± SE of four MHS patients. Lymphocytes from each patient were assayed two to five times in each condition.

however, the acute reactions that develop in the presence of halothane must be mainly due to release of calcium from the SR and not from influx of extracellular fluid calcium because dantrolene, a drug known to prevent release of calcium from the SR, is highly efficacious in treating acute MH reactions, while verapamil, diltiazem, and nifedipine — voltage-sensitive blockers of calcium influx from the extracellular fluid — are not efficacious in the management of MH crises.[45-47]

IV. RESULTS USING SINGLE WAVELENGTH SPECTROPHOTOMETRY AND FURA 2

Smiley et al.,[48] Ellis,[49] Heffron,[50] Ording,[51] and Fletcher[52] have been unable to reproduce the above difference between MHS and normal lymphocytes, although they have noted similar halothane-induced rises in cytoplasmic calcium concentrations in both normal and MHS lymphocytes. We are unable to comment on the latter three investigators' results because their work is as yet unpublished. In the report of Smiley, however, several points should be made. First, they used Fura 2, instead of Indo 1 or Quin 2. Second, their sample size was extremely small (only five normal and three MHS patients). Third, neither the clinical history nor the caffeine halothane contracture test results for the MHS patients was given. Fourth, they may have used an inappropriate syringe to transfer the halothane, and, finally, they may have waited too long after incubation before commencing and completing measurements.

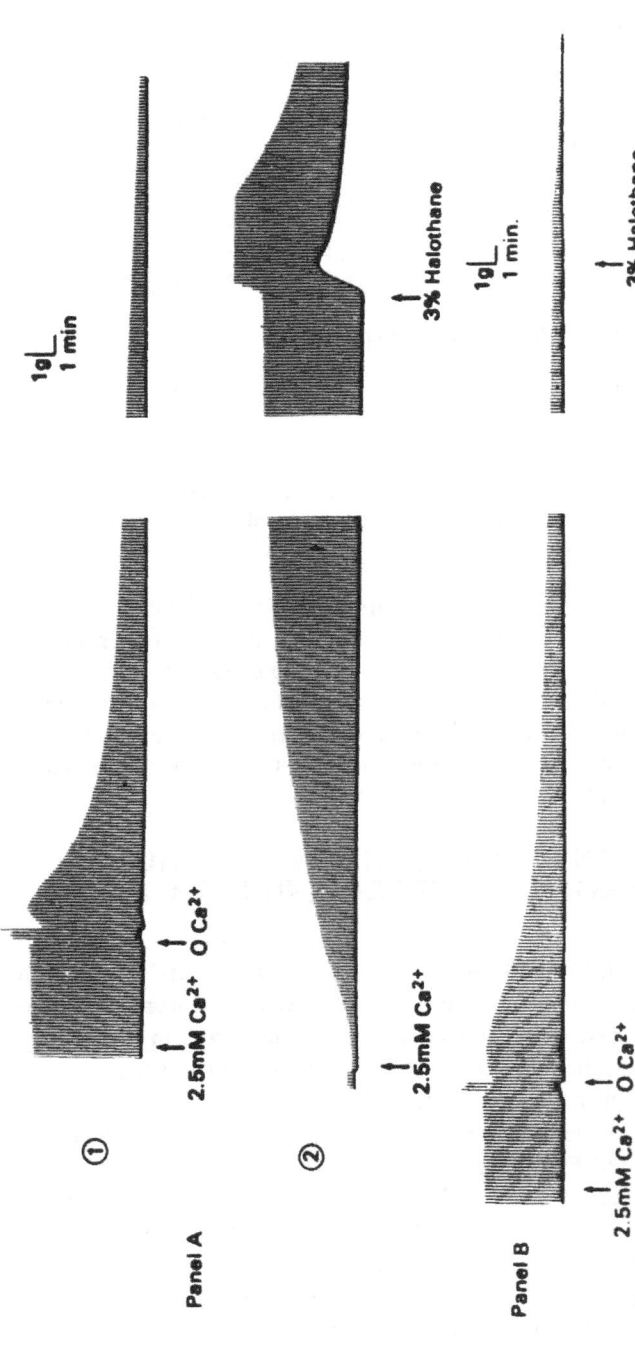

FIGURE 4. Reversible effects of incubating MH muscle in the absence of Ca²⁺. In panel A1, the
A2, the muscle was re-exposed to 2.5 m*M* Ca²⁺ solution, the twitch returns to control level and a ty
muscle was exposed to zero Ca²⁺ solution for 45 minutes at which time exposure to 3% halothane dic
Exp. Ther., 219, 107, 1981. With permission.)

V. RESULTS USING DUAL WAVELENGTH SPECTROPHOTOMETRY AND INDO 1

Recently O'Brien et al.[53] have performed lymphocyte studies on 10 MHS and 20 normal pigs. Their work has been carried out using a dual emission spectrofluorometry described by Grykiewicz et al.[42] and thereby has been able to monitor both free calcium and calcium bound to the fluorescent indicator Indo 1. This has the advantage of elimination of photo bleaching of the indicator and reduction of background fluorescence through use of the ratio of fluorescence of bound calcium to free calcium. Measurements are made at a 340-nm wavelength for excitation (0.9-nm slit width), 398-nm wavelength for emission (9-nm slit width) of the calcium bound form of the indicator, and 482-nm wavelength for emission (9-nm slit width) of the free form of the indicator.

The concentration of $(Ca^{2+})_i$ is calculated from the equation:

$$Ca = 240 \times (R - R_{min})/(R_{max} - R)$$

where R = complexed/uncomplexed fluorescent indicator; $R_{min} = 1/6 \ (R_{max} - R_{mn}) + R_{mn}$ and 240 is the dissociation constant of the calcium-Indo 1 complex in nanomoles per liter at 37°C. In contrast to the studies of Klip et al.[40] using fixed wavelengths of emission, the measurements at dual emission wavelength have been carried out at 37°C to better predict the lymphocyte calcium concentration at body temperature. Additionally, the fluorescence of the calcium-bound dye is divided by the fluorescence of the calcium-free dye to reduce artifact and increase sensitivity. Thus the percentage of increase in $(Ca^{2+})_i$ caused by the addition of halothane is calculated as $100 \times$ (nanomolar change from resting $(Ca^{2+})_i$/resting $(Ca^{2+})_i$). The halothane-induced increase in the rate of calcium accumulations is calculated as the ratio of the maximal slope of the fluorescence time graph in the presence of up to 2 mM/l halothane to the slope in the absence of halothane. Slopes are measured with a protractor and rounded off upward to the nearest degree.[53]

For the above study, a typical tracing of the halothane-induced changes in fluorescence of calcium-bound indicator and calcium-free indicator in MHS pig lymphocytes are shown in Figure 5. Examples of tracings of the ratioed (bound to free) calcium are given in Figure 6 (normal) and in Figure 7 (MHS). By this procedure it has been found that the cytoplasmic ionized calcium concentrations are lower in MHS than in normal pig lymphocytes (Table 7).[53,54] However, increasing the concentration of halothane reduces this difference so that by 2 mM/l halothane the calcium concentration is about the same in both groups of pigs (Table 7). Moreover, free calcium is increased at lower concentrations of halothane in the MHS than in the normal swine lymphocytes (Table 7).[53,54] Greater variability in calcium concentration occurs within the MHS pig lymphocytes (Table 7).

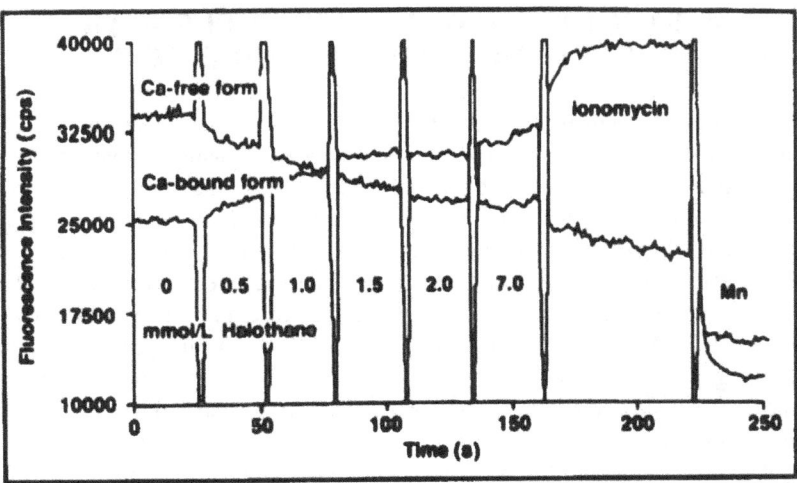

FIGURE 5. Dual-emission spectrofluorogram of halothane-induced increase in concentration of free calcium of lymphocytes from a pig susceptible to malignant hyperthermia. Transient increases in fluorescence to maximal or minimal values represent opening of the spectrofluorometer sample chamber to make drug additions. Changes in the calcium-free and the calcium-bound fluorescent dye were monitored simultaneously as halothane concentractions was increased. Addition of ionomycin indicates the maximal fluorescence, whereas addition of Mn displaces all calcium from the dye. As cytoplasmic calcium concentrations increased, the fluorescence of the calcium-bound dye increased, whereas the fluorescence of the calcium-free dye decreased proportionately. Fluorescence intensity is measured in counts per second (cps). (From O'Brien, P., et al., *Am. J. Vet. Res.*, 50, 132, 1989. With permission.)

The increase in calcium caused by the addition of halothane is greater in MHS than in normal lymphocytes (Table 8).[53,54] In particular $(Ca^{2+})_i$ increases at lower concentrations of halothane in the MHS than in the normal pig lymphocytes; at all concentrations of halothane, the percentage of increase in $(Ca^{2+})_i$ is 7- to 16-fold greater than for controls (Table 9 and Figure 8). $(Ca^{2+})_i$ increases at a slow rate in the absence of halothane, especially so for MHS lymphocytes (Figure 9). On the other hand, faster rates of calcium accumulation caused by exposure to up to 2 m*M*/l halothane occur in MHS than in normal lymphocytes (Figure 10). The percentage increase in rate of $(Ca^{2+})_i$ increase caused by exposure to halothane is 35-fold greater for MHS than for control pig lymphocytes and values for rates for the two groups of pigs do not overlap (Figure 11).

The finding that 0.5 and 1.0 m*M*/l halothane double and triple, respectively, the cytoplasmic calcium concentration of lymphocytes from MHS pigs yet has no effect on normal pig lymphocytes is in agreement with the results of Klip et al.[37-39] using Quin 2.

In contrast to the report of Klip et al.[40] O'Brien et al.[54] have observed an 80% lower free calcium concentration in lymphocytes from MHS pigs, compared with normals, but resting calcium concentrations of clinically normal

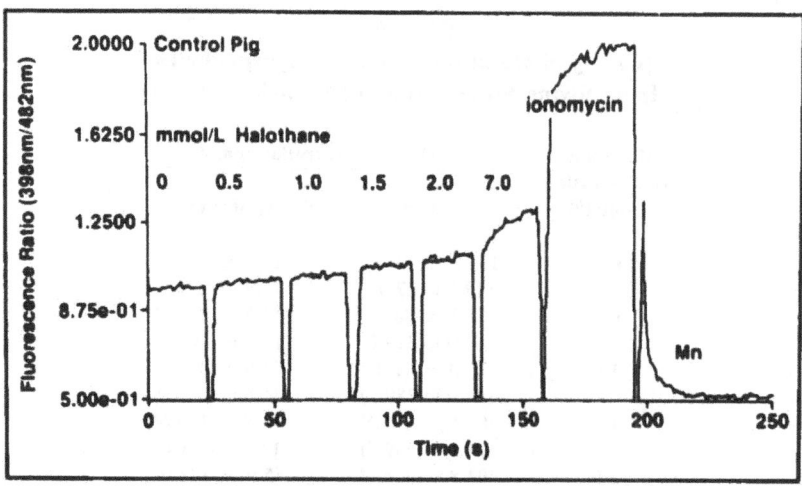

FIGURE 6. Rationmetric spectrofluorogram of halothane-induced increase in concentration of free calcium of lymphocytes from a control pig. The ordinate indicates the cytoplasmic concentrations of ionized calcium as indicated by the ratio of fluorescence of the calcium-bound dye to fluorescence of calcium-free dye. Fluorescence is measured in counts per second. There was a gradual increase in the cytoplasmic concentration of calcium of lymphocytes with additions of halothane until 7.0 mmol was achieved, at which time calcium accumulations was rapid. (From O'Brien, P., et al., *Am. J. Vet. Res.*, 50, 132, 1989. With permission.)

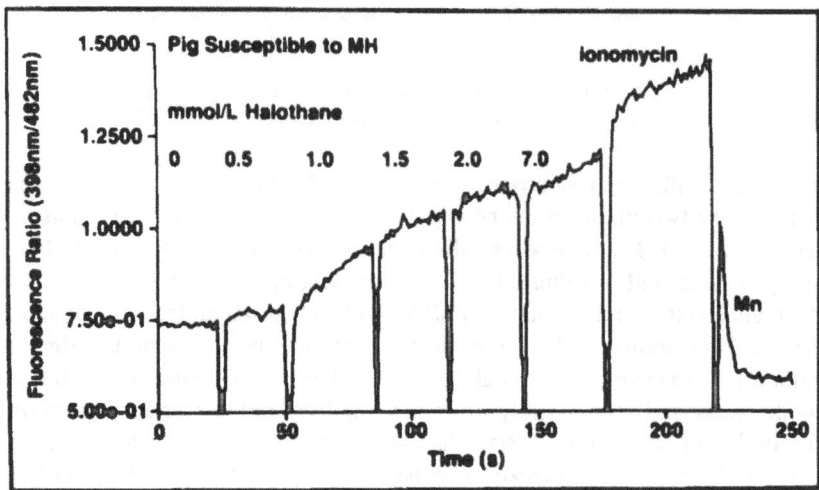

FIGURE 7. Rationmetric spectrofluorogram of halothane-induced increase in concentration of cytoplasmic free calcium of lymphocytes from a pig susceptible to MH. Concentrations of calcium in lymphocytes abruptly increased at 1 mmol/l halothane. The resting calcium concentration is lower than that for the control pig illustrated in Figure 8. (From O'Brien, P., et al., *Am. J. Vet. Res.*, 50, 132, 1989. With permission.)

TABLE 7

$[Ca^{2+}]_i$ of Halothane-Treated Lymphocytes
from Swine Susceptible to MH using Indo 1

Halothane concentration (mmol/l)	Calcium concentration (nmol/l)	
	Control	Susceptible to MH
0	185.3 ± 91.6 (49.5 to 377)	40.5 ± 38.8[a] (2.3 to 135.2)
0.5	207.3 ± 88.7 (60.0 to 399.0)	83.5 ± 90.9[a,b] (11.1 to 335.6)
1.0	225.0 ± 91.4 (54.0 to 389.2)	127.9 ± 81.3[a,b] (44.8 to 317.6)
1.5	265.5 ± 100.5[b] (81.3 to 439.7)	173.8 ± 110.6[a,b] (42.1 to 415.1)
2.0	303.8 ± 116.0[b] (86.1 to 543.9)	255.9 ± 182.0[b] (57.0 to 612.2)
7.0	856.8 ± 664.5[b] (183.2 to 2,655)	821.8 ± 836.4[b] (210.1 to 2,870)

Note: Data are expressed as mean concentration of free calcium ± SD (range) for 20 control Yorkshire and 10 Pietrain x Poland China MH-susceptible swine after exposure to various concentrations of halothane.

[a] Significantly different from controls (p < 0.05).
[b] Significantly different from resting calcium concentration (p < 0.05).

From O'Brien, P. J., Kalow, B. I., Brown, B. D. et al., *Am. J. Vet. Res.*, 50, 134, 1989. With permission.

swine are similar to those reported by Klip et al.[40] The cause for this difference between the two studies is unknown. It may reflect the use of a more sensitive technique by O'Brien. However, the variation in this parameter in the O'Brien study is large with resulting $(Ca^{2+})_i$ values ranging from 4 mM on. Another difference is that in the Klip study all blood had been taken from thiopentone-anesthetized animals who were clearly suffering no stress at the time of sampling. However, all animals in the O'Brien study have been sampled while awake and very possibly were suffering from mild stress due to handling during blood collection. O'Brien has suggested that the lower MHS $(Ca^{2+})_i$ that he observed may indicate increased calcium extrusion activity in lymphocytes from MHS pigs as a compensatory adaptation to hypersensitivity to stimuli such as stress that increases $(Ca^{2+})_i$. This would be analogous to the situation in muscle from MHS pigs whereby the calcium-sequestering activity of terminal cisternae is increased, compared with normals[34] and also analogous to the situation of erythrocytes from MHS dogs, in which the calcium-extrusion pump is increased twofold in activity compared with normals.[33] This

TABLE 8
Halothane-Induced Increase in $[Ca^{2+}]_i$ in nM of Lymphocytes from Swine Susceptible to MH using Indo 1

Halothane concentration (mmol/l) (nM)	nM Change in cytoplasmic calcium concentration	
	Control	Susceptible to MH
0.5	22.7 ± 17.2	43.1 ± 56.6[a]
	(0 to 56.2)	(2.3 to 200.4)
1.0	40.5 ± 26.4	87.6 ± 54.5[a]
	(0 to 88.4)	(21.8 to 182.4)
1.5	76.5 ± 44.0	144.2 ± 110.8[a]
	(0 to 177.9)	(22.7 to 339.4)
2.0	114.5 ± 66.4	216.8 ± 162.0[a]
	(0 to 241.1)	(44.3 to 521.0)
7.0	671.4 ± 640.4	779.6 ± 802.9
	(133.7 to 2515.0)	(207.8 to 2735.0)

Note: nM increase of $[Ca^{2+}]_i$ is from initial reading in absence of halothane. Data are expressed as mean nmol/l increase in calcium concentration ± SD (range) for 20 control Yorkshire swine and 10 Pietrain x Poland China MH-susceptible swine after exposure to various concentrations of halothane.

[a] Significantly different from controls (p <0.05).

From O'Brien, P. J., Kalow, B. I., Brown, B. D. et al., *Am. J. Vet. Res.*, 50, 134, 1989. With permission.

hypothesis is further supported by O'Brien's finding that lymphocytes from MHS pigs spontaneously accumulate calcium at only half the rate of normals.

In a more recent work, O'Brien and Lassaline[55] have found not only lower than normal $(Ca^{2+})_i$ in MHS lymphocytes but also a greater than normal extrusion rate of calcium from the MHS lymphocytes (Table 10 and Figure 12) and lesser rate of spontaneous calcium accumulation in the absence of halothane in the MHS lymphocytes (Table 11 and Figure 13). In this study calcium influx is eliminated by suspending the cells in a calcium free medium and by the addition of a calcium chelater. These abnormalities, as noted above, may be a compensatory mechanism for the increased calcium accumulation that occurs during MH reactions. In the case of pigs such reactions would most likely be of the stress-induced type that so frequently afflicts swine, rather than the halothane-induced type, because halothane is rarely administered to pigs and certainly almost never repeatedly.

TABLE 9

**Halothane-Induced Percent Increase in $[Ca^{2+}]_i$
of Lymphocytes from Swine Susceptible to MH
using Indo 1**

Halothane concentration (mmol/l) (%)	Change in cytoplasmic calcium concentration (%)	
	Control	Susceptible to MH
0.5	16.0 ± 15.0 (0 to 46.0)	129.0 ± 107.0[a] (16.0 to 383.0)
1.0	28.0 ± 21.0 (0 to 75.0)	440.0 ± 427.0[a] (56.0 to 1280.0)
1.5	51.0 ± 42.0 (0 to 160.0)	698.0 ± 791.0[a] (99.0 to 2640.0)
2.0	75.0 ± 60.0 (0 to 242.0)	1070.0 ± 1110.0[a] (282.0 to 3840.0)
7.0	403.0 ± 392.0 (100.0 to 1790.0)	2990.0 ± 2950.0 (876.0 to 9030.0)

Note: Percent increase of $[Ca^{2+}]_i$ is from initial reading in absence of halothane. Data are expressed as percentage of increase in calcium concentration ± SD (range) for 20 control Yorkshire swine and 10 Pietrain x Poland China MH-susceptible swine after exposure to various concentrations of halothane.

[a] Significantly different from controls ($p < 0.05$).

From O'Brien, P. J., Kalow, B. I., Brown, B. D. et al., *Am. J. Vet. Res.*, 50, 134, 1989. With permission.

This latter work of O'Brien[55] has been performed with a revised equation for the calculation of the concentration of ionized cytoplasmic calcium:

$$(Ca^{2+})_i = K_d \times G_{max}/G_{min} \times ((R - R_{min}) - dR)/(R_{max} - R) - dR$$

where k_d is the dissociation constant of the calcium-Indo 1 complex; $G_{max} = G_{min} + dG/dF (F_{max} - F_{min})$; G_{min} = the minimal value for the fluorescence of the calcium free form of Indo 1 at 482 nm at maximal cytoplasmic calcium concentration; dG/dF = the rate of change in G per rate of change; F_{max} and F_{min} are the maximal and minimal values for the fluorescence of the calcium-bound form of Indo 1 at 398 nm; R_{max} and R_{min} = the values for the ratio F/G at maximal and minimal cytoplasmic calcium concentration; and dR is the change in R due to Indo 1 leakage from cells.[56] This formula is independent of intracellular dye concentration, instrument sensitivity, lamp intensity fluctuations, and light path length and corrects for extracellular dye derived from rupture or leaky cells, background fluorescence, and manganese quenching of the G signal.

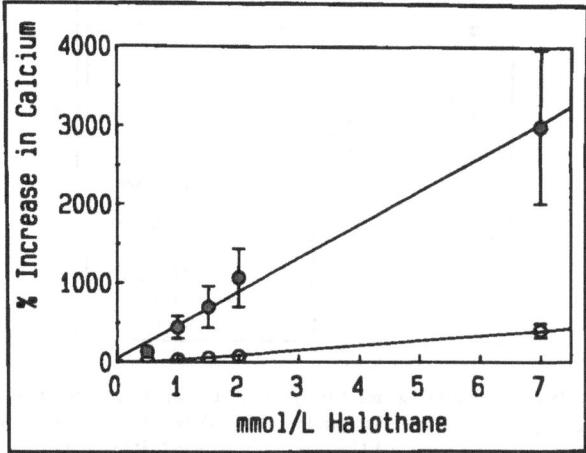

FIGURE 8. Dose-response curve of halothane-induced increase in concentration of cytoplasmic free calcium of lymphocytes from swine susceptible to MH and from control swine. Data are expressed as mean percentage increase ± SE of the mean for 20 control (open circles) and 10 swine susceptible to MH (solid circles). Values for the two groups are significantly different. (From O'Brien, P., et al., *Am. J. Vet. Res.*, 50, 132, 1989. With permission.)

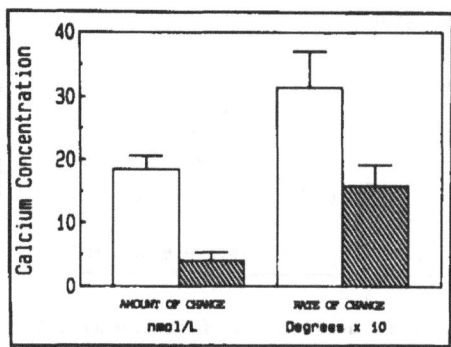

FIGURE 9. Increase in resting concentration of cytoplasmic calcium (see units along x axis) in lymphocytes of swine susceptible to MH. Data are expressed as mean ± SE of the mean for 20 control swine (open bars) and 10 swine susceptible to MH (diagonal bars). Rate of increase was determined by measuring the slope in degrees of the fluorescence-time graph before addition of halothane. Values for the two groups were significantly different. (From O'Brien, P., et al., *Am. J. Vet. Res.*, 50, 132, 1989. With permission.)

It should be noted that all the pigs used in the above studies were homozygous for the MH defect, while most, if not all, the humans are heterozygous. Differences between normal and MHS pig lymphocytes are, therefore, likely to be greater than those between normal and MHS human lymphocytes.

O'Brien et al.[57] have applied the lymphocyte test to a Border Collie suffering from canine distress syndrome. Canine distress syndrome occurs in

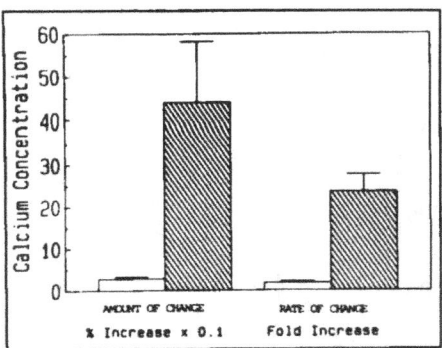

FIGURE 10. Halothane-induced increase in cytoplasmic calcium concentration (see units along x axis) of lymphocytes from swine susceptible to MH. Data are expressed as mean ± SE of the mean for 20 control (open bars) and 10 swine susceptible to MH (diagonal bars). The increase in rate of calcium accumulation is the ratio of the rate of calcium accumulation in the presence of 1 mmol/l halothane to the rate in the absence of halothane. (From O'Brien, P., et al., *Am. J. Vet. Res.*, 50, 132, 1989. With permission.)

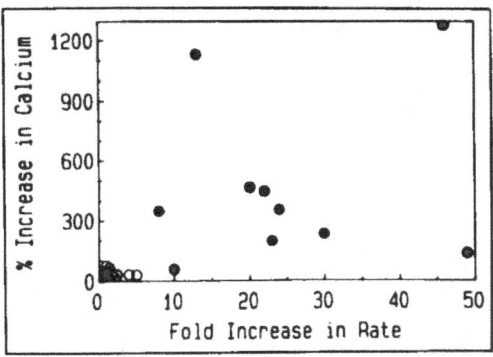

FIGURE 11. Scattergram for amount vs. rate of halothane-induced increase in accumulation of cytoplasmic free calcium. The increase in rate of calcium accumulation is the ratio of the rate of calcium accumulation in the presence of 1 mmol/l halothane to the rate in the absence of halothane. Data for 20 control swine (open circles) and 10 swine susceptible to MH (solid circles) are shown. Values for control swine are clustered in the lower left corner of the graph. There is no overlap in values for the two groups. (From O'Brien, P., et al., *Am. J. Vet. Res.*, 50, 132, 1989. With permission.)

some temperamentally hyperactive dogs. In these animals the stress of moderate exercise causes an MH-like syndrome with temperature rises of up to 42°C, apparent muscle cramping, dyspnea, and metabolic but not respiratory acidosis.[58] The condition can be identified by exercise challenge testing.[59] Caffeine causes calcium release from the muscle SR in greater than normal amounts and rates. As a result, a compensatory increase in calcium sequestration by the SR develops.[58] Muscle fascicles are excessively resistant to the contracture-producing effects of calcium in a manner similar to that observed

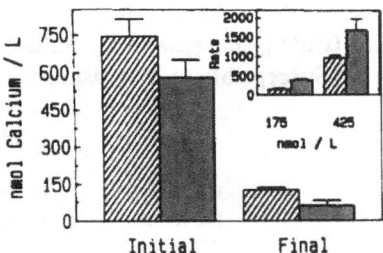

FIGURE 12. Calcium extrusion activity in lymphocytes from susceptible to malignant hyperthermia (MH). Calcium influx was eliminated by suspending the cells in calcium-free media and addition of calcium chelator. Data are expressed as mean ± SE of the mean for 3 control (diagonal bars) and 3 MH-susceptible (solid bars) swine for calcium concentration before and after extrusion. Determinations were done at 37°C to increase energy-dependent calcium extrusion activity and thereby optimize assay precision. The insert shows the calcium extrusion rates for these swine at two different concentrations of calcium, 175 and 425 nmol/l. Data for each animal are the average value for two experiments. Differences between groups are significant for final calcium concentrations and for rates of extrusion. (From O'Brien, P., et al., *Am. J. Vet. Assn.*, in press. With permission.)

TABLE 10
Rate of $[Ca^{2+}]_i$ Release from Lymphocytes of Swine Susceptible to MH using Indo 1

| | Calcium Concentration (nmol/l) | |
	Control	MHS
Initial	745 ± 119	583 ± 120
	(660 to 881)	(472 to 710)
Final	128 ± 15[b]	61 ± 36[a,b]
	(113 to 143)	(31 to 100)
Extrusion (nmol/l/min)	154 ± 36	408 ± 47[a]
(at 175 nmol/l)	(113 to 175)	(408 to 456)
(at 425 nmol/l)	972 ± 111	1690 ± 505[a]
	(846 to 1060)	(1170 to 2180)

Note: Data are expressed as mean value ± SD for three control Yorkshire and three Pietrain x Poland China MH-susceptible swine. Values for each pig were the average for two experiments. Calcium concentrations were determined 30 to 90 min after cell processing.

[a] Significantly different from controls ($p < 0.05$).
[b] Significantly different from initial calcium concentration (within group; $p < 0.05$).

From O'Brien, P. J. and Lassaline, L. A., *Am. Med. Vet. Assoc.*, 51, 1038–1043, 1990. With permission.

TABLE 11
Rate of [Ca²⁺]ᵢ Increase in Lymphocytes of Swine Susceptible to MH using Indo 1

	Control	MHS
Initial	370 ± 216	86 ± 40[a]
	(146 to 666)	(32 to 139)
Final	388 ± 239[b]	99 ± 54[a,b]
	(151 to 738)	(9 to 148)
Accumulation/min	127 ± 52	39 ± 16[a]
	(66 to 234)	(23 to 72)

Note: Data are expressed as mean value ± SD for seven control Yorkshire and seven Pietrain x Poland China MH-susceptible swine.

[a] Significantly different from controls (unpaired *t* test; p <0.05).
[b] Significantly different from initial calcium concentration (paired t test; p <0.05); within group.

From O'Brien, P. J. et al., *N. J. Vet. Res.*, 51, 1038–1043, 1990. With permission.

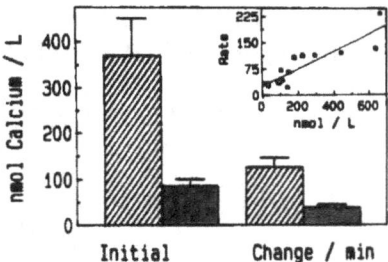

FIGURE 13. Calcium accumulation in resting lymphocytes from swine susceptible to malignant hyperthermia (MH). Data are expressed as mean ± SE of the mean for 7 control swine (diagonal bars) and 7 swine susceptible to MH (solid bars) for the initial ionized calcium concentration and the rate of increase in ionized calcium concentration occurring when lymphocytes are incubated in physiological saline with 1.5 m*M* CaCl₂. Determinations were done at 22°C to increase net calcium accumulation activity by decreasing energy-dependent calcim extrusion and thereby optimize assay precision. Values for the two groups are significantly different (P < 0.05). The insert shows the relationship between rate of calcium accumulation for 7 swine susceptible to MH (solid circles) and 7 control swine (open circles). The least squares regression line is drawn. (From O'Brien, P., et al., *Am. J. Vet. Assn.*, in press, 1990. With permission.)

in nonrigid MH humans.[60] This resistance is probably attributable to the increased calcium sequestration by the SR.[57] Lymphocyte studies on the above-mentioned Border Collie have produced results similar to those observed by O'Brien et al.[57,59] in pigs. Thus, the concentration of free cytoplasmic calcium is less than normal, and the lymphocytes exhibit a greater than normal ability to prevent calcium increase while halothane increases cytoplasmic free calcium by a greater than normal amount and rate.[57]

VI. CONCLUDING REMARKS

Can this test be used as a diagnostic test to complement or replace the CHC test or must it remain a screening test? O'Brien's experiments[54,55] would suggest that in homozygous pigs the test may be truly diagnostic because no overlapping between MHS and normal pig lymphocytes has been observed. Klip's[37,39] as well as our own[9] data, however, do show overlapping in human lymphocytes, which as noted above are probably heterozygous. For humans, therefore, at the present time this test must remain purely as a screening test and as a research tool. Furthermore, the test appears to be fraught with error, which makes it difficult to consistently perform correctly. For example, once the incubation is over, the cells remain viable for only a very few minutes and great care must be taken in transferring the halothane to prevent loss. Finally, the spectrofluorometer used by Dr. O'Brien costs in excess of $100,000 and thus likely would be unavailable in most hospital laboratories.

REFERENCES

1. **Ording, H. and Skovgaard, L. T.,** *In vitro* Diagnosis of susceptibility to malignant hyperthermia: evaluation of tests with halothane-caffeine, potassium chloride, suxamethonium and caffeine-suxamethonium, *Acta Anaesthesiol. Scand.,* 31, 462, 1987.
2. **Ellis, F. R., Halsall, P. J., and Harriman, D. G. F.,** The work of the Leeds Malignant Hyperpyrexia Unit, 1971–84, *Anaesthesia,* 41, 809, 1986.
3. **Ording, H., Ranklev, E., and Fletcher, R.,** Investigation of malignant hyperthermia in Denmark and Sweden, *Br. J. Anaesth.,* 56, 1183, 1984.
4. **Ranklev, E. and Fletcher, R.,** Investigation of malignant hyperthermia in Sweden, *Acta Anaesthesiol. Scand.,* 30, 693, 1986.
5. **Ranklev, E., Fletcher, R., and Blomquist, S.,** Static vs. dynamic tests in the *in vitro* diagnosis of malignant hyperthermia susceptibility, *Br. J. Anaesth.,* 58, 646, 1986.
6. **Rosenberg, H. and Reed, S.,** *In vitro* contracture tests for susceptibility to malignant hyperthermia, *Anesth. Analg.,* 62, 415, 1983.
7. **Melton, A. T., Martucci, R. W., Kien, N. D., and Gronert, G. A.,** malignant hyperthermia in humans — standardization of contracture testing protocol, *Anesth. Analg.,* 69, 437, 1989.
8. **Halsall, P. J. and Ellis, F. R.,** A screening test for the malignant hyperpyrexia phenotype using suxamethonium-induced contracture of muscle treated with caffeine, and its inhibition by dantrolene, *Br. J. Anaesth.,* 51, 753, 1979.
9. **Britt, B. A.,** Malignant hyperthermia — a review, in *International Encyclopedia of Pharmacology and Therapeutics. Thermoregulation: Pathology, Pharmacology and Therapy,* E. Schonbaum and P. Lomax, Eds., Pergamon Press, Oxford, 1990, 327.
10. **Britt, B. A.,** Dantrolene — *in vitro* studies in malignant hyperthermia susceptible (MHS) and normal skeletal muscle, *Can. Anaesth. Soc. J.,* 31, 180, 1984.
11. **Anderson, I. L. and Jones, E. W.,** Porcine malignant hyperthermia: effect of dantrolene sodium on *in vitro* halothane-induced contraction of susceptible muscle, *Anesthesiology,* 44, 57, 1976.

12. **Britt, B. A., Frodis, W., Scott, E., Clements, M. J., and Endrenyi, L.,** Comparison of the caffeine skinned fibre tension (CSFT) test with the caffeine halothane contracture (CHC) test in the diagnosis of malignant hyperthermia, *Can. Anaesth. Soc. J.,* 29, 550, 1982.

13. **Kalow, W., Britt, B. A., Terreau, M. E. et al.,** Metabolic error of muscle metabolism after recovery from malignant hyperthermia, *Lancet,* 2, 895, 1970.

14. **Britt, B. A., Kalow, W., Gordon, A., Humphrey, J. G., and Rewcastle, N. B.,** Malignant hyperthermia — an investigation of five patients, *Can. Anaesth. Soc. J.,* 20, 431, 1973.

15. **Ording, H.,** The European mH group: protocol for *in vitro* diagnosis of susceptibility to MH and preliminary results, in *Malignant Hyperthermia,* B. A. Britt, Ed., Martinus Nijhoff, Boston, 1987, 269.

16. **Britt, B. A.,** The North American caffeine halothane contracture test, in *Malignant Hyperthermia Current Concepts,* Nalda Felipe, M. A., Gottmann, S., and Khambatta, H. J., Eds., Normed Verlag, Bad Homburg, 1988, 53.

17. **Isaacs, H. and Heffron, J. J. A.,** Morphological and biochemical defects in muscles of human carriers of the malignant hyperthermia syndrome, *Br. J. Anaesth.,* 47, 475, 1975.

18. **Heffron, J. J. A. and Mitchell, G.,** Calcium uptake by sarcoplasmic reticulum of muscle of pigs susceptible to malignant hyperthermia (Abstr.), Proc. Int. Pig Veterinary Soc. Congr., Ames, Iowa, 1976.

19. **Dhalla, N. S., Sulakhe, P. V., Clinch, N. F., Wode, J. G., and Naimark, A.,** Influence of fluothane on calcium accumulation by the heavy microsomal fraction of human skeletal muscle: comparison with a patient with malignant hyperpyrexia, *Biochem. Med.,* 6, 333, 1972.

20. **Steward, D. J. and Thomas, T. A.,** Intracellular calcium metabolism and malignant hyperpyrexia, in *Int. Symp. Malignant Hyperthermia,* R. A. Gordon, B. A. Britt, and W. Kalow, Eds., Charles C. Thomas, Springfield, IL, 1973, 409.

21. **Britt, B. A., Endrenyi, L., and Cadman, D.,** Calcium uptake into muscle sarcoplasmic reticulum of pigs susceptible to malignant hyperthermia: *in vitro* and *in vivo* studies with and without halothane, *Br. J. Anaesth.,* 47, 650, 1975.

22. **Takagi, A.,** Increased release of calcium from sarcoplasmic reticulum (SR) by halothane in malignant hyperthermia (MH), *Hiroshima J. Anesth.,* 13, 155, 1977.

23. **Wood, D. S.,** Sarcoplasmic reticulum function and caffeine sensitivity in human malignant hyperthermia, presented at the IVth Int. Congr. Neuromuscular Diseases, Montreal, Quebec, 1978.

24. **Blanck, T. J. J., Gruener, R., Stern, L. Z., and Thompson, M.,** Malignant hyperthermia: the sarcoplasmic reticulum, *Anesthesiology,* 51, S246, 1979.

25. **Nelson, T. E. and Bee, D. E.,** Temperature perturbation studies of sarcoplasmic reticulum from malignant hyperthermia pig muscle, *J. Clin. Invest.,* 64, 895, 1979.

26. **Blanck, T. J. J., Gruener, R., Suffecool, S. L., and Thompson, M.,** Calcium uptake by isolated sarcoplasmic reticulum: examination of halothane inhibition pH dependence and Ca^{2+} dependence of normal and malignant hyperthermic human muscle, *Anesth. Analg.,* 60, 492, 1981.

27. **Nelson, T. E.,** Abnormality in calcium release from skeletal sarcoplasmic reticulum of pigs susceptible to malignant hyperthermia, *J. Clin. Invest.,* 72, 862, 1983.

28. **Nelson, T. E.,** Dantrolene does not block calcium pulse-induced calcium release from a putative calcium channel in sarcoplasmic reticulum from malignant hyperthermia and normal pig muscle, *FEBS Lett.,* 167, 123, 1984.

29. **Nelson, T. E.,** Skeletal sarcoplasmic reticulum in the malignant hyperthermia syndrome, in *Malignant Hyperthermia,* B. A. Britt, Ed., Martinus Nijhoff, Boston, 1987, 43.

30. **Yagi, S., Ishizuka, T., Horiuti, K., Endo, M., Koga, Y., and Amana, K.,** Ca-induced Ca release mechanism in the sarcoplasmic reticulum of the muscle from a malignant hyperthermia paltient, *Hiroshima J. Anaesth.,* 19, 71, 1983.

31. **Kim, D. H., Sreter, F. A., Ohnishi, S. T., Ryan, J. F., Roberts, J., Allen, P. D., Meszaros, L. G., Antoniu, B., and Ikemoto, N.**, Kinetic studies of Ca^{2+} release from sarcoplasmic reticulum of normal and malignant hyperthermia susceptible pig muscles, *Biochim. Biophys. Acta*, 775, 320, 1984.

32. **Kim, D. H., Sreter, F. A., and Idemoto, N.**, Kinetic and biochemical studies of Ca^{2+} release from sarcoplasmic reticulum of normal and malignant hyperthermic pig muscles, IVth Int. Malignant Hyperpyrexia Workshop, York, England, 1986.

33. **O'Brien, P. J.**, Porcine malignant hyperthermia susceptibility: increased calcium-sequestering activity of skeletal muscle sarcoplasmic reticulum, *Can. J. Vet. Res.*, 50, 329, 1986.

34. **MacLennan, D. H., Duff, C., Zorzato, F., Fujii, J., Phillips, M., Korneluk, R. G., Frodis, W., Britt, B. A., and Worton, R. G.**, The ryanodine receptor gene: a candidate gene for the predisposition to malignant hyperthermia, *Nature*, 343, 559, 1990.

35. **Lopez, J. R., Jones, D., Alamo, L., Papp, A. P., Gergely, J., and Sreter, F.**, $(Ca^{2+})_i$ in muscles of malignant hyperthermia susceptible pigs. Determined *in vivo* with Ca^{2+} selective microelectrodes, *Muscle Nerve*, 9, 85, 1986.

36. **Lopez, J. R., Allen, P. D., Alamo, L., Jones, D., and Sreter, F. A.**, Myoplasmic free (Ca^{2+}) during a malignant hyperthermia episode in Swine, *Muscle Nerve*, 11, 82, 1988.

37. **Klip, A., Britt, B. A., Elliott, M. E., Walker, D., Ramlal, T., and Pegg, W.**, Changes in cytoplasmic free calcium caused by halothane. Role of the plasma membrane and intracellular Ca^{2+} stores, *Biochem. Cell Biol.*, 64, 1181, 1986.

38. **Klip, A., Britt, B. A., Elliott, M. E., Pegg, W., Frodis, W., and Scott, E.**, Anaesthetic-induced increase in ionized calcium in blood mononuclear cells from malignant hyperthermic patients, *Lancet*, 1, 463, 1987.

39. **Klip, A. and Britt, B. A.**, Selective increase in cytoplasmic calcium by anesthetic in lymphocytes from malignant hyperthermia susceptible pigs, *Anesth. Analg.*, 66, 381, 1987.

40. **Klip, A., Mills, B. B., Britt, B. A., and Elliott, M. E.**, Halothane-dependent release of intracellular Ca^{2+} in blood cells in malignant hyperthermia, *Am. J. Physiol.*, 258, (*Cell. Physiol.*, 27), C495, 1990.

41. **Tsien, R. Y., Pozzan, T., and Rink, T. J.**, Calcium homeostasis in intact lymphocytes: cytoplasmic free calcium. New intracellularly trapped fluorescent indicator, *J. Cell Biol.*, 94, 325, 1982.

42. **Grykiewicz, G., Poeniue, M., and Tsien, R. Y.**, A new generation of Ca indicators with greatly improved fluorescence properties, *J. Biol. Chem.*, 260, 2330, 1985.

43. **Banrany, M., Chang, Y.-C., and Arus, C.**, Effect of halothane on the natural abundance ISC NMR spectrum of excised rat brain, *Biochemistry*, 24, 7911, 1885.

44. **Nelson, T. E.**, Abnormality in calcium release from skeletal sarcoplasmic reticulum of pigs susceptible to malignant hyperthermia, *J. Clin. Invest.*, 72, 862, 1983.

45. **Iwatsuki, N., Koga, Y., and Amaha, K.**, Calcium channel blocker for treatment of malignant hyperthermia, *Anesth. Analg.*, 62, 855, 1983.

46. **Harrison, G. G., Wright, I. G., and Morrell, D. F.**, The effects of calcium channel blocking drugs on halothane initiation of malignant hyperthermia in MH swine and on the established syndrome, *Anaesth. Intens. Care*, 16, 197, 1988.

47. **Gallant, E., Foldes, F., Rempel, W. M., and Gronert, G. A.**, Verapamil in porcine malignant hyperthermia, *Anesth. Analg.*, 64, 601, 1985.

48. **Smiley, R., Greenberg, S., and Silverstein, S. C.**, Anesthetics increase cytosolic calcium in mononuclear cells from normal and MH-susceptible patients, *Anesthesiology*, 69, A418, 1988.

49. **Ellis, F. R.**, Prediction of MH susceptibility by clinical signs, *Acta Anaesth. Scand.*, 33, 22, 1989.

50. **Heffron, J. A.**, personal communication.

51. **Ording, H. P.,** personal communication.
52. **Fletcher, J. E.,** personal communication.
53. **O'Brien, P. J., Kalow, B. I., Brown, B. D., Lumsden, J. H., and Jacobs, R. M.,** Porcine malignant hyperthermia susceptibility: halothane-induced increase in cytoplasmic free calcium in lymphocytes, *Am. J. Vet. Res.,* 50, 131, 1989.
54. **O'Brien, P. J., Klip, A., Britt, B. A., and Kalow, B. I.,** Malignant hyperthermia susceptibility: biochemical basis for pathogenesis and diagnosis, *Can. J. Vet. Res.,* 54, 83, 1990.
55. **O'Brien, P. J., Kalow, B. I., Ali, N., Lassaline, L. A., and Lumsden, J. H.,** Compensatory increase in calcium extrusion activity in untreated lymphocytes in swine susceptible to MH, *N. J. Vet. Res.,* 51, 1038–1043, 1990.
56. **O'Brien, P. J., and Ali, N.,** Lymphocyte calcium extrusion: kinetic and thermodynamic measurements using ratiometric dual-emission spectrofluorometry, *Mol. Cell Biochem.,* 96, 89–96, 1990.
57. **O'Brien, P. J., Pook, H. A., Klip, A., Britt, B. A., Kalow, B. I., Mclaughlin, R. N., Scott, E., and Elliott, M. E.,** Canine stress syndrome/malignant hyperthermia susceptibility: calcium-homeostasis defect in muscle and lymphocytes, *Res. Vet. Sci.,* 48, 124, 1990.
58. **O'Brien, P. J. and Rand, J. S.,** Canine stress syndrome, *J. Am. J. Vet. Res.,* 186, 432, 1985.
59. **Rand, J. S. and O'Brien, P. J.,** Exercise-induced malignant hyperthermia in a springer spaniel, *J. Am. Vet. Med. Assoc.* 190, 1013, 1987.

Chapter 17

A NONINVASIVE DIAGNOSIS OF MALIGNANT HYPERTHERMIA: DIRECT THERMOMETRY OF INTRAMUSCULAR TEMPERATURE

S. Tsuyoshi Ohnishi and Kenneth K. Sadanaga

TABLE OF CONTENTS

I.   Introduction 252

II.   Principle and Rationale 252

III.   Test with MH-Susceptible Pigs 253

IV.   Problems with the Temperature Method 255

References 256

0-8493-8093-6/94/$0.00 + $.50
© 1994 by CRC Press, Inc.

I. INTRODUCTION

The name malignant hyperthermia (MH) comes from the fact that the body temperature of a susceptible patient increases abnormally during inhalational general anesthesia. Although there were reports of cases where muscle rigor developed without a rise of body temperature, the increase of temperature is still an important symptom of this disease. The authors found that inhalational general anesthetics induce abnormal calcium release from the skeletal sarcoplasmic reticulum (SR) and that the release is abnormal in MH-SR.[1-8] This abnormal calcium release can cause muscle rigor and hypermetabolism, leading to a rise of body temperature. The rise of body temperature further enhances calcium release and hypermetabolism and results in a vicious cycle of increasing body temperature that becomes life threatening.[9] If so, can this abnormal temperature response of muscle to stimulating agents be used as a means of preoperative diagnosis? In this article, the authors discuss the possibility of developing a minimally invasive diagnostic method based upon the measurement of muscle temperature.

II. PRINCIPLE AND RATIONALE

Principle — The diagnostic principle is to apply a small amount of test agent and measure the rise of intramuscular temperature. Inhalational general anesthetics, such as halothane, may not be recommended to use as test agents, because they may induce an MH reaction; local anesthetics are believed to be safer to use with MH patients.[10] Because the action of local anesthetics is limited to the site of administration, it is less likely to cause widespread systemic effects. If a local anesthetic that causes abnormal calcium release from the skeletal SR could be found then it could be used for this test. Even though such a local anesthetic agent may enhance calcium release, it would not cause an MH reaction, because the effect is localized and the amount to be used for the test is extremely small (20 to 40 µl). The rise of body temperature can be measured by a needle-type thermistor probe connected to an appropriate thermometer.

Method of administration of test drugs — A temperature probe was developed in which a tiny thermistor is cemented inside a 13-gauge needle (Figure 1). A test drug can be delivered using the needle of the temperature probe itself.

Selection of an appropriate local anesthetic agent — Using a method of measuring the calcium-induced calcium release from the SR of skeletal muscle, the authors found that inhalational anesthetics such as halothane and enflurane release calcium from the SR,[1-9] and, local anesthetics were screened using this method. Because tetracaine and procaine have been found to inhibit calcium release,[1,2,6,8] the authors tested other local anesthetics and found that dibucaine enhances calcium release of skeletal SR and that the degree of

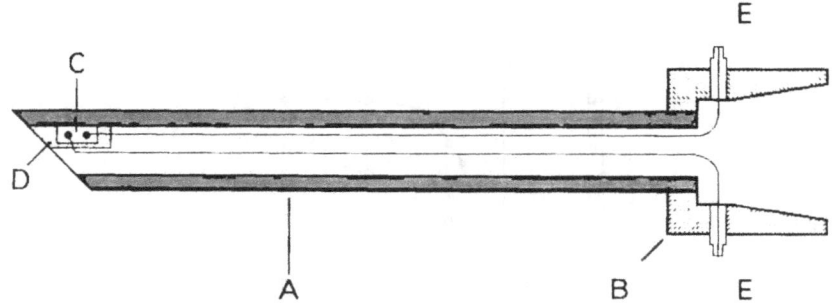

FIGURE 1. Schematic illustration of a needle-type thermistor probe: (A) 13-gauge needle; (B) plastic hub; (C) thermistor; (D) water-resistant cement; (E) electric connectors. (Not to scale.)

release in the MH-SR was much greater than that in the control SR (Figures 2 and 3).

III. TEST WITH MH-SUSCEPTIBLE PIGS

The feasibility of this method was tested using pigs. MH-susceptible pigs and control pigs were purchased from the Department of Animal Sciences, Iowa State University, and caged at the animal facility of the University of

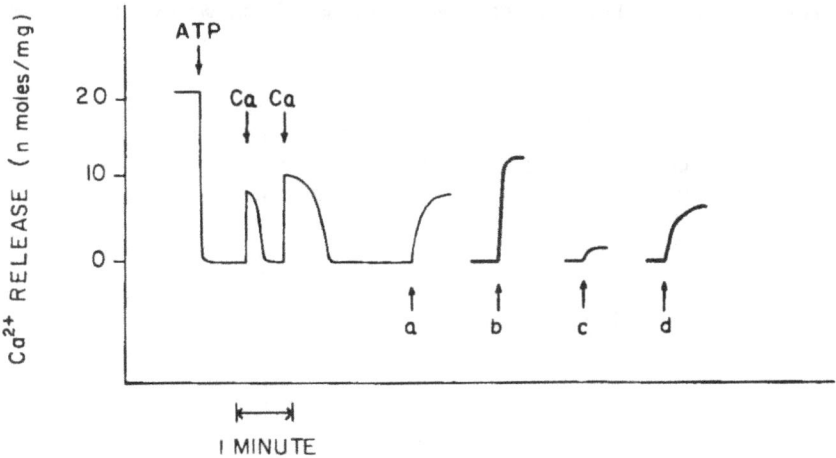

FIGURE 2. Calcium release from skeletal SR prepared from pigs induced by dibucaine. Additions of (a) and (b) are for MH-SR and those of (c) and (d) are for control SR. Concentrations of added agents: 0.5 mM ATP; 10 μM CaCl$_2$; 350 μM dibucaine (a and c); and 875 μM dibucaine (b and d). For traces of (b), (c), and (d), the initial portion of the trace that includes the additions of ATP and calcium are abbreviated. Experimental conditions: 150 mM KCl; 20 mM MES buffer (pH 6.8); 0.5 mM MgCl$_2$; 1.0 mg SR protein/ml; and 15 μM arsenazo III, 25°C.

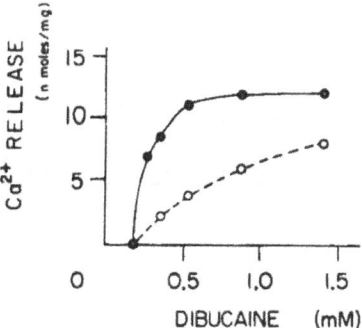

FIGURE 3. Dose-response relationship of calcium release from the MH-SR (filled circles) and control SR (open circles). Conditions are the same as those in Figure 2.

Pennsylvania School of Veterinary Medicine. Temperature is easily elevated if a pig is excited during the measurement; therefore, two methods were used to minimize this effect: (1) keeping a pig in a hammock-type sling restrainer and (2) anesthesizing the animal with an i.p. injection of pentobarbital (50 mg/kg).

The temperature probe was inserted 20 mm into the epaxial muscle. Then, 20 μl of a saline solution was injected. As shown in Figure 4A, the temperature fell once, but it recovered to the same temperature in both control and MH pigs. The probe was reinserted into a different location and delivered a 20-μl solution of 2% dibucaine (dissolved in saline). As shown by ΔT in Figure

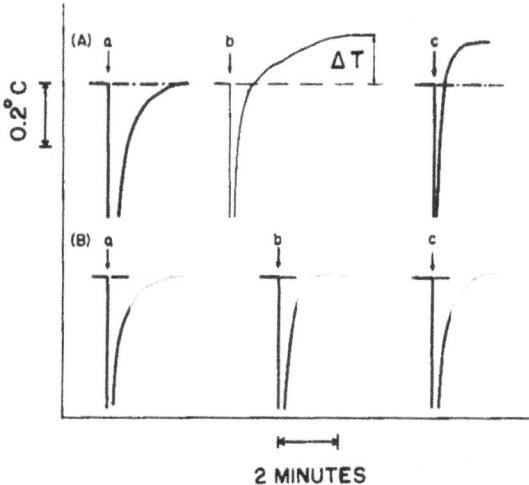

FIGURE 4. Examples of the measurement of intramascular temperature changes: (A) with an MH pig and (B) with a control pig. Injections of 20 μl of (a) normal saline, (b) 2% dibucaine, and (c) 1% caffeine. An arrow sign with ΔT indicates the final temperature change.

TABLE 1
Temperature Rises Induced by
Intramuscular Injection (20 μl) of
2% Dibucaine and 1% Caffeine

	Control pig	MH pig
Dibucaine	0.010 ± 0.022	0.178 ± 0.091
Caffeine	0.015 ± 0.021	0.118 ± 0.060

Note: Six measurements with two pigs (three measurements each). Values are shown in the mean ± SD. For both dibucaine and caffeine, the differences between control and MH pigs are statistically significant ($p < 0.05$).

4B, the authors observed a rise of 0.16°C in MH-susceptible pigs and 0.01°C in control pigs. Because caffeine also induces calcium release from the SR,[1-9] the effect of 20 μl of 1% caffeine (dissolved in saline) was tested. It had a similar effect as that of 2% dibucaine (Figure 4C).

Using two MH pigs and two control pigs, Three dibucaine and three caffeine measurements were done in each pig, always using a new location in their back muscle. The results are summarized in Table 1.

IV. PROBLEMS WITH THE TEMPERATURE METHOD

Although the temperature method provided some promising results, several problems existed. In the case of pigs, it was found that their intramuscular temperature was not stable. For example, when the needle probe was inserted into the epaxial muscle of conscious animals, they normally became excited and moved around in the sling. The size of the 13-gauge needle is quite large, producing discomfort in animals. This movement easily caused a temperature rise of 0.2°C, thereby interfering with our measurements. If pentobarbital was used, the animal was anesthetized and the temperature slowly lowered, again interfering with measurements. As shown in Figure 4, a flat baseline is essential before delivering an agent. If the muscle temperature is slowly drifting, the measurement cannot be performed. In pigs it was often difficult to achieve a stable muscle temperature.

Despite the inherent problems, this method is simple and may be worthwhile to pursue. Currently, the smallest needle in which a thermistor can be mounted is a 13-gauge needle. If a smaller thermistor could be mounted in an 18-gauge needle, this method may be applicable to humans. In the case of humans, body temperature may be more stable than in pigs, because a test subject is not usually excited by the insertion of needles. Researchers interested in further developing this method are encouraged to contact the authors.

REFERENCES

1. **Ohnishi, S. T.**, Calcium-induced calcium-release from fragmented sarcoplasmic reticulum, *J. Biochem.*, 86, 1147, 1979.
2. **Ohnishi, S. T.**, Calcium-induced calcium release as a gated calcium transport, in *Mechanism of Gated Calcium Transport Across Biological Membranes*, S. T. Ohnishi and M. Endo, Eds., Academic Press, New York, 1981, 275.
3. **Ohnishi, S. T., Taylor, S., and Gronert, G. A.**, Calcium-induced calcium-release from sarcoplasmic reticulum of pigs susceptible to malignant hyperthermia: the effect of halothane and dantrolene, *FEBS Lett.*, 161, 103, 1983.
4. **Kim, D. H., Ohnishi, S. T., and Ikemoto, N.**, Kinetic Studies of calcium release from sarcoplasmic reticulum *in vitro*, *J. Biol. Chem.*, 258, 9662, 1983.
5. **Kim, D. H., Streter, F. A., Ohnishi, S. T., Ryan, J. F., Roberts, J., Allen, P. D., Meszaros, L. G., Antoniu, B., and Ikemoto, N.**, The kinetic studies of calcium release from sarcoplasmic reticulum of normal and malignant hyperthermia susceptible pig muscles, *Biochim. Biophys. Acta*, 775, 320, 1984.
6. **Ohnishi, S. T., Waring, A. J., Fang, S. G., Horiuchi, K., Flick, J. L., Sadanaga, K. K., and Ohnishi, T.**, Abnormal membrane properties of the sarcoplasmic reticulum of pigs susceptible to malignant hyperthermia: modes of action of halothane, caffeine, dantrolene and two other drugs., *Arch. Biochem. Biophys.*, 247, 294, 1986.
7. **Ohnishi, S. T.**, Effects of alcohol and halothane on the structure and function of sarcoplasmic reticulum, *Ann. N.Y. Acad. Sci.*, 492, 138, 1987.
8. **Ohnishi, S. T.**, Effects of halothane, caffeine, dantrolene and tetracaine on the calcium permeability of skeletal sarcoplasmic reticulum of malignant hyperthermic pigs, *Biochim. Biophys. Acta*, 897, 261, 1987.
9. **Ohnishi, S. T. and Katsuoka, M.**, Why does halothane relax cardiac muscle but contract malignant hyperthermic skeletal muscle?, *Adv. Exp. Med. Biol.*, 301, 73, 1991.
10. **Britt, A. B., Ed.**, *Malignant Hyperthermia*, Martinus Nijhoff, Boston, 1987, 314.

Part V
New Developments in
Malignant Hyperthermia
Research and Molecular
Genetic Diagnosis of
Malignant Hyperthermia

Chapter 18

THE GENETIC BASIS OF MALIGNANT HYPERTHERMIA

David H. MacLennan, Michael S. Phillips, and Yilin Zhang

TABLE OF CONTENTS

I. Human Malignant Hyperthermia 260

II. Porcine Malignant Hyperthermia 260

III. Physiological Basis of Malignant Hyperthermia 261

IV. Ca^{2+} Release Channel *(RYR)* Genes 263

V. Genetic Basis of Porcine Malignant Hyperthermia 264

VI. Genetic Basis of Human Malignant Hyperthermia 266

VII. Concluding Remarks 268

Acknowledgments 269

References 269

I. HUMAN MALIGNANT HYPERTHERMIA

Malignant hyperthermia (MH) is an inherited, potentially lethal condition in which skeletal muscle rigidity, accompanied by hypermetabolism, high fever, and cellular ion imbalances are triggered in susceptible individuals by exposure to a combination of potent inhalational anesthetics and depolarizing skeletal muscle relaxants.[1] If therapy is not initiated immediately, the patient may die or suffer serious neurological kidney or liver damage. Monitoring for the early symptoms of an MH episode and responding to such symptoms by terminating the anesthetic process and infusing the clinical antidote, dantrolene, has lowered the death rate for these episodes from over 80% to less than 7% in recent years. Neurological or kidney damage, however, still contributes to the morbidity.

Statistical data, collected prior to concerted efforts to predict and prevent anesthetic-induced MH reactions, indicated that the incidence of MH episodes was about 1 in 15,000 anesthetics in children's hospitals and about 1 in 50,000 in adult hospitals. These figures underestimate the true genetic predisposition to the condition, however, because many fulminant MH episodes occur for the first time in patients who have previously undergone uneventful anesthesia. Most MH mutations seem to be inherited in families, suggesting that spontaneous occurrence is low.

MH does not pose a serious threat to susceptible individuals in their daily lives or in any way incapacitates most of them. Accordingly, a major goal of MH research has been to identify MH-susceptible individuals prior to administration of anesthetics. If MH susceptibility is known, use of specific alternate anesthetics and nondepolarizing muscle relaxants can be used that do not trigger MH episodes. To diagnose MH-susceptible individuals, *in vitro* caffeine halothane contracture (CHC) tests for MH susceptibility were developed.[2,3] The tests are invasive and expensive and, because of the potential danger of false-negative diagnosis, may err on the side of false-positive diagnosis.[4] Still, diagnostic testing over two decades has confirmed the autosomal dominance of inheritance of the human MH gene.

II. PORCINE MALIGNANT HYPERTHERMIA

MH also occurs in domestic animals such as swine.[5,6] Animals homozygous for the abnormality respond to stress with muscle rigidity, hypermetabolism, and high fever. The stress-induced death of such animals (porcine stress syndrome or PSS) leads to large economic loss due to the syndrome. The incidence of MH (PSS) in swine varies from breed to breed and from country to country. As many as 1 in 8 homozygotes die of PSS, and up to 50% of the meat from homozygotes can be devalued through the occurrence of pale, soft, exudative pork (PSEP) in large segments of the carcasses of these animals. Efforts to rid swine stocks of this apparently deleterious gene have not been successful, in part because the gene also has beneficial effects and, in part, because no suitable test for heterozygote carriers has been available.

The beneficial effects of the MH gene are associated with leanness and muscle hypertrophy, and appear to add to lean, dressed carcass weight.[7,8] By selecting breeding stock for leanness and heavy muscling, selection also is inadvertently being made for the MH gene. Recognition that the gene leads to PSS and contributes to PSEP[9] provided the stimulus for attempts to eliminate the MH gene from swine breeding stock. These efforts were frustrated until a diagnostic test able to detect heterozygous carriers with the accuracy required to eliminate the gene and within acceptable limits of cost was developed by the authors.[10]

III. PHYSIOLOGICAL BASIS OF MALIGNANT HYPERTHERMIA

The underlying cause of MH became apparent as the understanding emerged that the primary biochemical abnormalities associated with the syndrome occur in skeletal muscle[1,5] and that contraction, relaxation, and energy metabolism are regulated in skeletal muscle by Ca^{2+}. The sarcoplasmic reticulum (SR) is the major regulator of Ca^{2+} concentrations in skeletal muscle.[11,12] Ca^{2+} is pumped into the SR by a Ca^{2+} transport ATPase to initiate relaxation, stored in the junctional terminal cisternae in association with calsequestrin, and released through a Ca^{2+}-release channel to bind to troponin in the thin filament, initiating muscle contraction. Ca^{2+} also binds to phosphorylase kinase, activating glycolytic pathways and the resynthesis of ATP to replenish that used during contraction.

The Ca^{2+} release channel of the sarcoplasmic reticulum is a tetrameric protein complex constructed from four identical 565-kDa subunits.[12] Single channel measurements in planar bilayers have shown that Ca^{2+} release is mediated by a ligand-gated channel with a conductance greater than 100 pS in 50 mM Ca^{2+}.[13,14] Transmembrane sequences are located in the COOH-terminal fifth of each subunit[15,16] and the remainder of the subunit is probably cytoplasmic, bridging the gap between the SR and the transverse tubule (Figure 1). Transmembrane sequences in the tetramer probably combine to form the membrane-spanning pore of the Ca^{2+} release channel, and cytoplasmic sequences from each subunit appear to interact to enclose four extended channels that radiate from the central transmembrane channel and exit in peripheral vestibules.[17] Regulatory sequences may exist near the transmembrane sequences[15] or in the cytoplasmic domain.[16,18] Although it is not clear what signals open the channel in the muscle cell, Ca^{2+} and ATP act synergistically to open the channel in isolated vesicles and Mg^{2+} and calmodulin inhibit channel opening. Dantrolene, the clinical antidote for MH reactions,[1] inhibits halothane-induced[19] and Ca^{2+}-induced[20] Ca^{2+} release from

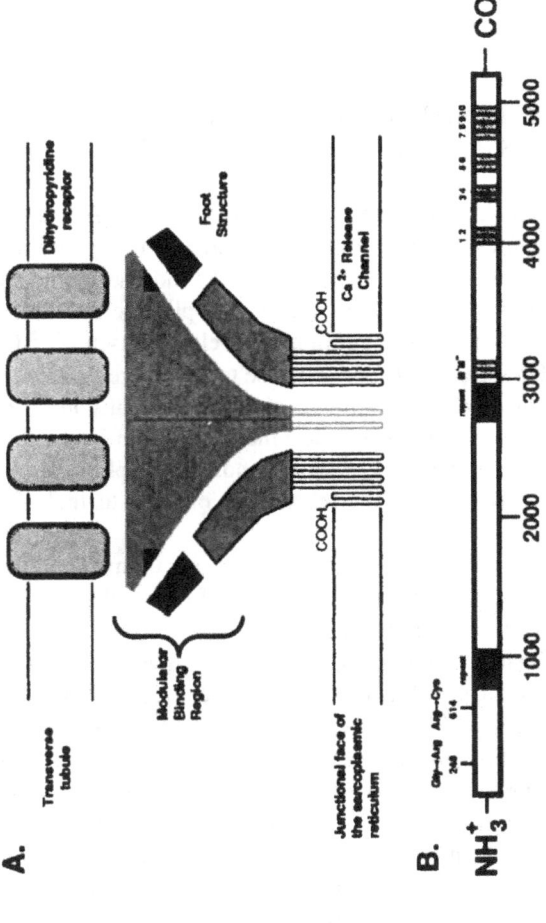

FIGURE 1. (A) Molecular model for the ryanodine receptor based upon predicted structure and hydropathy plot. Morphological studies suggest that most of the protein is located in the cytoplasmic space between the SR and transverse tubular membranes and is constructed as a homotetramer with internal channels radiating from a central transmembrane channel. The ryanodine receptor abuts the dihydropyridine receptors located in the transverse tubular membrane and may be functionally coupled to them. The cytoplasmic domain appears to contain MH mutations indicating potential regulatory domains. (B) The transmembrane domain is made up of 4 to 12 transmembrane sequences, of which 4 to 10 are located in the COOH-terminal 1/5 of the protein and 2 are more central. There are two tandem repeat sequences, but their function is unknown. Known MH mutations at positions 248 and 614 (615) are indicated. (From MacLennan, D. H., *Biophys. J.*, 58, 1355, 1990.)

SR preparations. In single Ca^{2+} release channels, dantrolene at 5 to 25 μM first activates and then inactivates the channel in planar lipid bilayers.[21]

The release of Ca^{2+} is the end result of a cascade of events including: depolarization of nerve, muscle, and transverse tubular membranes; charge movement associated with the slow Ca^{2+} channel of the transverse tubular membrane (the dihydropyridine receptor);[22] and opening of the Ca^{2+} release channel. An abnormality in regulation of Ca^{2+} within skeletal muscle could account for all of the symptoms of MH. In particular, contracture may result from the continued presence of Ca^{2+} within the cell, and enhanced glycolytic and aerobic metabolism might deplete ATP, glucose, and oxygen, produce excess CO_2, lactic acid and heat, and upset cellular and extracellular ion balances.

Because abnormalities in the regulation of the intracellular concentrations of Ca^{2+} that lead to MH might result from mutations in the Ca^{2+} release channel, investigators looked for abnormalities and found higher rates of Ca^{2+}-induced Ca^{2+} release, particularly at low levels of inducing Ca^{2+}, in preparations from both human[23] and porcine[19,24,25] muscle. The closing of single porcine MH channels at high Ca^{2+} concentrations was shown to be inhibited.[26] In comparable studies of humans, Ca^{2+} release channels with abnormally greater caffeine sensitivity were detected in MH individuals.[27] In SR from swine with MH, ryanodine binding, which is dependent on the open state of the Ca^{2+} release channel, is enhanced[28] and digestion with trypsin revealed an alteration in the amino acid sequence of the Ca^{2+} release channel in MH animals.[29]

IV. Ca^{2+} RELEASE CHANNEL *(RYR)* GENES

We have shown that two genes encode Ca^{2+} release channels of the SR by cloning full length cDNAs encoding the rabbit,[16] human,[16] and porcine[30] skeletal muscle isoforms *(RYR1)* and the rabbit[13] cardiac and brain isoform *(RYR2)*. More recently, a third *RYR* gene *(RYR3)* has been cloned.[31,32] *RYR1* encodes the Ca^{2+} release channel of both slow- and fast-twitch skeletal muscle; *RYR2* encodes a second Ca^{2+} release channel that is expressed in cardiac muscle and brain; and *RYR3* appears to be expressed most abundantly in brain and specific smooth muscles,[32] although it is also expressed in lung.[31] We have localized *RYR1* on human chromosome 19q13.1 (Figure 2)[33] and *RYR2* on human chromosome 1.[18] We also identified a series of restriction-fragment length polymorphisms (RFLPs) in *RYR1* that permitted us to study linkage between inheritance of one or more of these RFLPs and inheritance of MH, defined by CHC tests.[34] Cosegregation was found in 23 meioses in 9 families, with no recombinants, leading to a probability of about 16,000 to 1 that the two loci are linked.[34]

In studies of swine, linkage was demonstrated between inheritance of MH (the *HAL* gene) and polymorphisms in a linkage group consisting of

Sublocalization of the RYR 1 Gene on
Chromosome 19

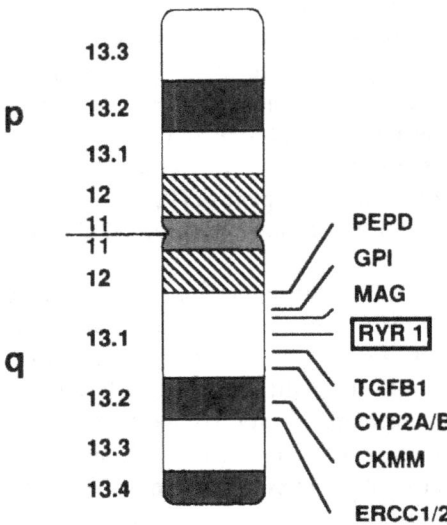

FIGURE 2. Sublocalization of the *RYR1* gene on human chromosome 19. (From Mackenzie, A. E. et al., *Am. J. Hum. Genet.*, 46, 1082, 1990.)

HAL, glucose phosphate isomerase *(GPI)*, 6-phosphogluconate dehydrogenase *(PGD)*, and α-1-B glycoproteins *(A1BG)* genes, the H blood group locus, and loci controlling the expression of the (A-O) blood groups, localized near the centromere of pig chromosome 6.[35] A similar region was identified on the long arm of human chromosome 19[36] in which a number of human markers, including *GPI*, were located. These human markers were then used to link MH to the region of human chromosome 19q12-13.2 where *RYR*1 was localized.[37]

V. GENETIC BASIS OF PORCINE MALIGNANT HYPERTHERMIA

In a comparison of *RYR*1 cDNA sequences from normal (Yorkshire) and MH (Pietrain) pigs, the authors observed a single deduced amino acid sequence difference.[30] The substitution of T for C1843 in the nucleotide sequence also leads to the substitution of Cys for Arg[615] in the amino acid sequence. Early studies indicated association of this mutation with MH in some 80 animals from five different breeds. The authors then went on to analyze linkage in backcrosses between British Landrace N/n and n/n animals.[38] In a study of 376 animals, including 338 informative meioses, complete linkage was observed between the presence of the nucleotide 1843 mutation and phenotypic diagnosis, based on the halothane challenge test and confirmed by *GPI* and *PGD* haplotype analysis. Cosegregation of the MH phenotype with the Cys for Arg[615] substitution led to an lod score (log of the odds favoring linkage) of 102 for a recombination fraction of 0.0.[38]

The same mutation was found in five breeds of pigs, suggesting that it might have originated in a founder animal. Analysis of three polymorphic sites across about 150 kbp within the *RYR*1 gene provided evidence for a common *RYR*1 haplotype in every MH animal tested, consistent with its origin in a founder animal.[30] Leanness and heavy muscling may be manifestations of the gene,[7,8] and these traits are readily selected by observant swine breeders. There is a physiological rationale for the contributions of the gene to leanness and heavy muscling. An abnormal Ca^{2+} release channel could stimulate spontaneous muscle contraction that would result in muscle hypertrophy and, because of greater energy utilization, in the limitation of fat deposition.

The substitution of T for C1843 in the porcine *RYR*1 gene deletes a *Hin*P1 restriction endonuclease site and creates an *Hgi*A1 restriction site.[30] By amplifying a segment of genomic DNA surrounding this site, an accurate diagnostic test was developed on the basis of analysis of the presence or absence of the *Hin*P1 or *Hgi*A1 sites.[10] The accuracy of tests based on restriction endonuclease digestion is greatly enhanced if a "built-in control" digestion site is present in that portion of the DNA that is amplified for digestion. Accordingly, the authors sequenced genomic DNA surrounding the variant site and found a constant or control *Hgi*A1 site 358 bp upstream from the variant site. We then amplified a 659-bp fragment that contained both control and variant *Hgi*A1 sites. Digestion of this fragment from normal animals yields two fragments, because only the control site is digested; DNA from homozygous MH animals yields three fragments, because control and variant sites are fully cleaved; and DNA from heterozygous animals yields four bands, because the control site is cleaved in both alleles, but the variant site is cleaved in only one allele. Thus the test readily distinguishes these classes and ambiguities arising from partial enzymatic digestion are eliminated.[10] The test is readily adapted to large scale commercial testing for the mutant gene (see Chapter 19).

For the swine industry, application of MH diagnostic testing is of enormous practical and economic importance. The test, which is accurate, noninvasive, and relatively inexpensive, detects the single mutation that has been found in all breeds. Swine breeders may choose to eliminate all carriers of the PSS gene from apex breeding stocks, freeing the entire porcine population of PSS and resulting in substantial savings to the industry by elimination of PSS deaths and reduction of PSEP. Alternatively, breeders might decide to take advantage of the apparent beneficial effects of the gene by, for example, establishing homozygous MH boar lines and normal sow lines for the purpose of producing heterozygous market animals.

VI. GENETIC BASIS OF HUMAN
MALIGNANT HYPERTHERMIA

Studies by the authors and other groups of a large number of MH families have demonstrated linkage between MH and *RYR*1.[34,37] We also identified a human Arg[614]-to-Cys mutation, corresponding to the porcine Arg[615]-to-Cys mutation, in a human family, where it segregated with MH (Figure 3).[39] Hogan et al.[40] have made similar observations. These observations, combined with the strong linkage of this mutation with MH in swine,[38] provide a very high degree of confidence that the Arg[614]-to-Cys mutation is causal of MH in those rare human families where it is found. We have also associated the mutation of Gly[248]-to-Arg with MH in an MH family, but have not proven its causal nature.[41]

Diagnosis of MH susceptibility is also possible through analysis of inheritance of polymorphisms in *RYR*1 or closely linked markers in families in which a large number of individuals have been diagnosed previously by the *in vitro* contracture test.[42] There is potential for error, however, if recombination should occur within the *RYR*1 gene or between *RYR*1 and flanking markers used in such a diagnosis.

In spite of these findings, it has not been possible to demonstrate linkage between MH and *RYR*1 in other studies involving several other families.[43-45] There is evidence that individuals with central core disease, (CCD)[46] King-Denborough syndrome,[47] Duchenne muscular dystrophy,[48] and other myopathies[46,49] are at risk for anesthetic-induced MH episodes. CCD, an autosomal dominant myopathy associated with proximal muscle weakness and hypotonia, is strongly associated with MH. Genetic linkage studies have provided lod scores as high as 11.8 for a recombination fraction of 0.0 for cosegregation of *RYR*1 and *CCO* (the central core disease gene).[50] Abnormalities in cellular Ca^{2+} regulation are probably secondary events in such myopathies. If these abnormalities were to lead to anesthetic-induced sustained chronic elevation of Ca^{2+} in the muscle, MH episodes could result.

It is possible that CCD and MH result from different functional mutations in *RYR*1. In MH, abnormalities in Ca^{2+} release within muscle cells may have little or no phenotype in absence of anesthetics, because the Ca^{2+} released is handled adequately by the system of Ca^{2+} pumps in the plasma membrane and SR, by the Na/Ca exchanger in the plasma membrane, or by mitochondria. Some forms of MH, for example, that are observed in swine, may lead to muscle hypertrophy due to muscle twitching arising from a leaky Ca^{2+} release channel. Those mutations causing CCD may, however, be more severe, leading to excessive Ca^{2+} leakage within the muscle cell. At the periphery, pumps and exchanger could handle the released Ca^{2+}, but in the center of the muscle cell (the core), mitochondria might take up the excess Ca^{2+} load, destroying themselves in the process and leading to central cores with low metabolic activity. Muscle weakness, sometimes observed in CCD, may result from

Human

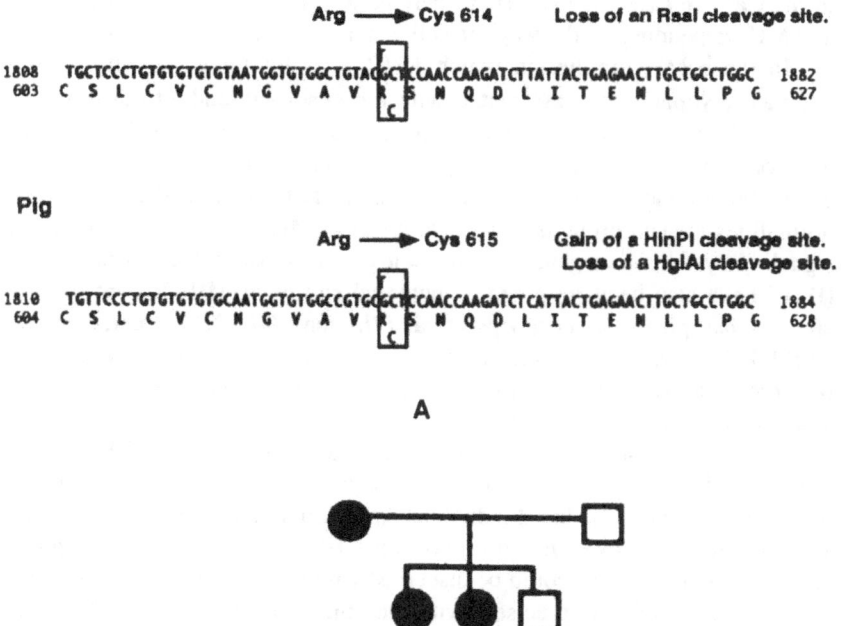

A

B

FIGURE 3. (A) Nucleotide and deduced amino acid sequences of the region of the *RYR1* gene surrounding the MH mutation site. In the human sequence, the replacement of C1840 with T results in the replacement of Arg[614] with His and in the loss of an *Rsa*l restriction endonuclease site. In the corresponding porcine sequence, the mutation of C1843 to T results in the mutation of Arg[615] to Cys and in the gain of an *Hin*Pl cleavage site and the loss of an *Hgi*Al cleavage site. (B) Detection of a C1840 → T alteration by detection of loss of an *Rsa*l restriction endonuclease site in the 74-bp PCR product amplified from genomic DNA from a chromosome 19-linked MH family. Cleavage of the 74-bp PCR product generates 41- and 33-bp fragments. Individuals 1, 2, and 3 carry the mutation and only one allele is cleaved. Individuals 4 and 5 are homozygous for the normal chromosome sequence and both alleles are cleaved. (From Gillard, E. F. et al., *Genomics,* 11, 751, 1991.)

damage to the muscle core due to Ca^{2+} leakage from a more severe defect in the Ca^{2+} release channel. There may be gradations between typical CCD and MH, depending on the way the cell is able to cope with the excess Ca^{2+}.

In those MH families in which *RYR*1 was not linked to MH,[43-45] no alternate myopathy was associated with the syndrome and, if one assumes that the diagnosis was accurate, the conclusion must be reached that genes additional to *RYR*1 or to known myopathic genes are causative of MH. Because excitation-contraction coupling requires the activity of several proteins, abnormalities in such proteins could also result in MH episodes. Alterations in signaling systems that generate fatty acids[51] and inositol 1,4,5-triphosphate (IP_3)[52] have also been proposed as potential causes of MH. Recent linkage analysis has placed a second potential *MH* gene (*MHS2*) on chromosome 17q11.2-24.[53] A sodium channel gene, previously linked to hyperkalemic periodic paralysis *(HPP)*,[54] is located in this region of chromosome 17 and is a candidate gene for *MHS2*.[55]

In one of our studies where lack of linkage between MH and *RYR*1 was reported,[56] MH status may, indeed, have been falsely diagnosed. In our study of a large French Canadian kindred, all individuals but one were classified as MH susceptible by standard criteria for CHC tests. Two clear groupings of diagnostic test results could be discerned within the family, however, with one of them correlating precisely with the inheritance of an *RYR*1 RFLP. If diagnostic limits for the various tests were altered in accordance with the different test groupings and with the genetic grouping, then linkage between MH and *RYR*1 polymorphisms was complete, the lod score favoring linkage being 3.84 for a recombination fraction of 0.0.

The accuracy of MH diagnosis by the CHC test is and will remain a serious problem in determining genetic heterogeneity in MH. In part, this potential error arises from the fact that muscle contracture is a multifactorial process in which a large number of protein polymorphisms, including mutations in *RYR*1, will contribute to the final contracture response. To illustrate this point, a plot of muscle responsiveness to caffeine and to caffeine plus halothane of almost 1200 patients, including large numbers of both MH-positive and -negative individuals, did not give rise to two clearly separated populations peaks, but rather to three to five peaks on a continuous background.[57] Accordingly, diagnostic cut-off points, allegedly discriminating between contracture responses of MH-susceptible vs. normal individuals, are not likely to be accurate for every individual in a large population.

VII. CONCLUDING REMARKS

MH is, at worst, a subclinical myopathy for heterozygous human carriers of abnormal genes and, accordingly, there is little urgency to effect a cure. The critical research goal is to be able to detect, in advance of anesthesia, the presence of any genetic abnormality that might predispose an individual to an MH episode. Accordingly, identification of all MH mutations and development of diagnostic tests for them is the highest priority both for the individual and for the health-care system. In MH families in which MH-susceptible individuals have been identified, all individuals are usually considered by the anesthetist to be predisposed to MH and anesthetic routines are altered at considerable expense to avoid a potential reaction. Management of an MH reaction in the operating room is expensive and, if death or morbidity occurs, can result in high medical or legal costs. Thus the availability of inexpensive and accurate diagnostic tests are eagerly awaited, first for accurate MH family analysis and, in the long run, for a large segment of the population undergoing anesthesia. In addition, knowledge gained from the study of MH mutations contributes greatly to our knowledge of structure/function relationships in the Ca^{2+} release channel.[30]

ACKNOWLEDGMENTS

Original research from Dr. MacLennan's laboratory was funded by grants from the Medical Research Council of Canada (MRC), the Muscular Dystrophy Association of Canada (MDAC), the Heart and Stroke Foundation of Ontario, and the Canadian Genetic Diseases Networks of Centers of Excellence. M. S. Phillips is a predoctoral fellow of the Heart and Stroke Foundation of Ontario; Yilin Zhang is an MRC/MDAC postdoctoral fellow.

REFERENCES

1. **Britt, B. A.,** Malignant hyperthermia: a review, in *Thermoregulation: Pathology, Pharmacology and Therapy*, E. Schonbaum and P. Lomax, Eds., Pergamon Press, New York, 1991, 179.
2. **Kalow, W., Britt, B. A., Terreau, M. E., and Haist, C.,** Metabolic error of muscle metabolism after recovery from malignant hyperthermia, *Lancet*, ii, 895, 1970.
3. **Ellis, F. R., Harriman, D. G. F., Keaney, N. P., Kyei-Mensch, K., and Tyrrell, J. H.,** *Br. J. Anaesth.*, 43, 721, 1971.
4. **Larach, M. G. and Landis, J. R.,** False positive diagnosis of malignant hyperthermia susceptibility in control subjects using the North American caffeine halothane contracture test, *Anesthesiology*, 73, A1013, 1990.
5. **O'Brien, P. J.,** Etiopathogenetic defect of malignant hyperthermia: hypersensitive calcium-release channel of skeletal muscle sarcoplasmic reticulum, *Vet. Res. Comm.*, 11, 527, 1987.
6. **Archibald, A.L.,** Inherited halothane-induced malignant hyperthermia in pigs, in *Breeding for Disease Resistance in Farm Animals*, J. B. Owen and R. F. E. Axford, Eds., CAB International, Wallingford, U.K., 1991, 449.
7. **Webb, A. J. and Simpson, S. P.,** Performance of British Landrace pigs selected for high and low incidence of halothane sensitivity. II. Growth and carcass traits, *Anim. Prod.*, 43, 493, 1986.

acid substitutions in the coding sequence of the ryanodine receptor (*RYR*1) gene in individuals with malignant hyperthermia, *Genomics*, 13, 1247, 1992.

42. **Healy, J. M. S., Heffron, J. J. A., Lehane, M., Bradley, D. G., Johnson, K.**, and **McCarthy, T. V.**, Diagnosis of malignant hyperthermia susceptibility with flanking DNA markers, *Br. Med. J.*, 303, 1225, 1991.

43. **Levitt, R. C., Nouri, N., Jedlicka, A. E., McKusick, V. A., Marks, A. R., Shutack, J. G., Fletcher, J. E., Rosenberg, H.**, and **Meyers, D. A.**, Evidence for genetic heterogeneity in malignant hyperthermia susceptibility, *Genomics*, 11, 543, 1991.

44. **Deufel, T., Golla, A., Iles, D., Meindl, A., Meitinger, T., Schindelhauer, D., DeVries, A., Pongratz, D., MacLennan, D. H., Johnson, K. J.**, and **Lehmann-Horn, F.**, Evidence for genetic heterogeneity of malignant hyperthermia susceptibility, *Am. J. Hum. Genet.*, 50, 1151, 1992.

45. **Iles, D. E., Segers, B., Heytens, L., Sengers, R. C. A.**, and **Wieringa, B.**, High-resolution physical mapping of four microsatellite repeat markers near the RYR1 locus on chromosome 19q13.1 and apparent exclusion of the MHS locus from this region in two malignant hyperthermia susceptible families, *Genomics*, 14, 749, 1992.

46. **Brownell, A. K. W.**, Malignant hyperthermia: relationship to other disease, *Br. J. Anaesth.*, 60, 303, 1988.

47. **Isaacs, H.** and **Badenhorst, M. E.**, Dominantly inherited malignant hyperthermia (MH) in the King-Denborough syndrome, *Muscle Nerve*, 15, 740, 1992.

48. **Brownell, A. K. W., Paasuke, R. T., Elash, A., Fowlow, S. B., Seagram, C. G. F., Diewold, R. J.**, and **Friesen, C.**, Malignant hyperthermia in Duchenne muscular dystrophy, *Anaesthesiology*, 58, 180, 1983.

49. **Heiman-Patterson, T., Rosenberg, H., Fletcher, J. E.**, and **Tahmoush, A. J.**, Malignant hyperthermia in myotonia congenita. Halothane-caffeine contracture testing in neuromuscular disease, *Muscle Nerve*, 11, 453, 1988.

50. **Mulley, J. C., Kozman, H. M., Phillips, H. A., Gedeon, A. K., McCure, J. A., Iles, D. E., Gregg, R. G., Hogan, K., Couch, F. J., MacLennan, D. H.**, and **Haan, E. A.**, Refined genetic localization for central core disease, *Am. J. Hum. Genet.*, 52, 398, 1993.

51. **Fletcher, J. E., Tripolitis, L., Erwin, K., Hanson, S., Rosenberg, H., Conti, P. A.**, and **Beech, J.**, Fatty acids modulate calcium-induced calcium release from skeletal muscle heavy sarcoplasmic reticulum fractions: implications for malignant hyperthermia, *Biochem. Cell Biol.*, 68, 1195, 1990.

52. **Foster, P. S., Gesini, E., Claudianos, C., Hopkinson, K. C.**, and **Denborough, M. A.**, Inositol 1,4,5-triphosphate deficiency and malignant hyperthermia in swine, *Lancet*, i, 124, 1989.

53. **Levitt, R. C., Olckers, A., Meyers, S., Fletcher, J. E., Rosenberg, H., Isaacs, H.**, and **Meyers, D. A.**, Evidence for the localization of a malignant hyperthermia susceptibility locus (MHS2) to human chromosome 17q, *Genomics*, 14, 562, 1992.

54. **Fontaine, B., Khurana, T. S., Hoffman, E. P., Bruns, G. A. P., Haines, J. L., Trofatter, J. A., Hanson, M. P., Rich, J., McFarlane, H., Yasek, D. M., Romano, D., Gusella, J. F.**, and **Brown, R. H.**, Hyperkalemic periodic paralysis and the adult muscle sodium channel alpha subunit gene, *Science*, 250, 1000, 1990.

55. **Olckers, A., Meyers, D. A., Meyers, S., Taylor, E. W., Fletcher, J. E., Rosenberg, H., Isaacs, H.**, and **Levitt, R. C.**, Adult muscle sodium channel α-subunit is a gene candidate for malignant hyperthermia susceptibility, *Genomics*, 14, 829, 1992.

56. **MacKenzie, A. E., Allen, G., Lahey, D., Crossan, M. L., Nolan, K., Mettler, G., Worton, R. G., MacLennan, D. H.**, and **Korneluk, R.**, A comparison of the caffeine halothane muscle contracture test with the molecular genetic diagnosis of malignant hyperthermia, *Anaesthesiology*, 75, 4, 1991.

57. **Kalow, W., Sharer, S.**, and **Britt, B. A.**, Pharmacogenetics of caffeine and caffeine-halothane contractures in biopsies of human skeletal muscle, *Pharmacogenetics*, 1, 126, 1991.

Chapter 19

DEMONSTRATION OF THE MUTATION ASSOCIATED WITH PORCINE STRESS SYNDROME

Xia Zhang, Hua Shen, C. Robert Cory, and Peter J. O'Brien

TABLE OF CONTENTS

I.   Introduction 274

II. Methods 275
     A.   PCR Protocol for Amplification and Detecton of
          the Gene Mutation Associated with PSS 275
          1.   Preliminary Notes 275
          2.   Isolation of Genomic DNA from
               Whole Blood 277
               a.   Principle 277
               b.   Materials 279
               c.   Procedure 279
     B.   Amplification of a DNA Target Sequence Using
          the Polymerase Chain Reaction 280
          1.   Principle 280
          2.   Materials 280
          3.   Procedure 282
     C.   RFLP Analysis of the PCR Product 282
          1.   Principle 282
          2.   Materials 283
          3.   Procedure 283
     D.   Agarose Gel Electrophoresis of DNA Restriction
          Fragments 283
          1.   Materials 283
          2.   Principle 284
          3.   Procedure 284
     E.   Diagnosis of the PSS Mutation Based on RFLP 286
          1.   Principle 286

III. Phenotyping of Swine Susceptible to PSS 286
     A.   Statistical Methods 287
     B.   Results 287
          1.   RFLP Analysis of the PSS Mutation 287
          2.   Comparison of DNA-Based Test with
               Hypersensitivity Tests 289
          3.   Costs of DNA-Based Test for PSS 289

0-8493-8093-6/94/$0.00 + $.50

IV.   Discussion 290

V.   Addendum 291

Acknowledgments 291

References...291

I. INTRODUCTION

Porcine Stress Syndrome (PSS) is an inherited neuromuscular disease analogous to malignant hyperthermia (MH) in humans. When triggered, PSS is characterized by the development of muscle contracture, hypermetabolism, and acidosis. In swine that are homozygous for this defect, the syndrome is triggered with the stress associated with transport, restraint, fighting, mating, vigorous exercise, and hot, humid weather. In addition, this syndrome is triggered by the anesthetic agents halothane and succinylcholine. The use of the halothane challenge (HC) test as the basis for diagnosis of swine homozygous for PSS gives rise to *HAL* as the name of the gene responsible for PSS.[1]

PSS is responsible for substantial revenue loss in the pork industry. In addition to stress mortality rates of approximately 10% among homozygotes, there is postmortem development of pale, soft, exudative pork (PSEP).[1] About 50% of the meat of homozygotes is PSEP, and revenue losses from these inferior carcasses occur through loss of weight from water exudation, decreased customer preference, and relegation of PSEP to less expensive products such as sausage. Despite the deleterious effects of the PSS gene, it has been inadvertently selected by swine breeders likely due to its association with increased muscularity and lean meat.

PSS susceptibility is the result of abnormal intracellular regulation of muscle calcium concentration. Muscle contraction and the requisite increase in metabolic activity are triggered by release of calcium through an ion-specific channel, the ryanodine receptor *(RYR)*, located in the terminal cisternae of the sarcoplasmic reticulum (SR). Functional assessment of the *RYR* from PSS animals has revealed that the release channel is hypersensitive to a variety of triggering agents[1,2] including caffeine, adenosine trisphosphate, and calcium at concentrations one order of magnitude lower than those required to open the normal channel.[1-4]

To date, diagnostic tests for the presence of PSS susceptibility have lacked specificity as evidenced by the fact that a low percentage of animals that are heterozygous for PSS will react to the commonly used HC test, whereas a small percentage of animals that are homozygous for PSS are HC nonreactors. In addition to the significant risk of misdiagnoses, HC tests, and other tests for PSS susceptibility such as the halothane and caffeine contracture tests are invasive and not cost effective for commercial breeding purposes.[1] Recently, the porcine ryanodine receptor *(RYR)* was cloned.[5] Sequence comparisons of *RYR* cDNA from PSS and normal pigs revealed 18 single nucleotide polymorphisms. At nucleotide position 1843, a replacement of C in the normal animal with T in the PSS animal led to the replacement of a cysteine with an arginine. Based on this mutation site, a DNA-based diagnostic test has been developed to identify swine that are normal, homozygous, or heterozygous for this mutation.

In this chapter, the authors describe in detail the procedure for a DNA-based diagnostic test for PSS (Figure 1). Additional[5] data showing a correlation between the presence of this mutation and susceptibility to PSS is provided. Genomic DNA is isolated from leukocytes and the region of the *RYR* gene containing the mutation site is amplified a millionfold. The amplified DNA is then subjected to restriction endonuclease digestion that cuts the DNA at the mutation site and a common control site. The fragments are then separated using agarose gel electrophoresis. Restriction-fragment length polymorphism (RFLP) analysis demonstrates three distinct banding patterns corresponding to normal, heterozygous, and homozygous for the PSS mutation. The RFLP pattern is visualized by staining the restriction fragments with a fluorescent dye.

This test is rapid, noninvasive, and can be applied to large numbers of samples. The occurrence of the mutation is shown to be highly correlated with PSS susceptibility as determined by PSS phenotyping based on halothane challenge, caffeine or halothane contracture tests, and controlled inbreeding. This definitive test provides a cost-effective opportunity for the elimination of PSS or the controlled expression of the PSS gene in commercial swine breeding programs.

II. METHODS

A. PCR PROTOCOL FOR AMPLIFICATION AND DETECTION OF THE GENE MUTATION ASSOCIATED WITH PSS

1. Preliminary Notes

The capacity of the polymerase chain reaction (PCR) to synthesize millions of DNA copies means that contamination of the sample reaction with products of a previous reaction or cross-contamination of the samples is a potential problem in providing a reliable and accurate diagnostic test. Meticulous laboratory technique is essential. Equipment and laboratory bench space

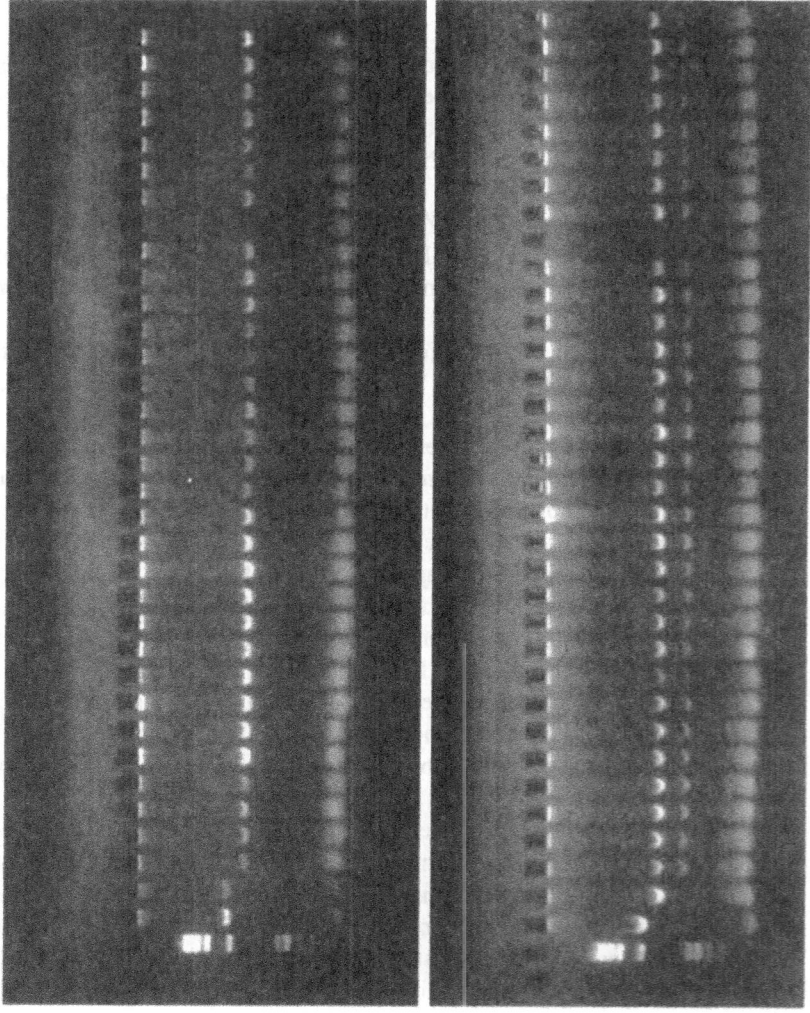

FIGURE 1. Test results for PSS susceptibility. The diagnosis of the susceptibility to PSS is made from a photograph of an agarose gel following electrophoresis of DNA restriction fragments. DNA was isolated from pig leukocytes, and a target sequence containing the PSS mutation site was amplified using PCR and cut with the restriction endonuclease *Bsi*HKA I. DNA in the gel is stained with ethidium bromide and visualized by UV transillumination. The direction of migration of the DNA is from the left to right of the figure. The photo on the left indicates the results for an experimental herd of swine that are normal, the photo in the middle is for an experimental herd of swine heterozygous for the PSS trait (plus one normal pig at bottom), and at right for a commercial herd with 6 heterozygotes, 27 normal, and 1 homozygote (third from bottom). The column at the far right indicates the RFLP for 2 heterozygotes and 3 PSS homozygotes from our experimental herds. At the bottom of each gel is a DNA standard and DNA that has not been cut by the endonuclease.

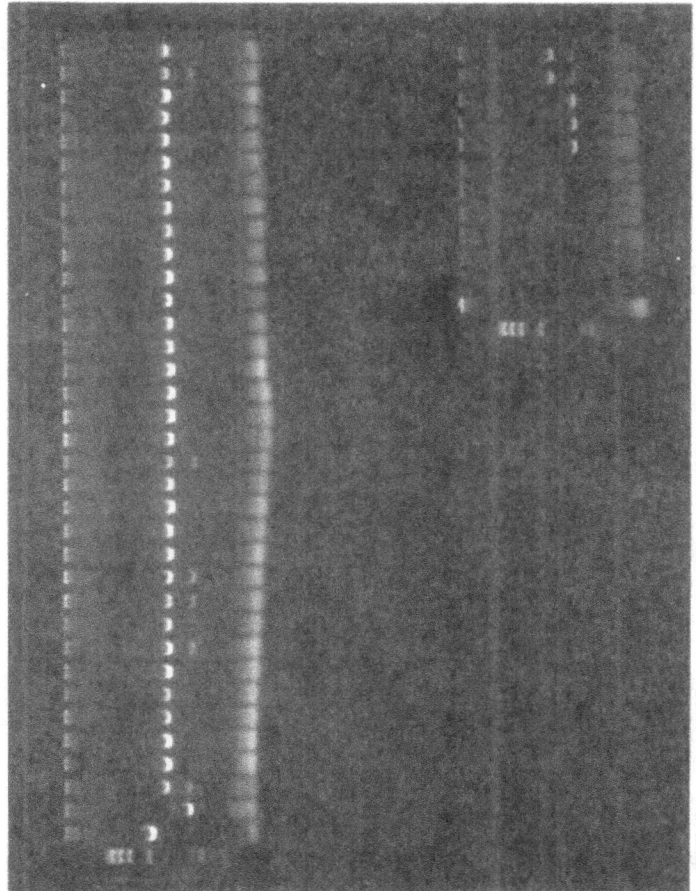

FIGURE 1. continued

used in the following methods are dedicated to this test. Whenever practical, solutions are prealiquoted. In addition, all tubes, pipette tips, and solutions (unless specifically stated) are autoclaved. All solutions are prepared using sterile, deionized distilled water. Reagents and chemicals were of the highest grade commercially available. A schematic diagram of the test procedure is shown in Figure 2.

2. Isolation of Genomic DNA from Whole Blood
a. Principle

Leukocytes isolated from whole blood are used as a source of genomic DNA. Erythrocytes are lysed and leukocytes are pelleted and washed free of red blood cell contamination. Genomic DNA is freed from associated protein by proteinase digestion.

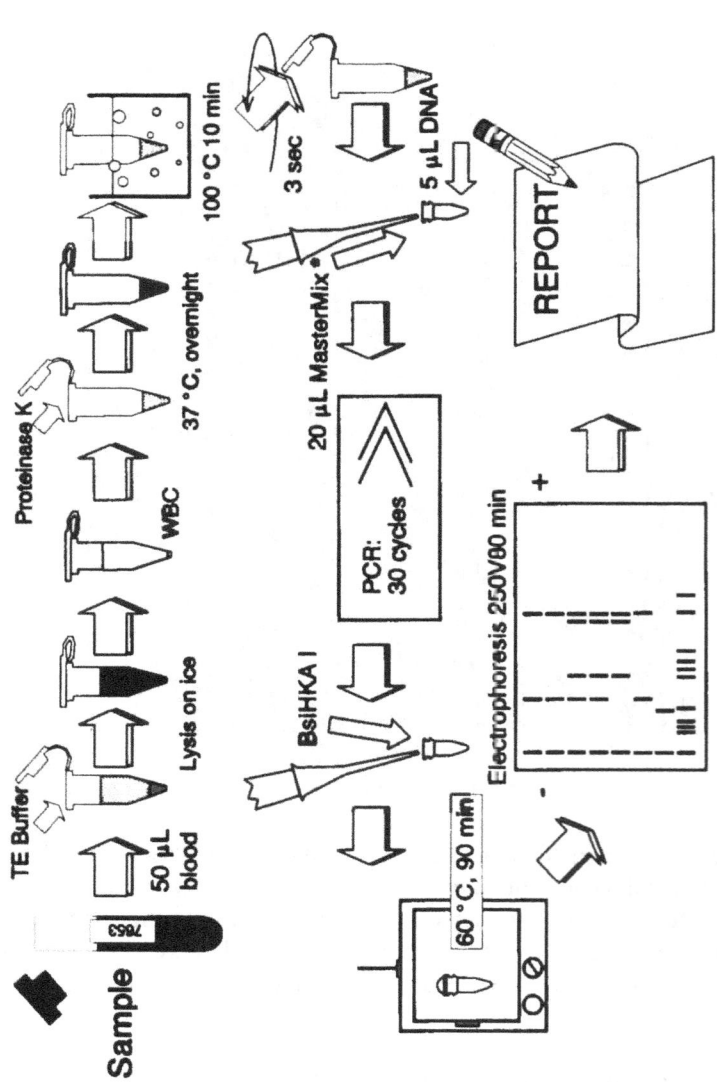

FIGURE 2. Flow chart of the DNA-based PSS test procedure. Thick arrows show the direction of the procedure, whereas thin arrows indicate the additions of the solution. For a more comprehensive explanation of the PCR, see Figure 3. (From O'Brien, P. J., et al., *J. Am. Vet. Med. Assoc.*, 203, 842, 1993. With permission.)

b. Materials

- Stock solutions, prepared using sterile distilled, deionized H_2O as follows: 0.5 M $Na_2EDTA \cdot 2H_2O$ (ethylenediamine tetra-acetic acid, disodium), pH 8.0; 1 M KCl; 1 M $MgCl_2 \cdot 6H_2O$; 1 M Tris-Cl [tris(hydroxymethyl)aminomethane], pH 8.0. The pH of all solutions is adjusted as shown. The solutions are autoclaved and stored at room temperature.

- Lysis buffer (10 mM Tris-Cl, 1 mM EDTA, pH 8.0): 5 ml of 1 M Tris-Cl stock is mixed with 1.0 ml of 0.5 M EDTA stock and brought to a final volume of 500 ml with deionized H_2O. The pH is adjusted to 8.0 and the solution is autoclaved.

- 20 mg/ml Proteinase K stock 20 mg of Proteinase K (Boehringer Mannheim Canada Ltd., Laval Que) in 1.0 ml of H_2O, stored at $-85°C$. The solution is mixed by gentle inversion and aliquoted in 200-µl volumes into microcentrifuge tubes. These aliquots may undergo several freeze thaw cycles with minimal losses in activity.

- Buffer A (50 mM KCl, 20 mM Tris-Cl, 2.5 mM $MgCl_2$, pH 8.3): 12.5 ml of 1 M KCl, 5.0 ml of 1 M Tris-Cl and 0.625 ml of 1 M $MgCl_2$ stock solutions are combined and brought to a final volume of 250 ml with deionized H_2O. The pH is adjusted to 8.3. The solution is autoclaved and stored at room temperature.

- Digestion buffer (buffer A containing 0.5% Tween-20,® and 100 µg/ml of Proteinase K): 99 µl of Buffer A mixed with 0.5 µl Tween-20® and 0.5 µl of 20 mg/ml freshly thawed Proteinase K stock. The solution is mixed thoroughly by gentle inversion. These volumes are multiplied by the number of samples to be digested plus 10% to allow for losses during pipetting. This buffer is used *immediately* after it is prepared.

c. Procedure

Step 1. Blood collection — 1 to 2 ml of whole blood is collected into sterile evacuated blood collection tubes (Vacutainer Brand, Canlab Scientific, Mississauga, ON) containing K_3EDTA anticoagulant. Other anticoagulants such as heparin are incompatible with this diagnostic test and should be avoided. Blood samples are immediately transported at room temperature to the test laboratory. If the testing is not performed immediately, the samples are refrigerated at 4°C for up to one week or placed at $-85°C$ for longer term storage. Upon receipt of the blood, each sample is assigned a laboratory identification number. The Laboratory identification number is placed on a corresponding *sterile* microcentrifuge tube. A record is made of animal identification number and the breed (provided by the breeder) and the laboratory identification number.

Step 2. Leukocyte isolation — The collection tubes containing the freshly collected blood sample are mixed on an orbital mixer (Adams Nutator, Becton

Dickinson Canada Ltd.) for at least 3 min. Red blood cells are lysed by adding 50 µl of mixed whole blood to a prelabeled, sterile 1.5-ml microcentrifuge tube containing 500 µl of lysis buffer. The sample is vortexed (Maxi Mix II, Thermolyne Inc.) for 3 s at the maximum setting and held on ice for 10 min. Leukocytes are pelleted by sedimentation in a table-top microcentrifuge (Eppendorf Model 5414) for 30 s at 13,000 rpm. The supernatant is gently decanted and any liquid clinging to the tube is removed by gentle blotting on a laboratory tissue. Care is taken not to disrupt the pellet. Using a sterile pipette tip, an additional 500 µl of lysis buffer is added to the microcentrifuge tube. The same pipette tip is used for all additions as long as it does not come into contact with any nonsterile surface or any part of the samples. The pellet is resuspended by vortexing at the maximum setting for 10 s or until the pellet is well dispersed. The centrifugation, RBC lysis, and washing steps are repeated three more times. In the event of persistent red blood cell contamination additional lysis and washing steps are added.

Step 3. Proteinase K digestion of leukocyte pellet — DNA is freed from protein in the washed pellet by Proteinase K digestion. Following the final wash the pellet is resuspended in 100 µl of digestion buffer. The sample is vortexed just long enough to resuspend the pellet (approximately 1 s) and placed on its side on an orbital mixer in a drying oven to incubate at 37°C overnight (15 to 18 h). Alternatively, an incubation at 56°C for 60 min is used for Proteinase K digestion of the pellet. Following digestion the Proteinase K is inactivated by placing the sample tube in a boiling water bath for 10 min. The sample is removed from the water and allowed to cool to room temperature. It is then centrifuged for 3 s at 13,500 rpm to pellet undigested material and to clarify the sample.

B. AMPLIFICATION OF A DNA TARGET SEQUENCE USING THE POLYMERASE CHAIN REACTION

1. Principle

The PCR is used to amplify a 659-bp DNA sequence flanking the PSS mutation site at position 1843 of the ryanodine receptor gene. Figure 3 shows the principle of PCR amplification of a sequence of a native DNA. The isolated genomic DNA is incubated in the presence of deoxynucleotides, Taq DNA polymerase, and two primer sequences of DNA complementary to nucleotide sequences upstream and downstream of the DNA target sequence. The PCR reaction involves a two-step sequence of heating and cooling cycles. These cycles permit the annealing of the complementary DNA primers with the DNA target, extension of the target sequence catalysed by the DNA polymerase, and melting of the synthesized double-stranded DNA to allow the cycle to repeat.

2. Materials

To prepare the PCR master mix, in a sterile microcentrifuge tube 16.55 µl of H_2O is combined with 2.5 µl of incubation buffer (supplied with Taq

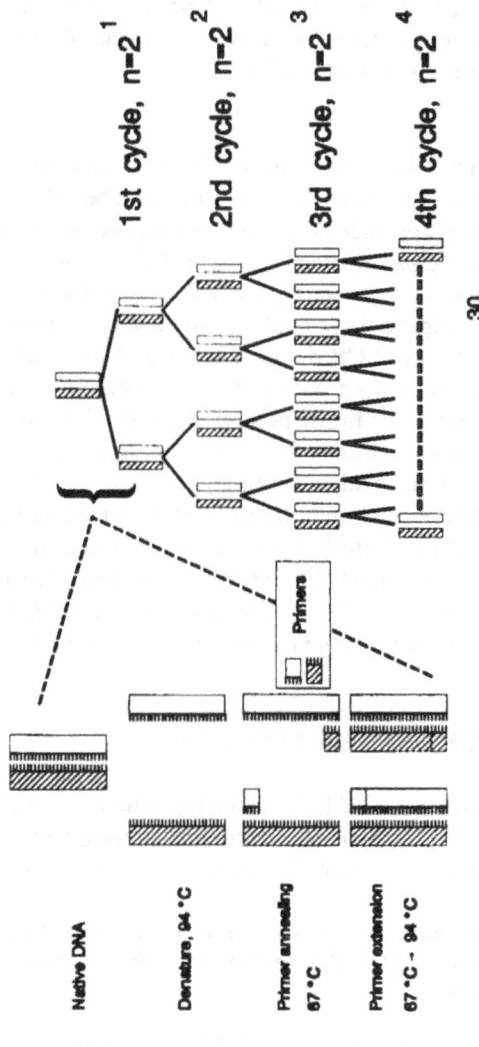

FIGURE 3. Principle of PCR. On the left side of the figure, a breakdown of one PCR cycle is shown. Double-stranded native DNA is denatured at 94°C for 10 s. The temperature is then reduced to 67°C for 80 s. The forward and reverse primers (shown as empty and shaded, respectively) anneal to complementary DNA sequences upstream and downstream from the mutation site. The DNA is then heated to 94°C for 10 s. During the thermal transition from annealing to denaturation the primer is extended in the forward and reverse direction catalyzed by Taq DNA polymerase. The schematic on the right side of the figure shows the amplification of a DNA sequence. Following 30 cycles of PCR the theoretical number of DNA copies is approximately 2^{30}. (From O'Brien, P. J., et al., *J. Am. Vet. Med. Assoc.*, 203, 842, 1993. With permission.)

DNA polymerase, Boehringer Mannheim, containing 500 mM KCl, 1 M Tris-Cl, 15 mM MgCl$_2$, and 10 mg/ml gelatin), 0.05 μl each of dATP, dCTP, dGTP, dTTP (200 μM final concentration), 0.25 μl each of the forward (5'-TCCAGTTTGCCACAGGTCCTACCA-3') and reverse (5'-TTCACCGGA GTGGAGTCTCTGAGT-3') primers (1 mg/ml final concentration), and 0.25 μl Taq DNA polymerase (Boehringer Mannheim, 5,000 U/ml). These volumes are multiplied by the number of samples to be run, allowing for 10% loss during pipetting. The master mix is prepared on ice and used immediately. The Taq DNA polymerase is stored at −20°C.

3. Procedure

Preparing a master mix reduces the volume of work, improves precision, and reduces the intersample variability. Sterile reaction tubes (MicroAmp,* Perkin Elmer Cetus) for PCR are loaded into custom-designed racks and placed on ice. While on ice 5 μl (approximately 0.2 μg/ml) of genomic DNA was added to the reaction tube. A separate pipette tip is used for each sample addition. The same sterile pipette tip is used as long as it does not touch any nonsterile objects. Then 20 μl of PCR master mix are added to each reaction tube after all the samples have been added and the tubes are capped. The solutions are thoroughly mixed by firmly holding the side of the sample tray with capped reaction tubes and placing the entire tray on a vortex mixer at maximal setting for 3 to 4 times with each duration of 1 s.

The sample tray is then loaded onto the thermal cycler (GeneAmp PCR System 9600,** Perkin Elmer Cetus). DNA amplification is immediately started using 30 cycles of a two-step PCR.*** In the first step DNA is melted at 94°C for 10 s. This is followed by an annealing step at 67°C for 80 s. Following the PCR run (which takes approximately 80 min) the samples are maintained at 4°C.

C. RFLP ANALYSIS OF THE PCR PRODUCT

1. Principle

The amplified target sequence of DNA is analyzed based on RFLP. The DNA sequence is cut into fragments using a restriction enzyme that recognizes a DNA sequence common to the normal gene and to a sequence in the mutated

---

* All PCR reaction tubes, caps, trays, and accessories are from Perkin Elmer Cetus. The tray permits the loading of up to 96 MicroAmp PCR reaction 96 tubes that are transferred directly in the rack to the thermal cycler.

** The use of the GeneAmp PCR System 9600 precludes the need for mineral oil as a vapor barrier or glycerol as a thermal transfer fluid because of the tight fit of the tubes in the block, the thin walls of the MicroAmp reaction tubes, and the heated cover of the instrument.

***In the 2-step PCR the extension time is completely eliminated for small target sequences since the Taq polymerase retains significant activity at lower temperatures and complete extension occurs during the thermal transition from annealing to denaturation.

gene containing the mutation site. The restriction fragments are separated using agarose gel electrophoresis and visualized with UV transillumination of ethidium bromide-stained DNA. Figure 4 shows the nucleotide sequence of part of the ryanodine receptor gene with about 16 amino acids on each side of the mutation site.

2. Materials

To prepare the cutting buffer, in a sterile microcentrifuge tube on ice 2.8 μl of NE Buffer 3 (New England Biolabs Ltd., Missisauga, ON*) containing (final concentrations) 100 mM NaCl, 50 mM Tris-Cl, 10 mM MgCl$_2$, and 1 mM DTT are combined with 0.28 μl BSA (100 μg/ml final concentration) and 0.50 μl of the endonuclease BsiHKA** (5 U/sample). The solution is mixed by gently inverting the tube several times. These volumes are multiplied by the number of samples to be analyzed, allowing for 10% loss during pipetting.

3. Procedure

Caps are removed from the PCR reaction tubes avoiding contact with nonsterile surfaces. The position of each row of caps is noted since they are reused. Using a separate tip for each addition, 3.58 μl of cutting buffer is added to each reaction tube for a final volume of 28.58 μl. This mixture is not added to tubes designated as "uncut controls." The tubes are recapped with the original cap and the entire set of tubes is briefly vortexed (three to four times for 1 s each at maximum setting). The sample tray is placed on an orbital mixer in a drying oven and the PCR product is digested at 56°C for 90 min. Following endonuclease treatment, DNA restriction fragments are separated using agarose gel electrophoresis.

D. AGAROSE GEL ELECTROPHORESIS OF DNA RESTRICTION FRAGMENTS
1. Materials

- Sample loading buffer: 40% glycerol (v/v), 5 mM Tris-Cl, 0.5 mM Na$_2$EDTA, 1% (w/v) sodium dodecylsulfate, and 0.125 mg% bromphenol blue, pH 8.0.
- TBE electrophoresis buffer: 89 mM Tris-Cl, 89 mM boric acid, 0.5 mM Na$_2$EDTA, pH 8.0.
- Ethidium bromide stock solution: 10 mg/ml ethidium bromide in H$_2$O. Ethidium bromide is a mutagen and an irritant. Gloves should always

---

* NE Buffer 3 is supplied by New England Biolabs as a 10 × concentrated stock solution with the restriction endonuclease BsiHKA I.

** BsiHKA I is an isoschizomer of HgiA I.

a) Normal gene   ↓

......GTGCTGGATGTCCTGTGTTCCCTGTGTGTGTGCAATGGTGTGGCCGTGCGGCTCCAAC
.   .   V   L   D   V   L   C   S   L   C   V   C   N   G   V   A   V   R   S   N

CAAGATCTCATTACTGAGAACTTGCTCCCTGGCCGCGAGCTT......
Q   D   L   I   T   E   N   L   L   P   G   R   E   L   .   .

b) Mutant gene   ↓

......GTGCTGGATGTCCTGTGTTCCCTGTGTGTGTGCAATGGTGTGGCCGTGTGCTCCAAC
.   .   V   L   D   V   L   C   S   L   C   V   C   N   G   V   A   V   C   S   N

CAAGATCTCATTACTGAGAACTTGCTCCCTGGCCGCGAGCTT......
Q   D   L   I   T   E   N   L   L   P   G   R   E   L   .   .

FIGURE 4. Nucleotide and deduced amino acid sequences of a porcine ryanodine receptor gene around the probable PSS mutation site (shown at the arrow). Only about 16 amino acids (48 bp) on each side of the probable mutation site are shown. The total length of the DNA amplified with this test is 659 bps. (From Fujii et al., *Science*, 253, 448, 1991. With permission.)

be worn to prevent exposure when gels or solutions containing the dye are handled. Solutions containing ethidium bromide are prepared in the fume hood.

2. Principle

The restriction fragments resulting from endonuclease treatment of the amplified DNA sequence are separated according to size using a 3% agarose gel and a high capacity electrophoresis system. DNA fragments are visualized by fluorescence of intercalated ethidium bromide using UV transillumination. Diagnosis of PSS is based on the number and size, relative to a DNA standard, of the restriction fragments visualized on the gel.

3. Procedure

Step 1. Casting the agarose gel — A 3% total agarose gel is prepared by melting 8.77 g of NuSieve GTG and 2.92 g Agarose NA* in 390 ml of TBE electrophoresis buffer and 0.38 μg/ml ethidium bromide on a hot plate with constant stirring. All steps in the preparation of the gel are performed in a fume hood to minimize contact with the ethidium bromide. Ethidium bromide is not added into the melted agarose until it is cooled to 55°C. After ethidium bromide is added, the gel is poured onto a 20 × 25 cm gel running tray.** Prior to casting the gel, the ends of the running tray are taped and

* NuSieve GTG is from FMC BioProducts, Rockland, ME. Agarose NA is from Pharmacia.

** The high capacity agarose gel electrophoresis (AGE) system is from Hoeffer Scientific Instruments (San Francisco, CA) and consists of a SuperSub 20 × 25 cm Submarine Gel Electrophoresis unit with 20 × 25 cm gel casting and gel running trays. The 20 × 25 cm gel accommodates three 36 well combs 3 mm thick × 3 mm wide for a total of 98 wells. Wells formed with these combs have a capacity of 8.9 μl/mm of gel depth.

the tray is leveled. The agarose is poured to a depth of 5 mm. Three combs are placed every 8 cm of gel length and the height is adjusted so that 1 mm of agarose remains between the bottom of the comb and the base of the gel running platform. Once the gel is hardened the tape and the combs are removed and the gel and the running tray are placed in the electrophoresis unit. A volume of TBE electrophoresis buffer is added to the unit sufficient to cover the gel to a depth of 1 mm. The electrophoresis unit is connected to a refrigerated circulation bath and the TBE buffer is maintained at a temperature of 4°C.

Step 2. Loading the samples — Following endonuclease digestion 7 μl of gel loading buffer is added to each PCR reaction tube for a total of 35 μl. The samples are mixed with the loading buffer by vortexing the entire tray at a 50% of the maximum speed for 2 to 3 s after all the tubes are added with the loading buffer. The entire sample is loaded into a well using a separate tip for each sample. Care should be taken to not disturb the TBE electrophoresis buffer as this may cause samples to be washed out of the wells. Standards and controls are included in each row of wells. An Hae III Digest of phage φX-174-RF DNA is used as a DNA molecular weight marker. A sample of DNA from a previously diagnosed pig heterozygous for the PSS mutation is used as a positive control and PCR product uncut by the endonuclease is the negative control for endonuclease activity. The electrophoresis unit is connected to the power supply (Bio-Rad Model 300Xi) and the samples are electrophoresed at 250 v constant for 80 min. The progress of DNA restriction fragment separation is monitored by the migration of the Bromphenol Blue. Sufficient separation is achieved when the dye front has migrated 5 to 6 cm from the origin.

Step 3. Photography of DNA in agarose gels — Following AGE the gel is gently removed from the running tray and placed on a UV transilluminator (Mighty Bright, Hoeffer Scientific). Latex gloves are worn to minimize contact with the ethidium bromide in the gel. The gel and the transilluminator are covered with a UV viewing box (The Benchtop Darkroom, Hoeffer Scientific) and the banding pattern is visualized. If necessary, background ethidium bromide fluorescence is reduced by destaining the gel under cold running tap water for 30 to 40 min. Once the background fluorescence is sufficiently reduced and the banding pattern is visually confirmed, the gel is photographed using a Polaroid film holder.* An orange filter is required to achieve a desirable film image of light transmitted by fluorescing DNA. Polaroid type 667 film (ASA 3000) offers ideal sensitivity, allowing as little as 1 to 10 ng of DNA to be detected on film after making adjustments of exposure time.

---

* The PhotoMan and Polaroid Direct Screen Camera System (Hoeffer Scientific Instruments) are used to photograph agarose gels. The camera is fitted with a Tiffen 40.5 mm # 15 orange filter and mounted on the PhotoMan bellows. The system fits directly over the UV transilluminator. Exposure settings are f16 for 1 s. Development time for the film is 40 s.

E. DIAGNOSIS OF THE PSS MUTATION BASED ON RFLP

1. Principle

Diagnosis of the mutation for PSS is based strictly on visualizing the RFLP banding pattern following restriction endonuclease digestion of an amplified DNA segment containing the mutation site. The amplified segment is 659 bp. If the sample has not been cut (uncut control), there is a bright band corresponding to the amplified 659 bp DNA segment. The RFLP banding pattern for normal pigs is a bright band at 524 bp and a fainter band at 135 bp. For swine that are heterozygous carriers of the mutation, the RFLP pattern shows in addition to the 524 and 135 bp a bright band at 358 bp and a relatively faint band of 166 bp demonstrating an addition of cut site resulting from the mutation at position 1843 of the ryanodine receptor gene. For the homozygous pig, the RFLP pattern shows a predominant band at 358 and 166 bp and an absence of the 524-bp "normal" band. In some cases the primer is visualized as a 24-bp band and also as primer dimers at 48 bp.

III. PHENOTYPING OF SWINE SUSCEPTIBLE TO PSS

The PSS susceptibility status was determined for 181 pigs in six breeds. Pietrain and Yorkshire swine were purebred and obtained from closed herds maintained at the Ontario Veterinary College, University of Guelph. These herds had been inbred for more than 10 years. The susceptibility for PSS was established using either the HC test or the halothane-specific contracture (HSC) test and the caffeine-specific challenge (CSC) test. In a typical HC test, 2- to 3-month-old pigs are physically restrained and forced to inhale 3 to 5% halothane in oxygen for several minutes. Those developing extensor muscle rigidity are susceptible to PSS. This test is known to detect more than 90% of homozygotes for the MH defect and less than 25% of heterozygotes for the PSS defect. In the HSC and CSC tests, muscle is excised, placed in oxygenated physiological saline, and connected to an isometric force transducer. Isometric tension is recorded on a polygraph during exposure to 5% halothane or progressively increasing amounts of caffeine. Swine are considered to be PSS susceptible if 5% halothane caused a greater than 0.5 g increase in force or if a 1-g increase in muscle tension occurred with less than 4 mM caffeine in the CSC test; normal if more than 7 mM caffeine was required to cause a 1-g increase in muscle tension and 5% halothane produced less than a 0.2 g increase in tension; and heterozygous if a 1-g increase in tension was produced by 5 to 6 mM caffeine.[6] Hypersensitivity of the Ca-release channel was directly demonstrated using isolated terminal cisternae of SR[5] for 10 of the swine homozygous for the PSS mutation.[3,5]

PSS-susceptible Pietrains and PSS-resistant Yorkshires were crossbred to produce a herd of pigs that were heterozygous for the PSS defect. All Yorkshires used had been shown to be negative for the halothane challenge test and to produce offspring that were also negative. PSS-susceptible Landrace and PSS-resistant Landrace were also crossbred to produce heterozygotes.

A. STATISTICAL METHODS

Following unequivocal diagnosis of PSS-susceptibility using HSC or CSC tests and the DNA-based test for the HAL-1843 mutation, swine homozygous, heterozygous, and normal were assigned a mutation dosage of 1, 0.5, and 0, respectively. Using a double-blind design Cochran's Q-test for agreement of categorical data was used to test the statistical significance for the agreement between diagnoses of PSS susceptibility. Similarly, correlations were determined in different swine breeds between estimates of PSS gene frequency made using halothane and caffeine contracture tests and diagnoses based on the DNA test. The p value for the correlation of estimates of PSS gene frequency using these methods was determined using David's r-test for correlation.[7]

B. RESULTS

The correlation data presented herein and demonstrating the relationship of DNA test results with caffeine or halothane hypersensitivity had been previously presented in part.[5] Additional data and detail are provided in Tables 1 and 2.

1. RFLP Analysis of the PSS Mutation

Photographs of agarose gel electrophoretograms showing the RFLP banding pattern of a 659-bp segment of porcine DNA flanking the HAL-1843 PSS mutation site are shown in Figure 1. Each lane running from left to right represents a DNA sample. The bottom lane of each gel contains an Hae III

TABLE 1
Agreement of Unequivocal Diagnoses of Susceptibility to PSS by Caffeine and Halothane Hypersensitivity Tests with Diagnoses by DNA-Based Test

Diagnosis	Number of swine tested	Number of tests performed	Log p value
Normal	9	12	
vs.			> -12
PSS	77	107	
Homozygous PSS	48	69	
vs.			> -4
normal or heterozygous PSS	93	104	
Heterozygous PSS	16	23	
vs.			> -7
normal or homozygous PSS	57	81	

Note: Log p values indicate the statistical significance for agreement of all diagnoses and as determined by Cochran's Q-test for agreement of categorical data.

TABLE 2
Correlation of Estimates of PSS Gene Frequency in Different Herds by Different Hypersensitivity Tests and the DNA-Based Test

| Herd | Number of swine tested | PSS gene-frequency estimate | |
		Hypersensitivity test	DNA-based test
Inbred Pietrain (P)	48	1.00	1.00
Normal Yorkshires	9	0.00	0.00
Heterozygous Yorkshires (Y)	2	0.50	0.50
P x Y crossbreeds	14	0.50	0.50
Y with no homozygous PSS pigs	43[a]	0.09	0.08
Halothane-reactive PSS Landrace	8	0.50–1.00	0.68
Halothane-resistant PSS Landrace	5	0.50	0.50
Duroc with no homozygous PSS but producing homozygous PSS pigs	31	0.05–0.15	0.10
Hampshire	20	0.00	0.00
Poland China	1	1.00	1.00

Note: Susceptibility status for PSS was determined on the basis of hypersensitivity to caffeine or halothane. The log of the p value for correlation of estimates of PSS gene frequency is > -12 as determined by David's r-test for correlation.

[a] Estimate of PSS gene frequency by caffeine hypersensitivity tests is based on 11 animals.

Digest of phage ϕX-174-RF DNA and is used as a restriction fragment size marker. The second lane from the bottom of each gel contains a 659-bp amplified segment of DNA from a normal swine that was not treated with endonuclease. In the gel on the far left, DNA from PSS-negative swine of our experimental control herd is shown following digestion with *Bsi*HKA I. The predominant bright band is now shifted from 659 to 524 bp with a fainter band at 135 bp. At the bottom of the last column of lanes in the gel to the far right, *Bsi*HKA I-treated DNA from three swine from our experimental herd of homozygotes for the PSS mutation is shown. The substitution of C at position 1843 with T on one allele results in the introduction of a second *Bsi*HKA I restriction site. As a result, the bands at 524 and 135 bp from the normal allele are joined by a bright band at 358 and a fainter band at 166 bp from the mutated allele. Amplified DNA from swine homozygous for PSS shows the loss of the normal 524-bp band; hence, only three bands are observed (358-, 166-, and 135-bp). Primers (24-bp) and primer dimers (48-bp) are seen as the diffuse bands at the bottom of the gel. Heterozygous carriers of the PSS mutation are shown in the second gel from the left. These animals had banding patterns identical to patterns derived from superimposition of the two homozygotes patterns, but with half the staining intensity. The gel on the right (second column from right) is for the breeding stock of a commercial herd with 27 normal stock, 5 heterozygotes, and 1 homozygote for the PSS mutation.

2. Comparison of DNA-Based Test With Hypersensitivity Tests

Table 1 shows the results of Cochran's Q-test for agreement between diagnoses made using caffeine and halothane sensitivity tests with diagnoses made using the DNA-based test. Regardless of cohort grouping, there was complete agreement between unequivocal diagnoses made using HSC and CSC tests with the identification of the HAL-1843 mutation.

Table 2 and Figure 5 show the results of PSS gene-frequency estimates made using caffeine and halothane sensitivity tests and the DNA-based test for the HAL-1843 mutation. The estimates of allele frequency based on phenotype analysis were highly correlated with genotype analysis (log p $> - 12$).

3. Costs of DNA-Based Test for PSS

Following recovery of costs of research and development, most costs of running the PSS test were attributable to the purchase of equipment. Approximately $40,000 was paid for a high-capacity PCR system, refrigerator and freezer, microcentrifuge, circulating water bath, mixers (vortexes, rotators, agitators), pipettors, heating/stirring plates, UV transilluminators, benchtop darkroom cabinet, instant copy camera with hood and filters, large format horizontal electrophoresis system, and incubators. A computer and fax machine were necessary for commercial application.

Costs of materials and supplies were less than $3 per assay. Most of these were attributable to the purchase of primers, Taq polymerase, nucleotides, proteinase, film for photographing gels, pipette tips, microcentrifuge tubes,

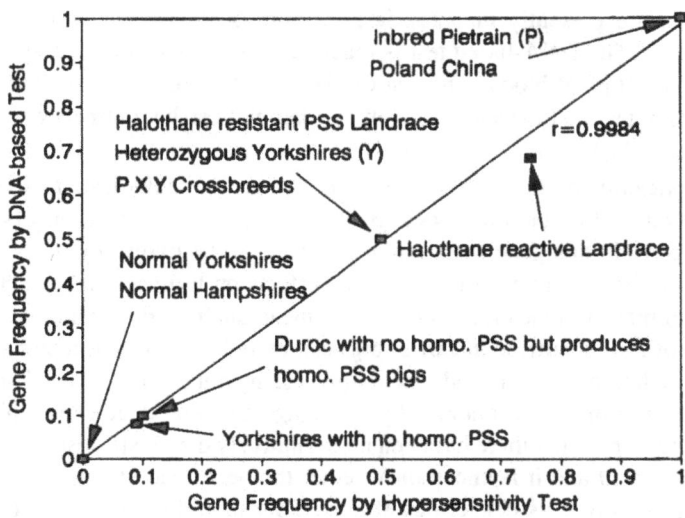

FIGURE 5. Correlations of PSS gene frequency in different breeds of swine estimated by classical hypersensitivity tests and the DNA-based test for the HAL-1843 gene mutation.

PCR reaction tubes and caps, disposable gloves, agarose, and DNA fragments standard.

Technician costs were also less than $3 per assay since 50 samples could be done per day by a skilled technician paid $20/h for a 7-h day. However, there were additional personnel costs of $3 to $4 per assay because of the need for a laboratory supervisor and secretarial assistance.

Final costs associated with performing the tests were dependent on the volume of samples analyzed. For an established diagnostic laboratory to perform the tests full time, direct total costs were less than $20 per assay.

IV. DISCUSSION

In this chapter the authors described a detailed method for a DNA-based blood test for the detection of PSS and a comparison of this test with the detection of PSS susceptibility using the classical halothane and CSC tests. The methods demonstrate that the DNA-based test is relatively easy to perform and is cost effective. PSS genotyping, based on the identification of the HAL-1843 mutation, was shown to be highly correlated with the phenotypic expression of PSS susceptibility based on halothane and CSC tests.

Despite the fact that the DNA-based blood test and the halothane and CSC tests are able to diagnose PSS, the former is more convenient for use in routine diagnoses. The halothane and CSC tests are invasive, require anaesthesia, are stressful to the animal, and time consuming. These qualities render them impractical for commercial use. Previously described blood tests[1,6] have not been sufficiently sensitive or specific for commercial use. Calcium transport tests for the biochemical defect of PSS, although useful for research purposes, are presently inappropriate for wide-scale screening for the PSS mutation.[3,9] The DNA-based test is much less invasive and can be applied to as little as 50 μl of blood. The test can be scaled up for batch analysis of up to 100 samples at a time and testing of 100 samples can be routinely completed within two days.

Application of this test in the swine industry could lead to the total eradication of PSS and the associated PSE.[10-13] Alternatively, it may be preferable to retain this gene mutation and to control the frequency of its occurrence in order to maximize its beneficial effects on leanness and muscularity and minimize its deleterious effects on meat quality. For example, if the amount of PSE occurring in carrier pigs can be reduced to an acceptable level by manipulation of swine and carcass processing conditions at the slaughterhouse, then it may be economically advantageous to produce carrier pigs for marketing. Until now there has been no definitively diagnostic test for carriers of the PSS trait and it is uncertain whether the beneficial effects of the gene mutation outweigh its deleterious effects. This should soon become clear as swine breeders identify the PSS susceptibility status of their pigs and monitor their live performance characteristics and carcass quality.

V. ADDENDUM

Licensing and performance of the test: The DNA-based test for the HAL-1843 mutation has been patented internationally[8] by the Universities of Toronto and Guelph, and licenses to perform the test are available from the Innovations Foundation, University of Toronto, 203 College Street, Suite 205, Toronto, Ontario M5T 1P9, Canada (telephone 416-978-5117) and from Hoffman LaRoche, who hold the patent rights for PCR technology.

ACKNOWLEDGMENTS

Primers were kindly provided by Dr. D. H. MacLennan of the University of Toronto. This work was supported by grants from the Ontario Ministry of Agriculture and Food, the Ontario Pork Producers Marketing Board, the Ontario Ministry of Colleges and Universities, the Ontario Heart and Stroke Foundation, and the Natural Sciences and Engineering Research Council of Canada. Peter James O'Brien is a Scholar of the Canadian Heart and Stroke Foundation.

REFERENCES

1. **O'Brien, P. J.**, Etiopathogenetic defect of malignant hyperthermia: hypersensitive calcium-release channel of skeletal muscle sarcoplasmic reticulum, *Vet. Res. Comm.*, 11, 527, 1987.
2. **O'Brien, P. J.**, Porcine malignant hyperthermia susceptibility: hypersensitive calcium-release mechanism of skeletal muscle sarcoplasmic reticulum, *Can. J. Vet. Res.*, 50, 318, 1986.
3. **O'Brien, P. J.**, Microassay for malignant hyperthermia susceptibility: hypersensitive ligand-gating of the Ca channel in muscle sarcoplasmic reticulum causes increased amounts and rates of Ca-release, *Mol. Cell. Biochem.*, 93, 53, 1990.
4. **O'Brien, P. J., Klip, A., Britt, B. A., and Kalow, B. I.**, Malignant hyperthermia susceptibility: biochemical basis for pathogenesis and diagnosis, *Can. J. Vet. Res.*, 68, 34, 1990.
5. **Fujii, J., Otsu, K., Zorzato, F., De Leon, S., Khanna, V. K., Weiler, J. E., O'Brien, P. J., and MacLennan, D. H.**, Identification of a mutation in the porcine ryanodine receptor associated with malignant hyperthermia, *Science*, 253, 448, 1991.
6. **O'Brien, P. J., Kalow, B. I., Brown, B. D. et al.**, Porcine malignant hyperthermia susceptibility: halothane-induced increase in cytoplasmic free calcium of peripheral blood lymphocytes, *Am. J. Vet. Res.*, 50, 131, 1989.
7. **Steel, R. G. D. and Torrie, J. H.**, *Principles and Procedures of Statistics with Special Reference to the Biological Sciences*, McGraw-Hill Book Company, Toronto, Canada, 1960.
8. **MacLennan, D. H. and O'Brien, P. J.**, Diagnosis for porcine malignant hyperthermia. Filed with British Patent Office for 45 countries of the Patent Corporation Treaty, Ireland, New Zealand, and South Africa on December 21, 1990 under serial No. 90 27869.8, on

May 24, 1991 under serial No. 91 110865.4, and on September 9, 1991 under serial No. 91 192500.

9. **O'Brien, P. J.**, Calcium-transport function tests for the detection of malignant hyperthermia susceptibility in swine and dogs, *Proc. Fourth Congr. Int. Soc. Anim. Clin. Biochem.*, University of California Press, Davis, 1990, 127.

10. **O'Brien, P. J. and MacLennan D. H.**, Application in the swine industry of a DNA-based test for porcine stress syndrome, *Proc. Am. Assoc. Swine Practitioners*, Nashville, TN, March 1992, 1992, 433.

11. **O'Brien, P. J. and MacLennan, D. H.**, DNA-based test for porcine stress syndrome, Ontario Swine Research Review, Ontario Agriculture College Publication #0292, 1992, 34.

12. **O'Brien, P. J. and MacLennan, D. H.**, Application of the DNA-based test for porcine stress syndrome in the swine industry., *Proc. Int. Pig Veterinarian's Soc. Meeting*, The Hague, The Netherlands, August 1992.

13. **O'Brien, P. J.**, DNA-based test for porcine stress syndrome: comparison of results with Ca sequestration activity of anoxia-challenged muscle from swine homozygous and heterozygous for defect, in State of the Art in Animal Clinical Biochemistry, A. Ubaldi, Ed., Boehringer Mannheim, Parma, Italy, 1992.

14. **O'Brien, P. J., Shen, H., Cory, C. R., and Zhang, X.**, Use of a DNA-based test for the mutation associated with porcine stress syndrome (malignant hyperthermia) 10,000 breeding swine, *J. Am. Vet. Med. Assoc.*, 203, 842, 1993.

Chapter 20

MOLECULAR GENETIC DIAGNOSIS OF HUMAN MALIGNANT HYPERTHERMIA

Kirk Hogan

TABLE OF CONTENTS

I. Introduction 294

II. Finding MH Genes 295

III. Candidate Regions Associated with
Chromosome Rearrangements.................................... 296

IV. Inheritance of Single Gene Mutations........................... 298

V. Candidate Genes by Disease Associations 300

VI. Linkage 300

VII. Linkage with RFLPs... 302

VIII. PCR and ASO 304

IX. MH and Linkage Analysis 305

X. From Linkage to Unknown Gene 306

XI. Candidate Genes.. 306

XII. Additional Animal MH Models 307

XIII. From Candidate Gene to Candidate Mutation 309

XIV. From Mutation to Causality.................................... 310

XV. Multifactorial Inheritance 311

XVI. Use of MH Markers and Mutations 311

Acknowledgments 313

References.. 313

0-8493-8093-6/94/$0.00 + $.50
© 1994 by CRC Press, Inc.

I. INTRODUCTION

A point mutation in the skeletal muscle calcium release channel, which is also called the ryanodine receptor or *RYR*1, was first found to be co-inherited with a predisposition to malignant hyperthermia (MH) in the pig.[1] The gene encoding the *RYR*1 protein is one of the largest and most complex known, consisting of over 250,000 nucleotide bases with more than 100 boundaries between coding (exon) and noncoding (intron) regions.[2] The search for a mutation in a gene this large was warranted by a substantial body of genetic[3-6] and biochemical[7-11] evidence pointing to a disorder of the *RYR*1 in pig MH. The discovery of the cytosine to thymine substitution at nucleotide 1843 was made by comparing the DNA sequences of the normal and mutant RYR1 alleles. The mutation, producing a cysteine for arginine substitution at position 615 of the *RYR*1 amino acid sequence (R615C), subsequently has been identified in over 450 pigs derived from six breeding strains, and thus far all pig MH can be traced to this alteration (Chapter 18).

Initial hopes that the genetic substrate of human MH would be similarly straightforward were heightened by linkage of MH susceptibility in 17 Canadian[12] and 3 Irish[13] families to a region of human chromosome 19 homologous to that of the pig containing the *RYR*1 gene. These hopes have not been fulfilled. The human mutation corresponding to the pig R615C substitution was found in only 1 of 35 MH pedigrees by Gillard et al.,[14] and in 1 of 62 families investigated in our laboratory.[15] Additional nucleotide substitutions giving rise to changes in the deduced amino acid sequence of the RYR1 protein that cosegregate with MH have recently been identified.[16] Because families with these mutations are small and no comparable animal models exist, it is not clear whether they represent causal mutations or non-pathogenic alleles. Interestingly, no *RYR*1 mutations have been reported in the families first demonstrating linkage to chromosome 19 markers, suggesting that in these families different mutations in the *RYR*1 or closely aligned genes await discovery. In turn, families with the R614C mutation have been too small to generate a high probability of linkage standing alone. Rather, the pathophysiologic significance of the human R614C mutation rests on its appearance in two species with MH. Owing to practical limitations of access to tissue, investigations using purified *RYR*1 protein from families demonstrating *RYR*1 linkage or mutations have not been undertaken to correlate genetic with biochemical alterations corresponding to experiments performed in the pig.

MH-like events or positive muscle contracture tests associated with distinct clinical diseases are well documented.[17,18] Moreover, numerous reports have appeared excluding linkage of human MH predisposition to chromosome 19 markers.[19-23] Reconciling these data, it is clear that MH in a highly selected inbred population of pigs is a genetically homogenous *disease* accounted for, at this writing, by a single mutation. By contrast, human MH is a genetically heterogenous *syndrome* with more or less identical phenotypes due to different mutations. In human MH, multiple mutations in large, randomly mating populations give rise to genetically disparate diseases each producing elevated myoplasmic calcium in the presence of depolarizing muscle relaxants and potent inhaled anesthetics. Human MH appears in single gene disorders demonstrating *allelic heterogeneity* (multiple disease mutations at a single locus, e.g., MH with central core disease (CCD) which is also linked to the *RYR*1 gene[24]) and *locus heterogeneity* (disease mutations at multiple loci, e.g., MH linkage to chromosome 17q[25]). Other mechanisms of MH genetic heterogeneity, including chromosomal abnormalities, multifactorial (polygenic), and non-Mendelian (mitochondrial) inheritance must also be anticipated.

The magnitude of causal heterogeneity in human MH makes it difficult to forsee a time when all patients about to undergo anesthesia will be screened with DNA-based techniques for MH predisposition. A more reasonable goal will be to estimate the risk of each individual in families with one or more affected members. Even with this more narrowly defined objective, the strengths and shortcomings of recombinant DNA diagnosis must be carefully weighed to predict MH susceptibility with exactitude. The intent of this chapter is to describe the clinical and pedigree data required to use recombinant DNA techniques, to survey the tools appropriate to unraveling the molecular genetic basis of human MH, and to temper over- and under-enthusiasm in their application.

II. FINDING MH GENES

The human genome is composed of roughly 3 billion nucleotide base pairs (bp). Individual genes vary in size from several hundred to 2 million bp. While the total number of genes in the human genome is not known, estimates fall within 50 to 100,000, of which no more than 5000 have been identified. DNA between transcribed genes (intergenic DNA) and noncoding DNA within genes (intronic DNA) comprise an estimated 98% of the total. The task of finding disease-associated mutations that may involve no more than a single base pair out of billions is tackled with a number of strategies, each dependent on the nature of the genetic information available at the outset. Specimens from patients in whom MH is joined with multiple congenital anomalies may be examined for chromosome rearrangements that could implicate specific chromosomal sites. If the apparent pattern of MH inheritance within a pedigree meets criteria for a single gene disorder, then disease associations, linkage analysis, and candidate proteins are employed in the identification of the mutant gene. MH mutations in additional animal models may recapitulate pig investigations of gene candidacy by homology. Finally, pedigree analysis may identify kindreds in which MH susceptibility reflects mechanisms of inheritance refractory to contemporary techniques developed for single gene disorders. Each of these circumstances will be considered below.

III. CANDIDATE REGIONS ASSOCIATED WITH CHROMOSOME REARRANGEMENTS

Syndromes characterized by growth delay, mental retardation, and a variety of somatic and structural abnormalities may be attributed on occasion to chromosome aberrations visible with light microscopy. Abnormal expression of multiple contiguous genes in the deleted, duplicated, or translocated chromosome segment explains these diverse features. If a hereditary trait such as MH is also associated with a syndrome produced by a cytogenetic abnormality, it is likely that the gene responsible for the trait resides in the aberrant segment and may also underlie the trait in families lacking the dysmorphic syndrome. Thus the retinoblastoma and dystrophin genes were assigned to their respective loci on chromosomes 13 and X[26,27] by changes in chromosome morphology detected in rare patients with multiply affected genes.

The karyotype, a chromosome photomicrograph (Figure 1), is prepared by treating anticoagulated blood with phytagglutinin to stimulate lymphocyte proliferation and agglutinate red blood cells. If specimens of fresh blood are not available, lymphoblast cultures immortalized with EB virus are suitable. Dividing cells are then stained in prometaphase with trypsin-Giemsa banding.[28] Light bands of euchromatin containing actively transcribed genes alternate with dark bands of heterochromatin made up of repetitive DNA. Chromosomes are identified by banding pattern, size, and centromere position. Up to 850 bands per haploid set of chromosomes are numbered and used for reference to the relative locations of genes, mapped markers, and rearrangements including inversions, interstitial deletions, rings, and translocations.

In most cases, MH reported in association with multiple congenital anomaly syndromes represents the coincidental occurrence of a rare syndrome with a rare disease at unrelated loci, e.g., a partial deletion of chromosome 4p in a patient with Wolf-Hirschhorn syndrome and MH.[29] However, MH associated with short stature, myopathy, micrognathia, low-set ears, and variable midline defects (cryptorchidism, pectus carniatum) in 15 children from the world's literature is recognized as a distinct entity known as King-Denborough syndrome. The high incidence of MH predisposition leads to the suspicion that the association is not fortuitous. While the clinical spectrum of King-Denborough syndrome appears compatible with a chromosomal rearrangement, we found that high-resolution karyotypes in one boy and one girl with this disorder were normal[30] and the R614C mutation was not found in either child. King-Denborough syndrome must therefore arise from a single abnormal gene with pleiotropic effects, or the chromosomal rearrangement exists at a submicroscopic level awaiting detection with molecular genetic techniques.

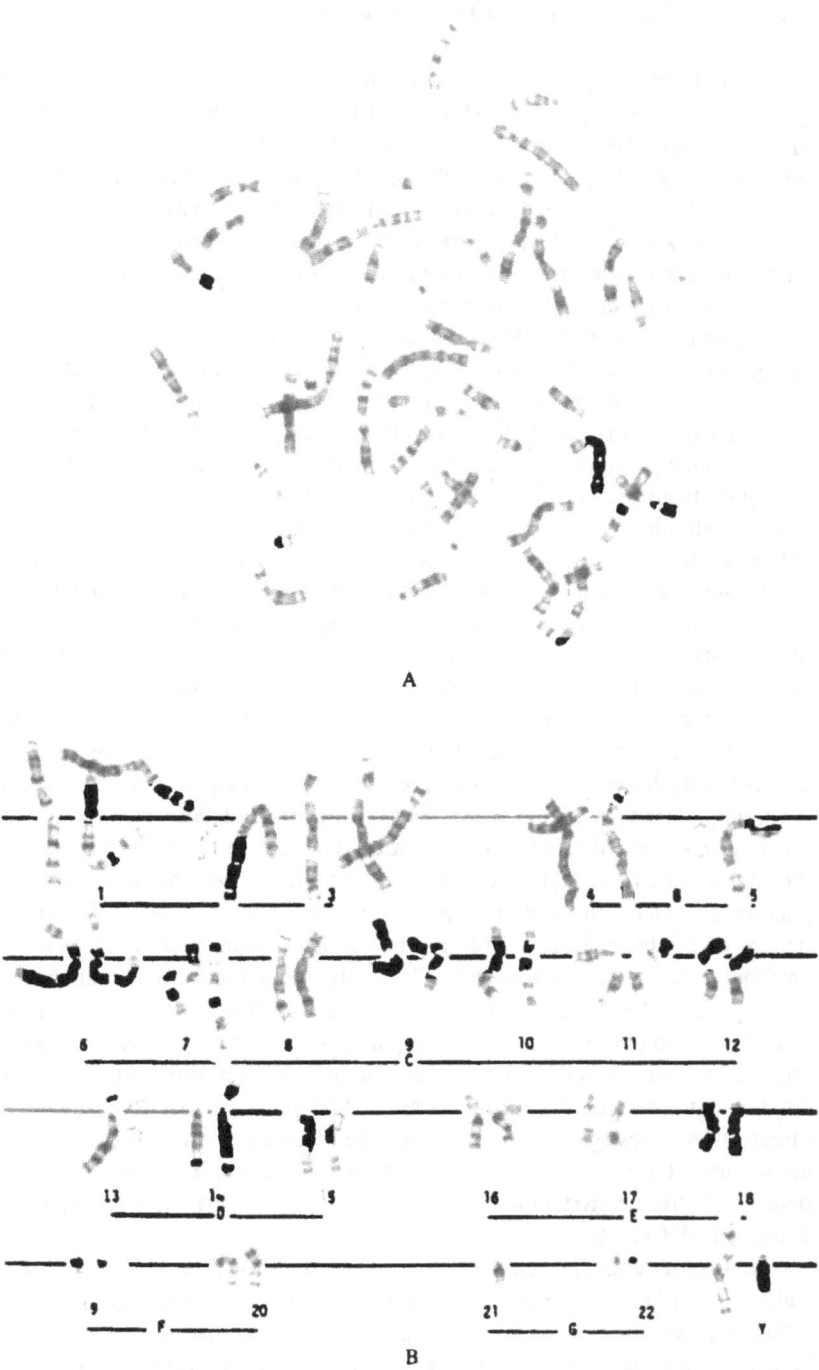

FIGURE 1. Karyotype of a child with King-Denborough syndrome showing normal chromosome morphology. (A) is a photomicrograph during prometaphase after staining with trypsin-Giemsa, and (B) is the karyotype after the chromosomes are grouped and sorted.

IV. INHERITANCE OF SINGLE GENE MUTATIONS

Recognition of karyotypic abnormalities depends on the occurrence of genetic events that may be extraordinarily rare. If the familial pattern of inheritance of MH is commensurate with predictions based on disordered function of a single gene product, molecular genetic techniques may be used to find the unknown gene without first identifying candidate proteins. About 4000 single gene disorders are known to be transmitted as autosomal dominant, autosomal recessive, sex-linked, or mitochondrial traits. Determination of the pattern of transmission is based not only on the presence or absence of a specific abnormal allele, but also is a function of both the genetic background in which the gene is expressed and the accuracy of the diagnostic technique. In the latter case, if the contracture test for MH discriminates the MH heterozygote from the homozygous normal patient, the trait appears to be autosomal dominant. Alternatively, inability to distinguish the MH heteozygote from the normal homozygote through contracture testing suggests that an individual must have two mutant alleles to be identified as affected. MH in such a pedigree would be interpreted as an autosomal recessive trait.

In autosomal dominant disorders, the presence of a single mutant allele is sufficient to recognizably alter the phenotype — the observed expression of a particular gene. Inspection of pedigrees exhibiting inheritance of single gene autosomal dominant traits reveals equal involvement of both sexes, that 50% of an affected parent's offspring are affected, unaffected parents do not transmit the disorder, and vertical inheritance is apparent. Dominant disorders that typically involve noncatalytic proteins, e.g., collagen and hemoglobin, frequently display variable expressivity with affected family members differing in the clinical signs of the disorder. The failure of obligate carriers of the mutant allele to express any sign of the mutant phenotype (incomplete penetrance) is a hallmark of many MH pedigrees fitting an autosomal dominant pattern of predisposition,[31] typifying autosomal dominant traits in which an environmental factor is required. Curiously, penetrance in human MH is inverted from the delayed onset seen in many other autosomal dominant disorders, with children in greatest jeopardy for MH episodes. While positive contracture tests in both parents of probands have been reported,[32] no clearcut homozygotes for dominant forms of MH have yet been confirmed by direct DNA investigations of the genotype. Homozygous dominant disease alleles almost always produce a more severely affected phenotype when compared with the heterozygote,[33] and it is conceivable that homozygosity for dominant MH is lethal.

Autosomal recessive inheritance arises in the offspring of two phenotypically normal heterozygotes. The disease is often confined to a single sibship rather than in multiple generations, and females and males are equally affected. Autosomal recessive MH predisposition has been described, but always in conjunction with other phenotypic features. Deficiency of carnitine palmitoyl transferase II (on chromosome 1), the enzyme that liberates long chain fatty acids on the inner mitochondrial membrane, is associated with rhabdomyolysis and MH-like episodes during anesthesia with trigger agents.[34] A positive contracture test has been reported in Brody myopathy, a deficiency of Ca^{2+} ATPase (on chromosome 12) responsible for sequestering unbound ionized calcium in the SR.[35] In both of these MH-related diseases the fundamental defect can be traced to deficient activity of a catalytic enzyme in common with many autosomal recessive disorders. Because pairs of mutant alleles are required at the same locus to manifest the disease phenotype, consanguinity is more prevalent in recessive inheritance. The mating of an individual homozygous for a recessive trait to a heterozygote will on average produce a 50/50 distribution of affected children. Termed pseudodominance, this union must be distinguished from autosomal dominant inheritance by wider scrutiny of the affected pedigree. Because many recessive disorders are sporadic, and family history may not be contributory, the frequency of the mutant allele and new mutation rate in the population are critical variables in estimating recurrence risk of recessive disorders.

Events resembling MH during anesthesia of otherwise normal children may be the first clinical sign of X-linked recessive Duchenne's muscular dystrophy, with the correct diagnosis disclosed at follow-up biopsy for contacture testing.[36] X-linked recessive traits are transmitted by both hemizygous males and heterozygous normal females, but only males are affected, and father to son transmission is never seen. Sex-limited traits in which the mutant gene is autosomal but clinical expression is influenced by X or Y genes (e.g., baldness), may be confused with X-linked recessive inheritance. In X-linked dominant inheritance all daughters of an affected male are affected. No instances of X-linked dominant or recessive inheritance of MH have been reported except as secondary manifestations of other genetic abnormalities.

A small number of neuromuscular and cardiac disorders have recently been mapped to mitochondrial DNA. Perturbed mitochondrial oxidative phosphorylation was an early hypothesis for MH etiology,[37] supported in part by the role of the mitochondria in buffering myoplasmic calcium. While most mitochondrial proteins are encoded by nuclear genes, approximately 40 genes are inherited in the 16,569 bp of circular DNA from maternal mitochondria.[38] Until the advent of recombinant DNA technology mitochondrial inheritance was confused with other modes of transmission. Myopathic phenotypes arising from mutations in mitochondrial DNA are characterized by an equal number of affected males and females, with transmission only from an affected female. Unlike genomic DNA, mitochondrial DNA is present in many copies per cell and is highly polymorphic due to a 5 to 10 times greater rate of evolution. Cases of MH in patients with mitochondrial myopathies have been described.[39,40] Confirmation of underlying alterations in mitochondrial DNA should be rapidly forthcoming if pedigrees exhibiting this pattern of MH susceptibility are available for genotyping.

V. CANDIDATE GENES BY DISEASE ASSOCIATIONS

Two distinct phenotypes occurring together more often than predicted by chance alone may provide clues to the whereabouts of altered genes. The association of Ca^{2+}-ATPase or CPTII deficiency with MH are examples of locus heterogeneity, raising the possibility that additional alleles at these mapped loci may produce MH in the absence of other intercurrent clinical illness. Early linkage maps of myotonic dystrophy, which carries MH pre-disposition,[41] placed the disorder close to the *RYR*1 gene on chromosome 19, hinting that myotonic dystrophy and at least one variant of human MH with homology to the pig disease were alleles at the same locus — allelic hetero-geneity. Subsequent mapping with high resolution markers clearly demon-strates that the two loci are distinct and that the shared sensitivity to anesthetic agents takes place in the pathophysiologic cascade, not at the genetic level.[42] A high proportion of patients with dominantly inherited CCD are susceptible to MH. Predisposition to this disorder, which is readily diagnosed in childhood by clinical and muscle biopsy criteria (central cores), maps very tightly to the *RYR*1 locus providing strong circumstantial evidence that it represents true allelic heterogeneity.[24] Mutations in the *RYR*1 have recently been shown to be co-inherited with CCD in two small families.[43] Other families with CCD lacked the mutations, indicating that this MH-associated malady is also ge-netically heterogenous. Mutations in genes for other disorders associated with MH that either have chromosomal assignment (e.g., autosomal dominant myotonia congenita on chromosome 17)[44] or remain to be mapped (e.g., chondrodystrophic myotonia (Schwartz-Jampel syndrome)[45] will expand the list of genetic alterations producing the MH syndrome.

VI. LINKAGE

Chromosomal rearrangements in the vicinity of MH-causing genes may be lethal or exiguous. Disease associations may account for only a small proportion of the MH syndrome. The homolog of the animal mutations may not exist in humans, or correlate with only a small proportion of human MH. An alternate strategy, linkage analysis, provides the means whereby human disease genes may be found despite the lack of clues based on chromosomal aberrations, disease associations, or animal models. Nothing needs to be known or surmised about the biochemical properties of the protein encoded by the disease gene, nor must specific gene probes be available to begin.

So long as transmission of MH susceptibility in the pedigree is compatible with a single gene disorder, inheritance of the phenotype of interest may be linked to co-inheritance of specific markers. The central concept of linkage analysis is that during meiosis reciprocal exchanges of segments occur between pairs of homologous parental chromosomes (Figure 2). The likelihood of segment exchange, termed recombination or crossing over, increases in

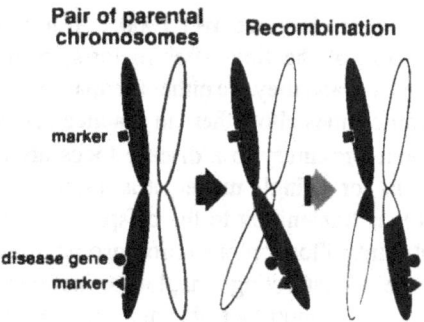

FIGURE 2. Crossing over or recombination of segments between a homologous pair of parental chromosomes is depicted. A marker (triangle) in close proximity to a disease gene (circle) cosegregates with the disease gene during meiosis, and its presence may therefore be used to infer the presence of the disease gene. An unlinked marker resides far from the disease gene (square), with a high frequency of crossing over between the two.

correlation to the distance between two loci on a chromosome. The closer together a pair of loci are on the same chromosome, the less will be the chance of crossing over between them. One to six recombinations per chromosome take place during each meiotic division so that the chromosome of the gamete is a hybrid of paternal and maternal segments, each consisting of many genes. The rate of crossing over, measured by the fraction of offspring with recombination between two loci along a chromosome divided by the total number of offspring, is an index of the intervening distance. A recombination fraction (θ) of 0.01 indicates that recombination takes place 1% of the time between the two loci. On average a 1% chance of a recombination between two loci during a meiotic event represents separation of the two by approximately 1 million base pairs. Referred to as the centiMorgan or cM, this is the standard unit of genetic distance.

Recombination between a marker and a disease locus demonstrated in one individual in a pedigree does not necessarily rule out linkage. If the pedigree is large and the marker is present in every other individual with the disease, the possibility exists that a crossover occurred between the marker and disease locus in the one individual purely by chance. The probability of chance recombination between two loci that are in fact quite close together can be statistically tested. By convention, the base 10 logarithm of the ratio of true linkage/apparent linkage by chance (LOD score) is calculated for a series of recombination fractions (0.00, 0.01, 0.05, 0.10, and 0.20). Hence,

$$\text{LOD score (Z)} = \log_{10} \frac{\text{likelihood data at } \theta}{\text{likelihood data} - \text{no linkage}}$$

A LOD score of 3.0 or higher is taken as evidence that the marker and disease loci are linked at a given recombination frequency and denotes that the odds against linkage by chance alone are over 1000:1. If alleles at two loci remain associated 50% or less of the time after meiosis, recombination occurs at random between the two, and they are either far apart on the same chromosome or on different chromosomes altogether. In practice several potential markers thought to be in close proximity to a disease locus are chosen, because if a parent is homozygous for a single maker, it is impossible to tell which of the two chromosomes was transmitted to the offspring. A group of alleles from two or more closely linked loci on one chromosome that is inherited as a unit is termed a haplotype. Constructing a haplotype incorporating markers flanking the disease gene is an important objective of linkage analysis.

Markers reflect allelic variation at a given locus. Ideally they exhibit a high degree of heteromorphism (many variants) and heterozygosity (each variant proportionally represented) in the general population so that alleles at a specific locus differ between each of a parent's two chromosomes and are different from those present on the other parent's chromosome at the same locus. Only by knowing which parent has transmitted the marker is it possible to know whether a specific marker allele and the disease gene are associated on the same chromosome or on opposite members of a homologous pair. In this way the phase of a marker is assigned. In general, markers have multiple alleles thereby increasing the likelihood of identifying the two parental chromosomes at a specific locus and discriminating between the two chromosomes of an affected individual. A marker linked to a disease phenotype in one family may be found in an individual from a second family without implying the presence of the disease. Only by investigation of the family taken as a whole can linkage data be interpreted. In the ideal setting for linkage analysis, expression of the disease is well defined, diagnosis is unequivocal with a standardized test, penetrance is high (everyone with the mutant allele can be diagnosed), there is clear-cut evidence of parent to child transmission, at least three living relatives from three generations are affected, and multiple families bearing close similarity have been identified.

Early markers were inferred by differences in expressed proteins. For example, MH in pigs was linked in 1977 to different variants of the enzyme glucose phosphate isomerase (GPI), each encoded by different alleles of the *GPI* gene on chromosome 6.[4] Expressed markers have notable limitations. Multiple assays (chemical, serologic, immunologic, etc.) are required, spacing of the marker loci is uneven throughout the genome, expressed traits are inherited as dominant and recessive phenotypes obscuring underlying variability, and the number of polymorphisms may be low. A revolution in human disease gene mapping arose from recombinant DNA techniques making it practical to directly identify numerous, widely spaced codominant (each allele can be distinguished) DNA sequence polymorphisms.

VII. LINKAGE WITH RFLPs

DNA polymorphisms appear in exons and introns of genes and in intergenic sequences of the human genome. This array of polymorphism first became available for the detection of disease genes by the use of restriction-fragment length polymorphisms (RFLPs). Present in bacteria to repel viral infection, restriction enzymes or endonucleases cut DNA at unique sites requiring an invariant sequence. Thus the restriction enzyme *ECOR*1 cleaves the DNA of viruses infecting *E. coli* at every occurrence of the sequence (GAATTC). Using restriction enzymes, DNA fragments from any source can then be compared for the presence or absence of the site. The fragment with the cleavage site will be cut into two smaller pieces, whereas the fragment lacking the recognition site will remain intact. The different sizes of the fragments can then be used to track the disease gene in a family.

The DNA fragments are sorted by size on an agarose electrophoretic gel and their relative positions measured by Southern blotting. In this technique DNA is transferred onto a nitrocellulose filter, denatured into single strands, hybridized to radiolabeled complementary DNA probes, and exposed on X-ray film. Probes are derived from genomic DNA and cDNA that have been previously cloned. Inheritance of differences in the electrophoretic pattern of DNA treated with identical enzymes and probes from normal and affected family members is strictly Mendelian, providing a marker for the disease locus if a sufficient number of individuals are heterozygous. In order to demonstrate linkage, the actual disease mutation need not be at the recognition site of the enzyme, just close enough to make the probability of recombination between the two remote. On occasion the mutation is at the recognition site by happenstance, or an enzyme specific for that site can be found once the mutation and its surrounding sequence is known (Figure 3).

The first step in linkage analysis is to isolate DNA from each family member's white blood cells. Restriction enzymes are used to digest the DNA that is then separated by size and Southern blotted. A LOD score is calculated for each marker and the disease phenotype at various recombination frequencies. Computer programs (LIPED, LINKAGE) perform the requisite calculations after the mechanism of inheritance, and estimates of penetrance and mutation rate are specified.[46] As the search narrows, higher LOD scores at lower recombination fractions may be generated by selection of other markers in the region.

VNTRs or variable number tandem repeats are a second type of genetic marker. These are DNA regions of up to 30 or more bp that are repeated in tandem arrays, with varying numbers of repeats on chromosome pairs at the same locus. Microsatellitte markers of 6 or fewer bp (e.g., CACACA-CACA. . . . CA) are widely distributed throughout the genome and easily detected.[47] RFLPs are dimorphic — the recognition site is either there or it is not. VNTRs are much more heteromorphic, having highly variable numbers of repeats at a single locus. A restriction enzyme that cleaves outside the VNTR produces fragments with lengths dependent on the size and number of the repeated segment. Because VNTRs are common and easily identified, they are invaluable as markers in linkage analysis. With techniques for amplifying DNA *in vitro*, VNTRs are also used for gene mapping.

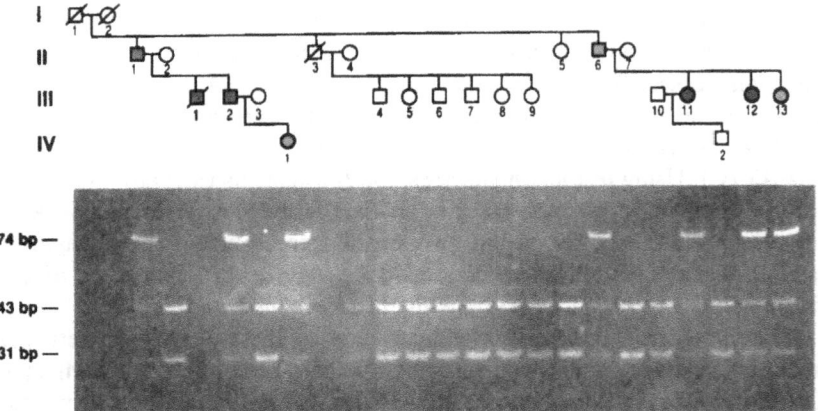

FIGURE 3. A four generation MH pedigree in which the R614C mutation is tracked by digestion of DNA fragments with *Rsa*I followed by separation on a 20% acrylamide gel. A solid symbol denotes affected individuals by clinical event or contracture test, and heterozygotes for the mutation are indicated by a shaded symbol. The normal gene is identified by the presence of the cleavage site (GTAC) creating 43- and 31-bp fragments. The 74-bp fragment is from the mutant allele, which lacks the final C of the recognition site (GTAT). Normal homozygotes have the site on each chromosome, each producing two bands. The MH heterozygote has three bands — 43- and 31-bp bands from the normal chromosome, and a 74-bp band from the mutant chromosome. Empty lanes are aligned beneath deceased individuals. (From Hogan, K., Couch, F., Powers, P., and Gregg, R., *Anesth. Analg.*, 75, 441, 1992. With permission.)

VIII. PCR AND ASO

If sequence information about a particular region is known, the polymerase chain reaction (PCR) may be used to amplify specific segments of DNA without cloning into bacteria for replication. As few as one to two copies of the sample DNA to be amplified are sufficient to initiate the reaction. First, primers 20 to 35 oligonucleotides long are made to be complementary to DNA sequences flanking the intervening 200 to 300-bp sequence of interest. Programmed cycles of *Taq* polymerase-mediated DNA synthesis, using single-strand DNA for the template, alternate with heat denaturation of the double to single strands, resulting in an exponential amplification in the amount of DNA in the region between the two primers (Figure 4).[48] DNA amplified by PCR may then be used for RFLP analysis described above, direct sequencing, or be assayed by allele-specific oligonucleotides (ASO) probes. Single base changes producing missense, nonsense, and frameshift mutations can be detected by hybridization of a tagged ASO complementary to the internal part of the PCR fragment. With any mismatch the ASO will not hybridize. The advantage of an ASO over RFLPs is the lack of dependence on a restriction site in the location to be tested. The disadvantage is that an ASO can detect only mutations that have previously been described.

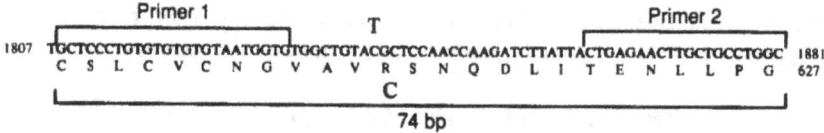

FIGURE 4. A region of *RYR*1 DNA amplified by PCR. Primers 1 and 2 amplify a 74-bp band in both genomic and cDNA. Beneath the middle base of each codon the corresponding amino acid is designated by its one-letter code. The MH C → T nucleotide substitution and the arginine to cysteine amino acid substitution are highlighted. (From Hogan, K., Couch, F., Powers, P., and Gregg, R., *Anesth. Analg.*, 75, 441, 1992. With permission.)

IX. MH AND LINKAGE ANALYSIS

Application of linkage analysis to estimation of MH genetic liability has many attractions. Most MH patients are otherwise normal; therefore, effective measures for presymptomatic diagnosis are life saving. Compared to many hereditary neuromuscular disorders, families with MH are relatively common; however, they often are too small to establish or exclude linkage. Furthermore, the genetic heterogeneity of the MH syndrome undermines efforts to generate high LOD scores calculated in aggregate by pooling data from separate families. At present it is impossible to know *a priori* if families pooled together for the purpose of linkage analysis in fact have the same disease. If they do not, interpretation of linkage data will be confounded.

Beyond these concerns, phenotypic uncertainty is the single greatest challenge facing MH linkage analysis. Clinical events are often poorly monitored and described. It is not uncommon that multiple trigger anesthetics are administered to an individual before an MH episode occurs, so that uneventful anesthetics in individuals at risk may be inconclusive indices of MH status. Because the contracture test is invasive, expensive, and of uncertain predictive value and interlaboratory reliability, it is rarely justifiable to phenotype all members at risk within a pedigree other than for research purposes. Even if enough family members are willing to undergo contracture testing, small adjustments of the cut-off point between normal and abnormal can profoundly affect the likelihood of linkage.[49] For these reasons it is essential that details of clinical events and contracture test methods and results be published in reports claiming or excluding MH linkage. Linkage analysis based on an erroneous diagnosis may be confused with nonpaternity (estimated at 5% in the general population), nonmaternity, intragenic recombination (crossing over within a gene), double recombinants (a second crossing over correcting the first event in part or in full), or a greater degree of genetic heterogeneity than may in fact be present. To partially counter these limitations, the Genetics Section of the European Malignant Hyperthermia Group has identified a small number of MH-susceptible families in which a large proportion of individuals have been diagnosed using a standardized version of the contracture test.[50]

Clearly, improvements will need to be made in the tissue and biochemical[51] diagnosis of MH for genetic progress to continue at its current pace.

X. FROM LINKAGE TO UNKNOWN GENE

Once linkage to a polymorphic marker is established, genetic diagnosis is feasible. However, optimal diagnosis and a complete understanding of the underlying pathophysiology relies on full characterization of the mutant allele(s) of the disease gene. Tightly linked markers may still be 1 to 5 cM from the disease locus, and several million nucleotides containing a few or many genes must be analyzed. Using the marker as a starting point, chromosome walking is begun by the isolation of a clone from a library of DNA fragments, which is known in advance to contain the marker. The goal is to build up a series of overlapping clones in phage, cosmid, or yeast libraries in order to define sequence further and further from the RFLP starting point, and closer to the disease gene. Smaller fragments of the cloned segment are then mapped and oriented so that overlapping regions are identified, and the clones aligned to reflect the original order of the fragments along the chromosome. By restriction enzyme mapping or direct sequencing, each new clone can be compared to the original clone and used to search the library for additional clones. Regions rich in repetitive DNA may be extremely difficult to clone, and methods are needed to cover the great length of DNA that may span a marker locus to disease gene. In chromosome jumping, rather than cloning and characterizing every fragment between the marker and disease loci, uninteresting regions of DNA are skipped or jumped by circularizing large DNA fragments with a selectable marker and bringing the two ends together in a loop. The loop is then ligated and the fragments containing the linked ends are cloned for screening with specific probes. With the ability to clone up to 1 Mb (10^6 nucleotides) of human DNA in yeast, chromosome walking with yeast libraries accomplishes the same objective as chromosome jumping, but with a substantial reduction in effort and time.

XI. CANDIDATE GENES

Linkage analysis and chromosome walking are laborious and expensive ways to find disease genes. Knowledge that a protein's structure and function are consonant with a possible etiologic role in a disease may foreshorten the gene search. Any of the numerous proteins responsible for the regulation of skeletal muscle calcium can be considered a candidate for human MH. Polymorphic markers within or near genes encoding these proteins can be used in linkage studies. Probes from the candidate gene can also be used in experiments to search for large deletions. If the animal or marker sequence is known, *in situ* hybridization with a probe tagged with silver, tritium, or fluorescent biotin may be used for chromosomal assignment. In this technique, metaphase chromosomes are denatured to single strands, excess tagged probe is applied and washed off, and a large number of chromosomes are examined to correct for background binding.

The skeletal muscle DHP-sensitive, voltage-dependent calcium channel is a heteropentameric T-tubule protein coupled to the calcium release channel of the sarcoplasmic reticulum (see Figure 1 in Chapter 18). To test the hypothesis that mutations of the component subunits of this channel cause human MH, we cloned their human genes and mapped their chromosomal locations by screening rodent-human somatic cell libraries for the presence of PCR-based intragenic markers. Libraries of somatic cell hybrids are created by fusion of human and rodent (mouse, hamster) cells, and cytogenetic techniques (described above) are used to identify which human chromosomes are present in a particular clonal line. Panels of hybrids that are commercially available may then be screened with the gene-specific probes. Hybrids not containing the target chromosome are negative for the probe, whereas all hybrids positive for the probe should contain the same chromosome. Analysis of many hybrids allows the chromosome on which the gene resides to be determined. To sublocalize the genes, we determined the inheritance of polymorphic PCR-based microsatellite markers on a panel of CEPH (Centre d'Etudes du Polymorphisme Humain, Paris) families. Computer comparison of the inheritance pattern of our markers with those in the database enables accurate chromosomal assignment. Using this approach, we have mapped the skeletal muscle DHP-sensitive VDCC subunit genes to the following chromosomes: α_1 to chromosome 1,[52] γ,[53] and β_1[54] to discrete loci on chromosome 17 (Figure 5). With additional markers in the vicinity of the mapped locus, the gene-specific marker may then be use for linkage analysis. Interestingly, the gene for the β_1-subunit maps into a region in which linkage data pooled from five families suggests a distinct MH locus.[25] In subsequent investigations, evidence for recombination between the β_1 subunit and MH in these pedigrees will be sought.

Other skeletal muscle proteins promising as candidate genes include triadin,[55] inositol trisphosphatases,[56] the inositol trisphosphate receptor,[57] the sodium channel α-subunit,[58] and enzymes integral to fatty acid metabolism.[59,60] While ongoing investigations of muscle calcium regulation and excitation-contraction coupling will undoubtedly suggest additional candidates, genetic investigations of human MH may correspondingly yield new genes encoding hitherto unknown proteins.

XII. ADDITIONAL ANIMAL MH MODELS

Porcine MH exemplifies the value of an animal model for the study of a human genetic disease. By controlled breeding, pedigree size need not limit the statistical power required for segregation analysis.[61] The mechanism of inheritance and number of disease loci are issues that can be addressed by

| | CACNLB1 sequence/ chromosome retention | | | | |
Chromosome	+/+	−/−	+/−	−/+	% Discordance
1	1	20	1	3	16
2	0	22	2	1	12
3	0	19	2	4	24
4	0	21	2	2	16
5	1	2	1	21	88
6	0	19	2	4	24
7	0	21	2	2	16
8	1	19	1	4	20
9	0	20	2	3	20
10	0	20	2	3	20
11	0	20	2	3	20
12	0	19	2	4	24
13	0	17	2	6	32
14	1	17	1	6	28
15	1	20	1	3	16
16	0	20	2	3	20
17	2	23	0	0	0
18	1	20	1	3	16
19	0	16	2	7	36
20	0	20	2	3	20
21	1	17	1	6	28
22	0	19	2	4	24
X	0	20	2	3	20
Y	0	19	2	4	24

FIGURE 5. Segregation of the β-subunit gene (CACNLB1) of the DHP-sensitive Ca^{2+} channel with human chromosomes in rodent-human somatic cell hybrids. +/+ indicates that both the PCR product and the chromosome were present. −/− indicates that both the PCR product and the chromosome were absent. +/− indicates that the PCR product was present and the chromosome was absent. −/+ indicates that the PCR product was absent and the chromosome was present. Numbers beneath each symbol indicate the number of cell lines in each category. The discordance percentage is calculated as the sum of +/− and −/+ divided by the total number of cell lines examined. (From Gregg, R. G., Powers, P. A., Hogan, K., *Genomics*, 15, 185, 1993. With permission.)

careful choice of breeding pairs and experimental backcrosses. Tissue for isolation of candidate proteins and appropriate messenger RNAs is plentiful. The risk of heavy investment in an animal model of human genetic disease is that the correspondence of animal disease alleles to those found in humans may be limited. Failure of pig MH to correlate with more than a rare variant of the human syndrome could be shared with additional species, although the scientific value of novel disorders of calcium regulation may be substantial.

Other than the pig, a canine model of MH is the most well defined.[62] MH events in a strain of Labrador retrievers consisting of tachycardia, hypercarbia, hyperthermia, and efficacious responses to dantrolene are inherited as an autosomal dominant trait in parallel with abnormal contracture tests.

Muscle rigidity and lactic acidosis are not pronounced. The authors have found that DNA isolated from a region spanning the porcine R615C mutation does not show the C1843→T mutation, indicating that MH in this canine strain represents a mutation distinct from that previously identified in all MH swine and several human kindreds (Figure 6). The next step will be to breed an obligate heterozygote and generate a colony with sufficient informative meioses to perform linkage analysis with markers from *RYR*1 and other candidate genes. If these fail to cosegregate with MH predisposition, a genome search with widely spaced markers will be conducted to identify regions with the highest likelihood of linkage in this animal model.

XIII. FROM CANDIDATE GENE TO CANDIDATE MUTATION

Any permanent and heritable change in the sequence of DNA can produce mutant alleles associated with human disease. Disease mutations may encode an abnormal protein (e.g., microdeletions, missense, nonsense, and frameshift mutations, interposition of termination codons, alterations in regulatory elements), or diminish the amount of a normal protein by interference with transcription, translation, or processing. Direct DNA sequencing is fundamental for the detection of these and other mutations. Even if details of gene structure, e.g., untranslated regions or exon/intron boundaries are unknown, sequencing DNA assembled with reverse transcriptase to be complementary (cDNA) to mRMA isolated from the disease tissue may be frutiful. The nucleotide sequence of a cDNA fragment is determined by chemical degradation (Maxam-Gibert) or enzymatic (Sanger) techniques.[62] In the latter more frequently employed method, a synthetic primer is hybridized to one end of a single strand of DNA to be sequenced, and the paired strand is synthesized with the addition of DNA polymerase, each of the four nucleotides, and a

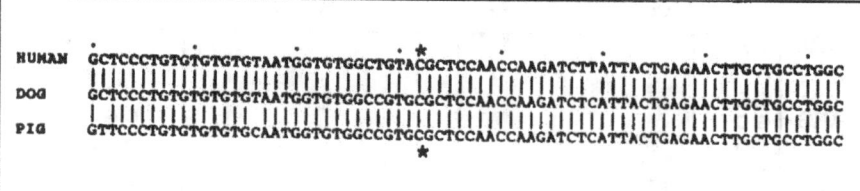

FIGURE 6. A comparison of the normal human, normal pig, and MH canine DNA sequences in a 74-bp fragment between nucleotides 1808 and 1881 of the *RYR*1. * indicates the site of the T for C substitution that cosegregates with MH in all pig lines and a subset of human families. MH dogs in this strain lack the R615C substitution, therefore, it is likely that they represent a second mutation in the *RYR*1 or other gene, which may also be shared with a variant of human MH.

small amount of their tagged dideoxy analogs. Extension of the growing strand is blocked by incorporation of the dideoxy nucleotide, so that in the reaction mixture strands of varying lengths will be present, each ending at its respective dideoxy base. After separation of the DNA products on a polyacrylamide gel and exposure of the gel to X-ray film, the sequence of the unknown fragment can be directly read (Figure 7). Up to 500 bp may be sequenced in a single set of reactions.

Direct sequencing of genes as large as the *RYR*1 in each individual likely to be manifesting a distinct mutation is not practical, and therefore more efficient techniques have been developed to narrow the search. Candidate regions for direct sequencing may be suggested by homology to regions mutated in related proteins or by specific regulatory domains of the molecule. Chemical mismatch, hetero-duplex denaturing gel, and single-strand conformation polymorphism (SSCP) techniques take advantage of changes in physical properties between mutant and normal sequences.[64] In SSCP, conformational changes alter mobility of short fragments of mutant DNA within a gel, and alleles associated with disease are rapidly discriminated from normal.[65] The exact mutation is then identified by direct sequencing of the mutant fragment. Using SSCP, large blocks of DNA can be excluded from the search for disease causing mutations without resort to tedious and costly sequencing.

XIV. FROM MUTATION TO CAUSALITY

The identification of a mutation of any type that is co-inherited with susceptibility to a disease suggests, but does not prove, that the mutation causes the disease. Many genetic alterations do not alter the phenotype, but may simply represent polymorphisms tightly linked to undetected causal mutations in the same gene or to a distinct but unknown disease gene in close proximity. The lack of the mutation in all unaffected members of a pedigree,

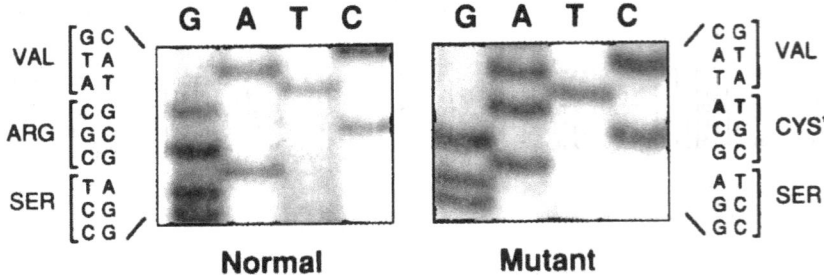

FIGURE 7. Autoradiogram of an *RYR*1 DNA sequencing gel. The sequence is from the antisense strand. The complementary sense strand is shown as is the amino acid sequence, which reads from top (amino terminus) to bottom (carboxy terminus). The C → T substitution (bold) in the sense strand results in a cysteine for arginine substitution * at position 614. (From Hogan, K., Couch, F., Powers, P., and Gregg, R., *Anesth. Analg.*, 75, 441, 1992. With permission.)

and in an unrelated population not known to have the disease, is presumptive albeit weak evidence of causality, based on the assumption that individuals from the population at large are truly normal in the absence of anesthetic complications or contracture test data. If it can be shown that purified preparations of the normal and mutant protein are qualitatively distinct in a magnitude consistent with the supposed disease pathophysiology (e.g., the mutant human *RYR*1 binding characteristics are in accord with increased open probability),[65] then the argument supporting causality is strengthened. Altered function of the normal and mutant proteins after transfer of their respective genes into transient expression systems (frog oocytes or CHO cells) provides complementary evidence in favor of causality by correlation of the effect of mutations at specific loci with functional properties of the molecule. However, differences in RNA splicing, post-translational modification or in the regulatory environment of the host cell may blur interpretation of this data. Observation of the identical disease-associated mutation in two separate species, as is the case for the MH R615C mutation, corroborates causality but is rare for most human disorders. In the absence of animal models of human disease at the molecular level, ultimate proof of causality relies on conferring the disease phenotype in a transgenic organism. For MH and other heterogenous disorders, it is unlikely that resources will be available to create transgenic animals for every mutation found by linkage analysis and DNA sequencing to cosegregate with susceptibility to the disease, and that varying degrees of uncertainty about the causality of each newly identified mutation will be unavoidable.

XV. MULTIFACTORIAL INHERITANCE

Traits and diseases that are not associated with chromosomal rearrangements or are not consistent with simple Mendelian inheritance may arise from the interaction of multiple genes, each with an additive effect. Multifactorial or polygenic inheritance, which is frequently apparent only in the setting of specific environmental factors, has been suspected in a subset of MH pedigrees.[31] In multifactorial genetic disease each first degree relative of an affected proband has roughly a 5% chance of being affected. At present, molecular genetic tools appropriate for mapping multiple genetic loci responsible for the inheritance of quantitative traits require controlled breeding of large sibships. Optimism for understanding the inheritance of multifactorial disease at the nucleotide level rests on the possibility that loci are shared between single and oligogenic disorders, and that animal models of human multifactorial disease can be discovered.

XVI. USE OF MH MARKERS AND MUTATIONS

The goal of molecular genetic diagnosis is disease prevention by presymptomatic detection of susceptible individuals. Identification of a mutation segregating in a family at risk appears on first glance to satisfy this objective, but it would be premature to counsel such a family without important caveats. First, linked markers including all mutations not proven causal, are dependent on correct phenotypic diagnosis to avoid diagnostic errors concealing or counterfeiting recombination between markers and the disease locus. Second, in a heterogenous disease such as MH the incidence of compound or double heterozygotes, that is, individuals heterozygous for disease alleles at one or more loci, may be fairly high, and until all mutations predisposing to MH are identified a second disease locus in the family cannot be ruled out. Ignorance of the new mutation rate (# of mutations/locus/gamete/generation) for any MH mutation means that an individual may not share the mutation present in a particular pedigree, but may manifest MH on the basis of an alteration at a second locus. In the worst case, MH could resemble disorders of the low density lipoprotein receptor in which most families have unique mutations not found in others. Appropriate use of DNA-based techniques for genetic counseling is no different than that for the use of nonrecombinant markers; assigning an individual's specific risk depends on estimates of the new mutation rate, penetrance, expressivity, and mechanism of inheritance for *each* mutation.[67]

For these reasons, it is unlikely that a method for screening human populations at risk for MH using recombinant DNA technology will be developed in the near future. For a subset of families genetic detection with linked markers, and in one instance a probable causal mutation owing to homology with the pig, is possible. However, individuals in these families who lack linked markers or the mutation cannot be considered to be at zero risk for the reasons outlined above. Contracture tests will continue to be performed both for differential diagnosis of complicated anesthetics and for characterizing pedigrees suitable for genetic investigation. Because human MH is a heterogenous syndrome rather than a homogenous disease, DNA-based tests will fail to detect some people who will develop MH. Conversely, because MH exhibits widely variable expression, the disorder may not always appear by clinical or contracture test data in individuals testing positive with markers or mutations. Nevertheless, steady progress in identifying the genetic basis of MH will lead to a cumulative improvement in predicting risk in specific pedigrees and have a deeper understanding of muscle physiology in health and disease as a consequence.

By referring patients to regional genetic centers clinicians are able to make contributions of inestimable value to the understanding of the molecular basis of MH. There immortalized lymphoblast cultures can be established for MH patients with multiple congenital anomaly syndromes, or other associated hereditary disease for future karyotyping and biochemical analysis. MH pedigrees with twins, or with children inheriting MH predisposition from both parents, should be recognized for their clinical and scientific importance. Physicians engaged in contracture testing should make every effort to test both parents, even if the first parent tested is found to be positive. Not testing the second parent on the assumption that gene frequency is low fails to test the assumption itself. Muscle from all patients having contracture tests should be preserved regardless of the test results, because sources of well-phenotyped human tissue for RNA isolation and protein analysis are extremely limited. Ideally, 100 mg of tissue would be collected before contracture testing, frozen immediately in liquid nitrogen without preservative and stored at −70°C. After contracture testing the specimens should be stored and not discarded. Blood should be collected from all probands, parents, and first degree relatives in ACD tubes, transferred to plastic tubes, and frozen. It is particularly important to collect specimens from elderly grandparents because a third generation is often crucial to assign phase to the disease chromosome. Finally, all MH patients in North America should be enrolled in the North American Malignant Hyperthermia Registry established for the purpose of coordinating clinical and contracture test data with ongoing investigations. In this way the consequences of identical or related mutations between unrelated pedigrees may be compared. Only by welding together observations at the bedside with those at the laboratory bench does recombinant DNA technology realize its full potential.

ACKNOWLEDGMENTS

This work was supported by a Merit Review grant from the Department of Veteran's Affairs and by the University of Wisconsin Anesthesia Research Foundation. I am indebted to T. Nelson for provision of canine MH specimens, and to R. Pauli, R. Gregg, and J. Kreul for insight and criticism.

REFERENCES

1. Fujii, J., Otsu, K., Zorzato, F., de Leon, S., Khanna, V. K., Weiler, J. E., O'Brien, P. J., and MacLennan, D. H., Identification of a mutation in the procine ryanodine receptor associated with malignant hyperthermia, *Science*, 253, 448, 1991.
2. MacLennan, D. and Phillips, M., Malignant hyperthermia, *Science*, 256, 789, 1992.
3. Andresen, E. and Jensen, P., Close linkage established between the Hal locus for halothane sensitivity and Phi(phosphohexose isomerase) locus in pigs of Danish Landrace breed, *Nord. Vet. Med.*, 29, 502, 1977.
4. Voegli, P., Stranzinger, G., Schneebli, H., Hagger, C., Kunzi, N., and Gerwig, C., Relationships between the H and A-O blood types, phosphohexose isomerase and 6-phosphogluconate dehydrogenase red cell enzymes and halothane sensitivity, and economic traits in a superior and inferior selection line of Swiss Landrace pigs, *J. Anim. Sci.*, 59, 1440, 1984.
5. Davies, W., Harbitz, I., Fries, R., Stranzinger, G., and Hauge, J., Porcine malignant hyperthermia carrier detection and chromosomal assignment using a linked probe, *Anim. Genet.* 19, 203, 1988.

6. Harbitz, I., Chowdhary, B., Thomsen, P. P., Davies, W., Kaufmann, U., Kran, S., Gustavsson, I., Christensen, K., and Hauge, J. G., Assignment of the procine calcium release channel gene, a candidate for the malignant hyperthermia locus, to the 6p11 → q21 segment of chromosome 6, *Genomics,* 8, 243, 1990.

7. Mickelson, J., Gallant, E., Litterer, L., Johnson, K., Rempel, W., and Louis, C., Abnormal sarcoplasmic reticulum ryanodine receptor in malignant hyperthermia, *J. Biol. Chem.,* 263, 9310, 1988.

8. Fill, M., Coronado, R., Mickelson, J. R., Vilven, J., Ma, J. J., Jacobson, B. A., and Louis, C. F., Abnormal ryanodine receptor channels in malignant hyperthermia, *Biophys. J.,* 50, 471, 1990.

9. Knudson, C., Mickelson, J., Louis, C., and Campbell, K., Distinct immunopeptide maps of the sarcoplasmic reticulum Ca^{2+} release channel in malignant hyperthermia, *J. Biol. Chem.,* 265, 2421, 1990.

10. Kim, D., Sreter, F., Ohnishi, S. et al., Kinetic studies of Ca^{2+} release from sarcoplasmic reticulum of normal and malignant hyperthermia susceptible pig muscles, *Biochem. Biophys. Acta,* 775, 320, 1984.

11. O'Brien, P., Procine malignant hyperthermia susceptibility: hypersensitive calcium-release mechanism of skeletal muscle sarcoplasmic reticulum, *Can. J. Vet. Res.,* 50, 318, 1986.

12. MacLennan, D., Duff, C., Zorzato, F., Fujii, J., Phillips, M., Korneluk, R. G., Frodis, W., Britt, B. A., and Worton, R. G., Ryanodine receptor gene is a candidate for predisposition to malignant hyperthermia, *Nature,* 343, 559, 1990.

13. McCarthy, T., Healy, J., Heffron, J., Lehane, M., Deufel, T., Lehmann-Horn, F., Farrall, M., and Johnson, K., Localization of the malignant hyperthermia susceptibility locus to human chromosome 19q12–13.2, *Nature,* 343, 562, 1990.

14. Gillard, E., Otsu, K., Fujii, J., Khanna, V. K., de Leon, S., Derdemezi, J., Britt, B. A., Worton, R. G., and MacLennan, D. H., A substitution of cysteine for arginine 614 in the ryanodine receptor is potentially causative of human malignant hyperthermia, *Genomics,* 11, 751, 1991.

15. Hogan, K., Couch, F., Powers, P., and Gregg, R., A cysteine-for-arginine substitution (R614C) in the human skeletal muscle calcium release channel co-segrates with malignant hyperthermia, *Anesth. Analg.,* 75, 441, 1992.

16. Gillard, E. F., Otsu, K., Fujii, J., Duff, C., De Leon, S., Khanna, V. K., Britt, B. A., Worton, R. G., and MacLennan, D. H., Polymorphisms and deduced amino acid substitutions in the coding sequence of the ryanodine receptor *(RYR1)* gene in individuals with malignant hyperthermia, *Genomics,* 13, 1247, 1992.

17. Brownell, A., Malignant hyperthermia: relationship to other disease, *Br. J. Anaesth.,* 60, 303, 1988.

18. Heiman-Patterson, T. D., Rosenberg, H., Fletcher, J. E., and Tahmoush, A. J., Halothane-caffeine contracture testing in neuromuscular diseases, *Muscle Nerve,* 11, 453, 1988.

19. Levitt, R., Nouri, N., Jedlicka, A., McKusick, V. A., Marks, A. R., Shutack, J. G., Fletcher, J. E., Rosenberg, H., and Magers, D. A., Evidence for genetic heterogeneity in malignant hyperthermia susceptibility, *Genomics,* 11, 543, 1991.

20. Stewart, A., Hall, J., Taylor, G. et al., Genetic linkage analysis using microsatellites in human malignant hyperthermia, *Cytogenet. Cell Genet.,* 58, 2025, 1991.

21. Deufel, T., Meitinger, T., Golla, A., Iles, D., Meindl, A., Meitinger, T., Schindelhaver, D., DeVries, A., Pongratz, D., MacLennan, D. H., Johnson, K. J., et al., Evidence for genetic heterogeneity of malignant hyperthermia susceptibility (MHS), *Am. J. Hum. Genet.,* 50, 1151, 1992.

22. Fagerlund, T., Islander, G., Ranclev, E., Harbitz, I., Hauge, J. G., Møkleby, E., and Berg, K., Genetic recombination between malignant hyperthermia and calcium release channel in skeletal muscle, *Clin. Genet.,* 5, 270, 1992.

23. Iles, D. E., Segers, B., Heytens, L., Sengers, R. C., and Wieringa, B., High-resolution physical mapping of four microsatellite repeat markers near the RYR1 locus on chromosome 19q13.1 and exclusion of the MHS locus from this region in two malignant hyperthermia susceptible families, *Genomics*, 14(3), 749, 1992.

24. Mulley, J. C., Kozman, H. M., Phillips, H. A., Gedeson, A. K., McCure, J. A., Iles, D. E., Gregg, R. G., Hogan, K., Couch, F. J., MacLennan, D. H., and Haan, E. A., Refined genetic localization for central core disease, *Am. J. Hum. Genet.*, 52, 398, 1993.

25. Levitt, R. C., Olckers, A., Meyers, S., Fletcher, J. E., Rosenberg, H., Isaacs, H., and Meyers, D. A., Evidence for the localization of a malignant hyperthermia susceptibility locus (MHS2) to human chromosome 17q, *Genomics*, 14, 562, 1992.

26. Lee, W., Bookstein, R., Hong, F., Young, L., Shew, J., and Lee, E., Human retinoblastoma susceptibility gene: cloning, identification, and sequence, *Science*, 235, 1394, 1987.

27. Francke, U., Ochs, H., de Martinville, B., Giacalone, J., Lindgren, V., Disteche, C., Pagon, R. A., Hofker, M. H., van Omnen, G. J., Pearson, P. L., et al., Minor Xp21 chromosome deletion in a male associated with expression Duchenne muscular dystrophy, chromosome granulomatous disease, retinitis pigmentosa, and McLeod syndrome, *Am. J. Hum. Genet.*, 37, 250, 1985.

28. deGrouchy, J., and Turleau, C., *Clinical Atlas of Human Chromosomes*, 2nd ed., John Wiley & Sons, New York, 1984, 94.

29. Ginsburg, R. and Purcell-Jones, G., Malignant hyperthermia in the Wolf-Hirschhorn syndrome, *Anaesthesia*, 43, 386, 1988.

30. Hogan, K., Gregg, R., Saul, R., Steenson, A., and Sekhon, G., Cytogenetic analysis of a male and female with malignant hyperthermia associated with King syndrome, *Anesth. Analg.*, 70(Suppl.), S162, 1990.

31. McPherson, E. and Taylor, C. A., The genetics of malignant hyperthermia: evidence for heterogeneity, *Am. J. Med. Genet.*, 11, 273, 1982.

32. Mauritz, W., Sporn, P., and Steinbereithner, K., Malignant hyperthermia susceptibility confirmed in both parents of probands, *Acta Anaesthesiol. Scand.*, 32, 24, 1988.

33. Pauli, R. M., Dominance and homozygosity in man, *Am. J. Med. Genet.*, 16, 455, 1983.

34. Vladutiu, G., Hogan, K., Saponara, I., Tassini, L., and Conroy, J., Carnitine palmitoyl transferase deficiency in malignant hyperthermia, *Muscle Nerve*, 16, 485, 1993.

35. Karpati, G., Charuk, J., Carpenter, S., Jablecki, C., and Holland, P., Myopathy caused by a deficiency of Ca^{2+}-adenosine triphosphatase in sarcoplasmic reticulum (Brody's disease), *Ann. Neurol.*, 20, 38, 1986.

36. Kefler, H. M., Singer, W. D., and Reynolds, R. N., Malignant hyperthermia in a child with Duchenne muscular dystrophy, *Pediatrics*, 71, 118, 1983.

37. Brucker, R. F., Williams, C. H., Popinigis, J., Galvez, T. L., Vail, W. J., and Taylor, C. A., in *Int. Symp. Malignant Hyperthermia*, R. A. Gordon, B. A. Britt, and W. Kalow, Charles C. Thomas, Springfield, IL, 1973, 338.

38. Tritschler, H. J. and Medori, R., Mitochondrial DNA alterations as a source of human disorders, *Neurology*, 43, 280, 1993.

39. Ohtani, Y., Miike, T., Ishitsu, T., Matsuda, I., and Tamari, H., A case of malignant hyperthermia with mitochondrial dysfunction, *Brain Dev.*, 7, 249, 1985.

40. Vladutiu, G., Saponara, I., Mitsumoto, H., DeBoer, G., and Conroy, J., Mitochondrial myopathies in patients contracture tested for malignant hyperthermia, *Pediatr. Res.*, 33, 377A, 1993.

41. Saidman, L. J., Havard, E. S., and Eger, E. I., Hyperthermia during anesthesia, *JAMA*, 190, 1029, 1964.

42. MacKenzie, A. E., Korneluk, R. G., Zorzato, F., Fujii, J., Phillips, M., Iles, D., Wieringa, B., Leblond, S., Bailly, J., Willard, H. F., Duff, C., Worton, R. G., and

MacLennan, D. H., The human ryanodine receptor gene: its mapping to 19q13.1, placement in a chromosome 19 linkage group, and exclusion as the gene causing myotonic dystrophy, *Am. J. Hum. Genet.*, 46, 1082, 1990.

43. Quane, K., Healy, J., Keating, K., Manning, B., Couch, F., Palmucci, L., Doriguzzi, C., Fagerlund, T., Berg, K., Ording, H., Bendixen, D., Mortier, W., Linz, U., Muller, C., and McCarthy, T., *Nature Genet.*, in press.

44. Ptacek, L., Johnson, K., and Griggs, R., Genetics and physiology of myotonic muscle disorders, *N. Eng. J. Med.*, 328, 482, 1993.

45. Seay, A. R. and Ziter, F. A., Malignant hyperpyrexia in a patient with Schwartz-Jampel syndrome, *J. Peds.*, 93, 83, 1978.

46. Lathrop, G. M., Lalouel, J. M., Julier, C., and Ott, J., Strategies for multilocus linkage analysis in humans, *Proc. Natl. Acad. Sci. U.S.A.*, 81, 3443, 1984.

47. Weissenbach, J., Gyapay, G., Dib, C., Vignal, A., Morissette, J., Millasseau, P., Vaysseix, G., and Lathrop, M., A second-generation linkage map of the human genome, *Nature*, 359, 794, 1992.

48. Innis, M., Gelfand, D., Sninsky, J., and White, T., *PCR Protocols: A Guide to Methods and Applications*, Academic Press, San Diego, 1990.

49. MacKenzie, A. E., Allen, G., Lahey, D., Crossan, M. L., Nolan, K., Mettler, G., Worton, R. G., MacLennan, D. H., Korneluk, R., A comparison of the caffeine halothane muscle contracture test with the molecular genetic diagnosis of malignant hyperthermia, *Anesthesiology*, 75(1), 4, 1991.

50. Ball S. P. and Johnson, K. J., The genetics of malignant hyperthermia, *J. Med. Genet.*, 30, 89, 1993.

51. Hogan, K., Valdivia, H., El-Hayek, R., Wedel, D., and Coronado, R., A scorpion venom that activates normal and inhibits malignant hyperthermia susceptible pig and human ryanodine receptors, *Biophys. J.*, 64, A150, 1993.

52. Gregg, R. G., Couch, F., Hogan, K., and Powers, P. A., Assignment of the human gene for the α_1-subunit of the skeletal muscle DHP-sensitive Ca^{2+} channel (CACNL1A3) to chromosome 1q31-q32, *Genomics*, 15, 107, 1993.

53. Powers, P., Liu, S., Hogan, K., and Gregg, R., Molecular characterization of the gene encoding the γ subunit of the human skeletal muscle 1,4-dihydropyridine-sensitive Ca^{2+} channel (CACNLG), cDNA sequence, gene structure, and cromosomal location, *J. Biol. Chem.*, 268(13), 9275-9279, 1993.

54. Gregg, R. G., Powers, P. A., and Hogan, K., Assignment of the human gene for the β subunit of the voltage-dependent calcium channel (CACNLB1) to chromosome 17 using somatic cell hybrids and linkage mapping, *Genomics*, 15, 185, 1993.

55. Brandt, N. R., Caswell, A. H., Brunschwig, J. P., Kang, J. J., Antoniu, B., and Ikemoto, N., Effects of anti-triadin antibody on Ca^{2+} release from sarcoplasmic reticulum, *FEBS Lett.*, 229, 1, 57, 1992.

56. Foster, P., Gesini, E., Claudianos, C., Hopkinson, K., and Denborough, M., Inositol 1,4,5,-trisphosphate phosphatase deficiency and malignant hyperpyrexia in swine, *Lancet*, 2(8655), 124, 1989.

57. Valdivia, C., Valdivia, H., Potter, B., and Coronado, R., Ca^{2+} release by inositol-trisphosphorothioate in isolated triads of rabbit skeletal muscle, *Biophys. J.*, 57, 1233, 1990.

58. Olckers, A., Meyers, D., Meyers, S., Taylor, E., Fletcher, J., Rosenberg, H., Isaacs, H., and Levitt, R., Adult muscle sodium channel α-subunit is a gene candidate for malignant hyperthermia susceptibility, *Genomics*, 14, 829, 1992.

59. Fletcher, J., Tripolitis, L., Erwin, K., Sanson, S., and Rosenberg, H., Fatty acids modulate calcium-induced calcium release from skeletal muscle heavy sarcoplasmic reticulum fractions: implications for malignant hyperthermia, *Biochem. Cell Biol.*, 68, 1195, 1990.

60. Levitt, R., McKusick, V., Fletcher, J., and Rosenberg, H., Gene candidate, *Nature*, 345, 297, 1990.

61. **Emery, A.**, Segregation analysis, in *Methodology in Medical Genetics*, Churchill Livingstone, Edinburgh, 1976, 35.
62. **Nelson, T. E.**, Malignant hyperthermia in dogs, *J. Am. Vet. Med. Assoc.*, 198, 989, 1991.
63. **Chen, E., Kuang, W., and Lee, A.**, Overview of manual and automated DNA sequencing by the dideoxy chain termination method. "DNA sequencing", *Methods: A Companion to Methods in Enzymology*, 3:1, 3, 1991.
64. **Rossiter, B. and Caskey, C.**, Molecular scanning methods of mutation detection, *J. Biol. Chem.*, 265, 12753, 1990.
65. **Orita, M., Suzuki, Y., Sekiya, T., and Hayashi, K.**, Rapid and sensitive detection of point mutations and DNA polymorphisms using the polymerase chain reaction, *Genomics*, 5, 874, 1989.
66. **Valdivia, H., Hogan, K., and Coronado, R.**, Altered binding site for Ca^{2+} in the ryanodine receptor of human malignant hyperthermia, *Am. J. Physiol.*, 261, C237, 1991.
67. **Holtzman, N.**, *Proceed with Caution: Predicting Genetic Risks in the Recombinant DNA Era*, Johns Hopkins University Press, 1989.

Index

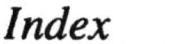

INDEX

A

Acetic acid, 226
Acetylcholine, 125
Acetylpromazine, 108
N-Acetyltransferase, 24
Acidosis, 33, 39, 74, 107, 120, 244, see also specific types
Actin, 88
Adenylate cyclase, 124
Adipose tissue, 134
Agarose gel electrophoresis, 275, 283–285
Aldehyde oxidase, 153
Aldehydes, 153, see also specific types
Allele-specific oligonucleotide (ASO) probes, 304
Allelic heterogeneity, 295
Althesin, 97
Amethocaine, 99
Amides, 98, see also specific types
Amoxapine, 123
Anaerobiasis, 39, 88
Animal models, 25, 26, 29–42, see also Dogs; Swine; specific types
   breeding of, 36–37
   discovery of MH in, 30–35
   early studies of, 37–41
   genetics and, 35–37
   molecular genetic diagnosis and, 307–309
   selection of, 36–37
Anticholinergic effects, 123, see also specific types
Antidepressants, 123, 125, see also specific types
Antimycin A, 214
Antioxidants, 153, 156, 158–159, 160, 161–162, 165, see also specific types
Antipirazo III, 49
Arachidonic acid, 155
Argon, 135
Arsenazo III, 49, 50
ASO, see Allele-specific oligonucleotide
Aspartate transaminase (AST), 106, 110
AST, see Aspartate transaminase
Autonomic activation, 120
Autosomal dominant disorders, 298, see also specific types
Awake triggering of MH, 78

B

"Barnyard test", 84
Basal ganglia, 124
Bicarbonate, 107
Biochemical accompaniments of MH, 86–87
Blood cell membrane defects, 108–112
BMHA, see British Malignant Hyperthermia Association
British Malignant Hyperthermia Association (BMHA), 18–19
Britt, Beverley A., 24, 25, 26
Brody myopathy, 299
Bruning, Anna, 4

C

Caffeine, 26, 39, 212
   in canine MH, 106
   in CHC test, see Caffeine halothane contracture (CHC) test
   CICR and, 200, 204, 206, 207
   hypersensitivity to, 287
   lymphocyte test and, 244
   porcine stress syndrome and, 274
   sarcoplasmic reticulum calcium release channel and, 51
Caffeine contracture test, 134, 275, see also Caffeine halothane contracture (CHC) test
Caffeine-contracture test, 180
Caffeine halothane contracture (CHC) test, 171–193, 226, 260
   anesthesia and, 173
   CICR and, 206, 207
   drug addition in, 178–179
   drug effects in, 188–190
   fascicle subdivision in, 176
   microscopy associated with, 172–173
   muscle selection for, 173
   muscle strip mounting in, 176–177
   muscle strip stimulation in, 177–178
   muscle transport from operating room to laboratory in, 174–176
   patient selection for, 172
   surgical excision of muscle for, 173–174
   temperature effects on, 186–188
   termination of, 179–180

timing of, 172–173
Caffeine-specific concentration (CSC), 109,
   179, 183, 286, 287, 290
Calcein, 55
Calcium
  active transport of, 163
  bound, 237
  in CHC test, 188
  contracture-producing effects of, 244
  cytoplasmic, 228, 231, 234, 238
    assays of, 226
    free, 112, 231, 246, 247
    ionized, 242
  in damaged muscle fibers, 139–140
  Debye-Huckel activity coefficient of, 135
  efflux of, 164
  excessive, 226, 231
  exogeneous, 231
  extracellular, 231, 235
  extrusion of, 241
  fluorescence of, 112, 237
  free, 237
    cytoplasmic, 112, 231, 246, 247
    intracellular, 164
    myoplasmic, 87, 91
  halothane and, 112, 226, 235, 237, 238
  influx of, 235
  intracellular, 127, 134, 145, 163, 164
  isolation of from sarcoplasmic reticulum,
    127–128
  lipid peroxidation and, 162–164
  loading of, 203, 205
  low intracellular, 163
  measurement of, 202–208
  mitochondrial uptake of, 214
  myoplasmic, 87, 91, 147, 152
  regulation of, 128, 145, 274
  releasable, 231
  release of, 39, 145, 231, 232
    inhibition of, 252
    through ion-specific channels, 274
    by sarcoplasmic reticulum, 164, 178,
      226, 244, 252, see also Calcium
      release channel from sarcoplasmic
      reticulum
        calcium-induced, see Calcium-
          induced calcium release (CICR)
  resting, 147, 237
  sarcolemma uptake of, 214
  sarcoplasmic reticulum accumulation of,
    163, 211–222
    diminished, 216

    experimental procedures for study of,
      213–214
    results of study of, 214–220
  sarcoplasmic reticulum release of, 164,
    178, 226, 244, 252, see also Calcium
    release channel from sarcoplasmic
    reticulum
    calcium-induced, see Calcium-induced
      calcium release (CICR)
  sarcoplasmic reticulum uptake of, 145
  in skeletal muscle, 128, 133–147, 212
    methods of study of, 134–138
    microelectrodes and, 135
    results of study of, 138–142
  in steady-state condition, 143
  transport of, 47, 128, 163, 231
  uptake of, 54, 145, 214
Calcium channel blockers, 99, 164, 235, see
    also specific types
Calcium channels, 152, 163, 164
Calcium chloride, 98
Calcium-dependent ATPase, 127
Calcium-dependent contractile processes in
    skeletal muscle, 122
Calcium-free media, 127
Calcium indicators, 47, 226, see also
    specific types
Calcium-induced calcium release (CICR),
    50–53, 127, 164, 199–209
  considerations for determination of, 201
  discovery of, 200
  enhancement of, 207
  inhibition of, 208, 261
  measurement of, 202–208
  rate of, 206, 209
  skinned fiber preparation and, 201–202
  thermometry and, 252
Calcium pump protein, 200
Calcium pumps, 62, 127
Calcium release channel from sarcoplasmic
    reticulum, 45–65, 261, see also
    Sarcoplasmic reticulum, calcium
    release by
  calcium-induced, 50–53
  cardiac muscle and, 59–63
  discovery of abnormality of in MH, 53–58
  dual-wavelength spectrometry and, 46–48,
    49, 54, 55
  murexide method and, 46–48, 49
  porcine MH and, 92
  skeletal muscle and, 59–63
Calcium release channel genes, 263–264

Calcium-selective microelectrodes, 127, 135, 142–145, 213
Calcium-sodium exchange, 62, 145
Calcium-transport ATPase, 109
Calmodulin-dependent phospholipase A, 94
Canine MH, 105–114
  blood cell membranes and, 108–112
  molecular genetic diagnosis and, 308
  muscle and, 108–112
Canine MHS, 106–108, 109, 110, 111
Canine stress syndrome (CSS), 105, 108, 243, see also Dogs
Capture myopathy, 96
Cardiac muscle, 59–63, 152
Carnitine palmitoyl transferase II, 298–299
Carnosine, 156
Catalase, 156, 165
Catecholamines, 87, 95, 96, 107, 120, 128, see also specific types
CCD, see Central core disease
Central core disease (CCD), 172, 266, 295, 300
Central nervous system (CNS) manifestations of MH, 76–77, 124–125
Centrifugation, 280, see also specific types
Ceruloplasmin, 165
CHC, see Caffeine halothane contracture
Chloroform, 26
Chlorpromazine, 127
Cholinergic receptors, 127, see also specific types
Cholinesterase, 23
Chromosome rearrangements, 296, 306
CICR, see Calcium-induced calcium release
CK, see Creatine kinase
Clinical features of MH, 69, 71–77, see also specific types
  hypermetabolic syndromes compared to, 120–121
CNS, see Central nervous system
Cocaine, 123
Cochran's Q-test, 289
Connective tissue, 134
Contractile proteins, 94–95, see also specific types
Contracture testing, 121, see also specific types
  caffeine, 134, 275, see also Caffeine halothane contracture (CHC) test
  halothane-induced, 222
  in vitro, 83
  molecular genetic diagnosis and, 313

skeletal muscle, 121
Creatine kinase, 110, 158, 159, 160, 161, 162, 172
Creatine phosphokinase, 75
CSC, see Caffeine-specific concentration
CSS, see Canine stress syndrome
Cyanosis, 74, 84, 87
Cyclopropane, 97
Cytoplasmic calcium, 228, 231, 234, 238
  assays of, 226
  free, 112, 231, 246, 247
  ionized, 242
Cytosolic esterases, 226, see also specific types

D

Dantrium, 9
Dantrolene, 3, 5, 41, 55, 212, 260, 261, 263
  calcium and, 235
  canine MH and, 107, 108
  in CHC test, 173, 190, 193
  CICR and, 208
  effects of, 142, 144
  hypermetabolic syndromes and, 121
  inhibitory effects of, 142, 144
  porcine MH and, 98
David's r-test, 287
Davison, Owen, 10
Debye-Huckel activity coefficient, 135
Denborough, Michael A., 5, 23, 24, 25
Depolarization, 127, 164
Diagnosis, see also specific methods
  antioxidants and, 161–162
  caffeine halothane contracture test in, see Caffeine halothane contracture (CHC) test
  calcium-induced calcium release in, see Calcium-induced calcium release (CICR)
  CHC test in, see Caffeine halothane contracture (CHC) test
  CICR in, see Calcium-induced calcium release (CICR)
  direct thermometry in, 251–255
  erythrocyte lipid peroxidation and, 168
  false-negative, 260
  false-positive, 260
  of hypermetabolic syndromes, 121–123
  intramuscular temperature thermometry in, 251–255

lymphocyte test in, see Lymphocyte test
of malignant hyperthermia susceptibility,
    211–222
    experimental procedures for study of,
        213–214
    results of study of, 214–220
membranes and, 161–162
molecular genetic, see Molecular genetic
    diagnosis
pharmaco-, 26
of porcine stress syndrome, 284, 286
Diazepam, 108
Dibucaine, 252
DIC, see Disseminated intravascular
    coagulation
Dienes, 158, see also specific types
Diethyl ether, 97
Digitalis, 98
Diltiazem, 99, 235
Dimethoxysulfoxide, 231
Dinitrophenol, 25, 26
Direct thermometry, 251–255
Disseminated intravascular coagulation
    (DIC), 76
DNA fluorescence, 285
DNA photography, 285
DNA polymerases, 282
DNA probes, 303
DNA restriction fragments, 283–285
DNA sequencing, 309
DNA target sequence, 280–282
Dogs, see also Animal models
    malignant hyperthermia in, 105–114
        blood cell membranes and, 108–112
        molecular genetic diagnosis and, 308
        muscle and, 108–112
    malignant hyperthermia susceptibility in,
        106–108, 109, 110, 111
    stress syndromes in, 105, 108, 243
Dopamine activity, 123
Dopamine agonists, 124, see also specific
    types
Dopamine antagonism, 124
Dopamine antagonists, 123, see also specific
    types
Dopamine hypothesis, 123–124
Dopamine-receptor antagonism, 119
Dopamine-receptor antagonists, 124, see also
    specific types
Dopamine receptors, 123, 124, see also
    specific types
Droperidol, 108, 119

Drugs, see also specific types
    calcium channel blocking, 99, 164, 235
    in CHC test, 188–190
    hypermetabolic syndromes induced by, see
        Hypermetabolic syndromes
    neuroleptic, 119, 124, 126, 128
    psychedelic, 123
    psychotropic, 118, 119
    screening of, 97–99
    serotonergic, 125
Dual-wavelength spectrometry, 46–48, 49,
    54, 55
    lymphocyte test and, 237–247
Duchenne's muscular dystrophy, 266, 299
Dyspnea, 244

E

ECC, see Excitation/contraction/coupling
Electrophoresis, 275, 283–285, see also
    specific types
Endoplasmic reticulum (ER), 153
End-tidal carbon dioxide elevation, 72–73
Enflurane, 51, 73, 107, 189
Enzymes, 120, 158, 303, see also specific
    types
Epidemiology, 118–120
ER, see Endoplasmic reticulum
Erythrocytes, 152, 159, 165, 168, 277, 280
Ethrane, 97
European Malignant Hyperthermia Group,
    305
Excitation/contraction/coupling (ECC), 91,
    93, 95, 97, 98, 128

F

Fatty acids, 94, 152, 153, 155, 158, 165,
    see also specific types
Fenfluramine, 125
Fentanyl droperidol, 108
FFAs, see Free fatty acids
Flavin dehydrogenase, 153
Fluorescence, 112, 227, 228, 232, 237, 242,
    284, 285
Fluorescent calcium, 112, 237
Fluorescent conjugates, 153
Fluphenazine, 126
Formaldehyde, 226
Free fatty acids (FFAs), 94, see also specific
    types
Free radicals, 151–165

antioxidants and, 153, 156, 158–159, 160, 161–162, 165
  calcium and, 162–164
  formation of, 153–155
  halothane and, 155–156, 160–161
  lipid peroxidation and, 152–153, 154, 155, 156, 158
    calcium and, 162–164
  membrane abnormalities and, 161–162
  stress and, 159–160
Fructose 1,6-diphosphate, 89
Fructose recycling, 89
Fura 2, 60, 235

G

GABA, 125
Gallamore, Suellen Long, 10–13
Gel electrophoresis, 275, 283–285
Genetic diagnostic methods, 65, see also specific types
Genetics, 35–37, 64–65, 259–269, 311
  of human MH, 266–268
  molecular, see Molecular genetic diagnosis
  of porcine MH, 82–84, 260–261, 263, 264–265
Genomic DNA, 277–280
Glucose, 263
Glucose-6-phosphate dehydrogenase, 23, 165
Glucose phosphate isomerase, 264, 302
Glutathione, 156
Glutathione peroxidase, 156, 165
Glycogen depletion, 39
Glycogenolysis, 87
Glycolysis, 39, 87
Gordon, R. A., 24, 25
GPI, see Glucose phosphate isomerase
Gross acidosis, 39

H

Haber-Weiss reaction, 153
HAL gene, 263–264, 290, 291
Haloperidol, 126
Halothane, 24, 26, 168, see also Caffeine halothane contracture (CHC) test
  in animal models, 36, 38, 39
  calcium and, 112, 226, 232, 235, 237, 238
  calcium release channel from sarcoplasmic reticulum and, 50, 51
  calcium SR accumulation and, 212, 213, 217, 218, 219

canine MH and, 106, 109, 112
  in CHC test, see Caffeine halothane contracture (CHC) test
  CICR and, 200, 206, 207
  clinical features of MH and, 73
  depolarization and, 164
  discontinuation of, 107
  effects of, 160–161
  fatty acids and, 155
  free radicals and, 155–156, 160–161, 164
  hypersensitivity to, 287
  in vitro effects of, 160–161
  in vivo effects of, 160–161
  lymphocyte test and, 228, 229, 230, 231, 232, 233, 234, 237, 241
  negative inotropic effect of, 50
  neuroleptic malignant syndrome and, 128
  porcine MH and, 83, 84, 97
  thermometry and, 252
Halothane challenge (HC) test, 274, 275
Halothane-specific contracture (HSC) test, 222, 286, 287, see also Caffeine halothane contracture (CHC) test
HC, see Halothane challenge
Heart muscle, 59–63, 152
Hemolysis, 23
High-performance spectrophotometry, 49
History of malignant hyperthermia, 23–26, 70–71
Hotline, MHAUS, 9, 11
HSC, see Halothane-specific contracture
Hybridization, 306, 307
Hydrocarbons, 153, see also specific types
Hydrogen, 135, 152, 155
Hydrogen peroxide, 155, 156, 158, 168
Hydrolysis, 87, 164
Hypercapnia, 86, 120
Hypercatecholemia, 107
Hyperkalemia, 75, 107
Hyperlactemia, 108
Hypermetabolic syndromes, 117–129, see also specific types
  clinical manifestations of, 120–121
  diagnostic testing for, 121–123
  disorders related to, 123
  epidemiology of, 118–120
  pathogenesis of, 123–128
  skeletal muscle and, 126–128
  treatment of, 121
Hyperpolarizing pulse, 137
Hypoxia, 120

I

Imidazole chloride, 214
Indo 1, 226, 227
    dual wavelength spectrophotometry and,
        237–247
    single wavelength spectrofluormetry and,
        232–235
Indo 1-acetoxy methyl ester, 226
Inositol-1-phosphatase, 125
Inositol triphosphate, 164
Inositol trisphosphatases, 307
Inositol trisphosphate receptor, 307
In situ hybridization, 306
Intracellular calcium, 127, 134, 145, 163,
    164
Intramuscular temperature, 251–255
In vitro contracture testing (IVCT), 83
Ionomycin, 228, 231, 232
Iron, 164
Irreversibility of MH, 93–94
Ischemia, 153
Isoflurane, 97, 189
Isoniazid, 24
IVCT, see *In vitro* contracture testing

K

Kalow, Werner, 23–26
Ketamine, 97
Kidney damage, 260
Kidney failure, 77
Kinase-linked phosphorylation, 145
King-Denborough syndrome, 266, 296
Krebs Ringer solution, 176, 178, 234

L

Lactacidosis, 86
Langendorf's perfused heart model, 61
Larberg, John, 13
Laser diffraction, 136
Leukocyte isolation, 279–280
Levodopa, 123
Lewis, Jerry and Lila, 13
Ligand-gated channels, 261
Lignocaine, 98
Linkage analysis, 300–303, 305–306
Linoleic acid, 155
Linolenic acid, 155
Lipid hydroperoxides, 153, 156
Lipid peroxidation, 158

calcium and, 162–164
detection of, 154
of erythrocytes, 168
free radicals and, 152–153, 154, 155, 156
initiation of, 155
measurement of, 154
Lithium, 123
Liver damage, 260
Liver transplants, 30
Local anesthetics, 98, 134, 252, see also
    specific types
Locus heterogeneity, 295
LSD, see Lysergic acid
Luckritz, Robert T., 10
Lymphocytes, 152
Lymphocyte test, 225–247
    Fura 2 and, 235
    Indo 1 and, 226, 227
        dual wavelength spectrophotometry and,
            237–247
        single wavelength spectrofluorometry
            and, 232–235
    Quin 2 and, 226, 227, 229–232, 234, 238
    single wavelength spectrofluorometry and,
        229–235
Lysergic acid (LSD), 125
Lysis, 280

M

Magnesium, 127, 135, 206, 261
Malignant Hyperthermia Association of the
    United States (MHAUS), 5, 9, 10–13
Malignant Hyperthermia Association of the
    United States (MHAUS) Hotline, 9,
    11
Malignant hyperthermia markers, 311–313
Malignant hyperthermia susceptibility (MHS)
    calcium in skeletal muscle and, 133–147
        methods of study of, 134–138
        microelectrodes and, 135
        results of study of, 138–142
    CHC test and, 174, 185, 189, 190
    defined, 226
    diagnosis of, 211–222
        experimental procedures for study of,
            213–214
        results of study of, 214–220
    in dogs, 106–108, 109, 110, 111, 240
    free radicals and, 161
    hypermetabolic syndromes and, 122
    lymphocyte test and, 226, 231, 232, 233

in swine, 30–42, 82, 83, 84, 85, 92, see
    also Porcine MH
  breeding of, 36–37
  calcium and, 212, 213
  capture myopathy in, 96
  CHC test and, 180
  creatine kinase and, 161, 162
  defined, 212, 226
  diagnosis of, 212, 213
  drug screening in, 97–99
  early studies of, 37–41
  free radicals and, 158, 159, 160, 161,
    162, 164
  genetics of, 35–37
  glutathione peroxidase and, 165
  halothane and, 36–37
  irreversibility and, 93
  lymphocyte test and, 226, 231, 233,
    237, 238, 240, 241, 243
  membranes and, 95
  mitochondria and, 94
  muscle and, 109, 111
  pathogenesis and, 87, 89
  phospholipase A and, 164
  sarcolemma and, 94
  sarcplasmic reticulum and, 91, 92
  selection of, 36–37
  sympathetic nervous system of, 95, 96
  thermometry and, 253–255
  triggering of MH in, 96–97
  vitamin E and, 158, 159, 162
Manganese, 242
Manganese chloride, 228
Martin, Betty L., 3–6
Martin, Francie, 4, 5
Martin, Jack, 4
Massik, Daniel, 7–9
Massik, George, 7–9, 10–13
Maxam-Gibert technique, 309
Membrane potential microelectrodes, 137
Metabolic acidosis, 33, 74, 120, 244
Metallochromic indicators, 47, see also
  specific types
Methoxyflurane, 97, 107, 189
Metoclopramide, 123
MHAUS, see Malignant Hyperthermia
  Association of the United States
MHS, see Malignant hyperthermia
  susceptibility
Michaelis constant, 145
Microelectrodes, 127, 135, 137, 142–145,
  213, see also specific types

Mitochondria, 39, 94, 111, 153, 163, 214
Mitochondrial DNA, 299
Molecular genetic diagnosis, 293–313
  allele-specific oligonucleotide probes and,
    304
  animal models and, 307–309
  chromosome rearrangements and, 296,
    306
  goals of, 311
  linkage analysis and, 300–303, 305–306
  mutations and, 309–313
  polymerase chain reaction and, 304, 307
  RFLPs and, 302–303
  single gene mutations and, 298–299
Monoamine oxidase inhibitors, 125, see also
  specific types
Monocytes, 152
Mottling of skin, 74
Multifactorial inheritance, 311
Murexide method, 46–48, 49
Muscle, see also specific types
  biopsy of, 111, 134, 212, 213
  calcium in, 139–140, 174
  canine MH and, 108–112
  cardiac, 59–63, 152
  in CHC test, 173–179
  chlorpromazine and, 127
  contracture of, 142, see also Contracture
    testing
  cramping of, 108, 244
  damaged, 139–140
  pain in, 172
  rigidity of, 73, 120, 172, 185, 260
  skeletal, see Skeletal muscle
  smooth, 152
  surgical excision of, 173–174
  trismus of, 73, 106
Muscle contracture test, see Contracture
  testing
Muscle enzymes, 120, 158, see also specific
  types
Muscle relaxants, 134, 260, see also specific
  types
Muscular dystrophy, 172, 266, 299
Mutations, 273–291, see also specific types
  DNA-based tests and, 289–290
  molecular genetic diagnosis and, 309–313
  polymerase chain reaction and, 278–283,
    290, 291
  RFLPs and, 263, 266, 275, 282–283,
    287–288
RYR, see *RYR* gene

single gene, 298–299
Myocytes, 60
Myoplasmic calcium, 87, 91, 147, 152
Myosin, 88
Myotonia congenita, 300
Myotonic dystrophy, 300

N

Napolitano, Vincent, 13
Negative inotropism, 50, 61
Neuroleptic drugs, 119, 124, 126, 128, see
        also specific types
Neuroleptic malignant syndrome (NMS),
        118–123, 172
    clinical manifestations of, 120–121
    epidemiology of, 118–120
    pathogenesis of, 123–128
    risk for, 125
    skeletal muscle and, 126–128
    systemic factors in, 125–126
Neurological damage, 77, 260
Neuromuscular blockade, 94
Neuromuscular pathology, 120
Neuromuscular systems, 124
Neurotransmitters, 125, see also specific
        types
Nifedipine, 235
Nitrogen, 135
Nitrous oxide, 97
NMS, see Neuroleptic malignant syndrome
Non-anesthetic related MH, 77–78
Nondepolarizing muscle relaxants, 260, see
        also specific types
Nondepolarizing neuromuscular blockade, 94
Non-operating room MH, 77–78
Norepinephrine, 125
North American Malignant Hyperthermia
        Registry, 313
Nucleotide hydrolysis, 87

O

Oleic acid, 155
Oxidative phosphorylation, 39, 89, 127, 159
Oxygen, 263
Oxygen radicals, 153–155, see also specific
        types
Oxygen uptake, 153
Oxymorphone, 108

P

Pale, soft, exudative pork (PSEP), 36, 82,
        83, 260, 261, 265, 274, 290
Pathogenesis
    of malignant hyperthermia, 87–95
    of neuroleptic malignant syndrome,
        123–128
Pathophysiology of MH, 118
PCR, see Polymerase chain reaction
Pentane, 159
Peroxidation, 159, 161, 165
    lipid, see Lipid peroxidation
Pharmacodiagnosis of MH, 26
Pharmacological assays, 26
Phenolic compounds, 123, see also specific
        types
Phenotyping, 275, 286–290, 313
Phosphatidylinositol 4,5-biphosphate, 164
6-Phosphogluconate dehydrogenase, 264
Phosphoinositide, 125, 128
Phospholipase A, 94, 164
Phospholipids, 156, see also specific types
Phosphorylation, 39, 89, 127, 145, 159, see
        also specific types
Physiological basis of MH, 262–263
Pifedipine, 99
Pigs, see Swine
Plasma membrane, 145
Platelets, 152
PMH, see Porcine MH
Polymerase chain reaction (PCR), 278–283,
        290, 291
    DNA target sequence and, 280–282
    molecular genetic diagnosis and, 304, 307
    principle of, 280
    products of, 282–283
Polymerases, 282, 289, 304, see also
        specific types
Polymorphisms, 268, 310
    restriction-fragment length, see
        Restriction-fragment length
        polymorphisms (RFLPs)
Polyunsaturated fatty acids (PUFAs), 152,
        153, 158, see also specific types
Porcine MH, 36, 81–99, see also Malignant
        hyperthermia susceptibility (MHS), in
        swine; Swine
    biochemical accompaniments of, 86–87
    capture myopathy and, 96
    clinical syndrome of, 84–85
    contractile proteins and, 94–95

drug screening and, 97–99
free radicals and, 161
future directions in study of, 99
genetics of, 82–84, 260–261, 263,
    264–265
identification of, 82–84
irreversibility of, 93–94
membranes and, 95
mitochondria and, 94
molecular genetic diagnosis and, 307
myoplasmic free calcium and, 87, 91
pathogenesis of, 87–95
sarcolemma and, 94
sarcoplasmic reticulum and, 91–92
sympathetic nervous system and, 95–96
triggering of, 96–97
Porcine stress syndrome (PSS), 36, 82, 120,
    126, 260, 261
    characteristics of, 274
    clinical syndrome of, 84–85
    defined, 274
    diagnosis of, 284, 286
    DNA-based tests for, 289–290
    free radicals and, 152
    mutations and, 273–291
        agarose gel electrophoresis and, 275,
            283–285
        diagnosis of, 286
        DNA-based tests and, 289–290
        phenotyping and, 275, 286–290
        polymerase chain reaction and,
            278–283, 290, 291
        RFLPs and, 263, 266, 275, 282–283,
            287–288
    phenotyping of, 275, 286–290
    susceptibility to, 286–290
Post, Frederick, 4
Potassium, 75, 188
Primaquine, 23
Procaine, 39, 99, 127, 206, 252
Propofol, 98
Prostaglandins, 125
Proteinases, 277, 279, 280, see also specific
    types
Proteins, 94–95, 200, 268, 313, see also
    specific types
PSEP, see Pale, soft, exudative pork
PSS, see Porcine stress syndrome
Psuedodominance, 299
Psychedelic drugs, 123, see also specific
    types
Psychotic states, 124

Psychotropic drugs, 118, 119, 123, see also
    specific types
PUFAs, see Polyunsaturated fatty acids
Pyruvate kinase, 158, 161, 162

Q

Quin 2, 226, 227, 229–232, 234, 238
Quin 2 tetra-acetyoxy methyl ester, 231

R

Recombinant DNA technology, see
    Molecular genetic diagnosis
Recording procedures, 137–138
Recrudescence, 75–76
Releasable calcium, 231
Renal damage, 260
Renal failure, 77
Respiratory acidosis, 74, 244
Resting calcium, 147, 237
Resting tension, 147
Restriction enzymes, 303, see also specific
    types
Restriction-fragment length polymorphisms
    (RFLPs), 263, 266, 275, 282–283,
    287–288
    molecular genetic diagnosis and, 302–303
Reverse transcriptase, 309
RFLPs, see Restriction-fragment length
    polymorphisms
Rhabdomyolysis, 75, 120, 172
Rigor mortis, 87
RNA isolation, 313
Rosenberg, Henry, 10
Rotenone, 214
Ruthenium red, 51
Ryanodine, 133–147
    calcium in control muscle and, 140
    in CHC test, 190
    effects of, 140–141, 147
    methods of study of, 134–138
    microelectrodes and, 135
    muscle contracture induced by, 142
    results of study of, 138–142
Ryanodine receptors, 226, 274
RYR genes, 263–264, 265, 266, 268, 275
    molecular genetic diagnosis and, 294,
    300, 311

S

Salicylates, 123, see also specific types

Sanger technique, 309
Saponin, 202
Sarcolemma, 39, 87, 94, 214
Sarcoplasmic reticulum (SR), 39, 261
    calcium accumulation in, 163, 211–222
        diminished, 216
        experimental procedures for study of,
            213–214
        results of study of, 214–220
    calcium concentration in, 127
    calcium-induced calcium release in, see
        Calcium-induced calcium release
        (CICR)
    calcium isolated from, 127–128
    calcium release from, 164, 216, 226, 235,
        244, 252
        calcium-induced, see Calcium-induced
            calcium release (CICR)
    calcium release channel from, see Calcium
        release channel from sarcoplasmic
        reticulum
    calcium transport in, 47
    calcium uptake by, 145
    canine MH and, 109
    depolarization of, 164
    free radicals and, 163
    instability of, 213
    malignant hyperthermia susceptibility and,
        134
    porcine MH and, 91–92
    terminal cisterne of, 274
Schwartz-Jampel syndrome, 300
Second messenger systems, 124
Selenium, 156, 168
Serotonergic drugs, 125, see also specific
        types
Serotonin, 125
Serum metabolites, 212
Sevoflurane, 97
SIDS, see Sudden infant death syndrome
Single gene mutations, 298–299
Single-strand conformation polymorphism
    (SSCP), 310
Single wavelength spectrofluorometry,
    229–235
Skeletal muscle, 59–63, 96
    calcium in, 128, 133–147, 212
        methods of study of, 134–138
        microelectrodes and, 135
        regulation of, 145
        results of study of, 138–142
    calcium-dependent contractile processes
        in, 122

calcium regulation in, 145
    CHC test and, 190
    dysfunction of, 128
    in frogs, 147
    hypermetabolic syndromes and, 124,
        126–128
    intracellular calcium regulation in, 145
    metabolic processes in, 122
    neuroleptic malignant syndrome and,
        126–128
    rigidity of, 260
Skeletal muscle contracture test, see
        Contracture testing
Skin mottling, 74
SL, see Sarcolemma
Smooth muscle, 152
SOD, see Superoxide dismutase
Sodium, 135, 145
Sodium-calcium exchange, 62, 145
Sodium channels, 307
Sodium exchange, 127
Southern blotting, 303
Spectrofluorometry, 226, 227, 229–235
Spectrometry, dual-wavelength, see
        Dual-wavelength spectrometry
Spectrophotometry, 168, see also specific
        types
    high-performance, 49
    lymphocyte test and, 237–247
SR, see Sarcoplasmic reticulum
SSCP, see Single-strand conformation
        polymorphism
State-related factors, 124
Stimulants, 123, see also specific types
Stress-induced MH reaction, 172
Stress syndromes, see also specific types
    clinical syndrome of, 84–85
    in dogs, 105, 108, 243
    free radicals and, 159–160
    porcine, see Porcine stress syndrome
        (PSS)
    in swine, see Porcine stress syndrome
        (PSS)
Striation spacing, 136
Succinylcholine, 23, 26, 39, 73, 83, 98
    calcium and, 226
    canine MH and, 107
    in CHC test, 180, 189
Sudden infant death syndrome (SIDS), 172
Superoxide anions, 153
Superoxide dismutase (SOD), 155, 165
Swine, see also Animal models; Porcine MH

lymphocytes of, 226, 231, 237, 238, 240, 241, 243
malignant hyperthermia susceptibility in, see Malignant hyperthermia susceptibility (MHS), in swine
stress syndromes in, see Porcine stress syndrome (PSS)
Sympathetic nervous system, 95–96

T

Tachydysrhythmias, 73–74
Taylor, Claude, 5
TBARS, see Thiobarbituric acid reactive substances
Tetracaine, 51, 134, 252
Tetramethyl murexide, 50
Thamylal, 108
Theophylline, 188
"Thermic stress syndrome", 122
Thermometry, 251–255
Thermoregulatory systems, 124
Thiobarbituric acid reactive substances (TBARS), 158, 159, 160
Thiopentone, 97, 240
α-Tocopherol acetate, 158
Treatment, 121, see also specific types
Triadin, 307

Trichloroethylene, 97
Tricyclic antidepressants, 123, 125, see also specific types
Trismus of muscle, 73, 106
Troponin, 88, 164

U

Ultraviolet transilluminators, 289

V

Variable number tandem repeats (VNTRs), 303
Verapamil, 99, 235
Vitamin C, 156
Vitamin E, 156, 158, 159, 162, 168
VNTRs, see Variable number tandem repeats

W

Winks, Alison, 15–18
Winks, John, 15
Winks, Tracey, 15
Wolf-Hirschhorn syndrome, 296

X

Xanthine oxidase, 153